CALVERT'S DESCRIPTIVE PHONETICS AND TRANSCRIPTION WORKBOOK

4th Edition

Pamela G. Garn-Nunn, PhD
Professor Emeritus
School of Speech-Language Pathology and Audiology
The University of Akron
Akron, Ohio

Thieme

New York • Stuttgart • Delhi • Rio

Executive Editor: William Lamsbeck
Managing Editor: Elizabeth Palumbo
Editorial Assistant: Mohammad Ibrar
Production Editor: Barbara A. Chernow
International Production Director: Andreas Schabert
International Marketing Director: Fiona Henderson
Director of Sales, North America: Mike Roseman
International Sales Director: Louisa Turrell
Senior Vice President, Editorial and E-Product
Development: Cornelia Schulze
Senior Vice President and Chief Operating Officer: Sarah Vanderbilt
President: Brian D. Scanlan
Cover design: Thieme Publishing Group
Typesetting by Carol Pierson, Chernow Editorial Services, Inc.

Library of Congress Cataloging-in-Publication Data

Garn-Nunn, Pamela G., author.
  [Calvert's descriptive phonetics]
  Calvert's descriptive phonetics and transcription workbook /
Pamela G. Garn-Nunn. — 4th edition.
      p. ; cm.
  Descriptive phonetics
  Preceded by Calvert's descriptive phonetics / Pamela G. Garn-Nunn,
James M. Lynn. 3rd ed. c2004.
  Includes bibliographical references and index.
  ISBN 978-1-60406-651-7 (hardback) — ISBN 978-1-60406-652-4 (eISBN)
I. Title. II. Title: Descriptive phonetics.
[DNLM: 1. Phonetics. 2. Speech. WV 501]
PE1135
414—dc23   2014023193

© 2015 Thieme Medical Publishers, Inc.
Thieme Publishers New York
333 Seventh Avenue, New York, NY 10001 USA
+1 800 782 3488, customerservice@thieme.com

Thieme Publishers Stuttgart
Rüdigerstrasse 14, 70469 Stuttgart, Germany
+49 [0]711 8931 421, customerservice@thieme.de

Thieme Publishers Delhi
A-12, Second Floor, Sector-2, Noida-201301 Uttar Pradesh, India
+91 120 45 566 00, customerservice@thieme.in

Thieme Publishers Rio, Thieme Publicações Ltda.
Argentina Building 16th floor, Ala A, 228 Praia do Botafogo
Rio de Janeiro 22250-040 Brazil
+55 21 3736-3631

Printed in the United States of America by Sheridan Books   5 4 3 2 1

ISBN 978-1-60406-651-7
Also available as an e-book: eISBN 978-1-60406-652-4

Important note: Medicine is an ever-changing science undergoing continual development. Research and clinical experience are continually expanding our knowledge, in particular our knowledge of proper treatment and drug therapy. Insofar as this book mentions any dosage or application, readers may rest assured that the authors, editors, and publishers have made every effort to ensure that such references are in accordance with the state of knowledge at the time of production of the book.

Nevertheless, this does not involve, imply, or express any guarantee or responsibility on the part of the publishers in respect to any dosage instructions and forms of applications stated in the book. Every user is requested to examine carefully the manufacturers' leaflets accompanying each drug and to check, if necessary in consultation with a physician or specialist, whether the dosage schedules mentioned therein or the contraindications stated by the manufacturers differ from the statements made in the present book. Such examination is particularly important with drugs that are either rarely used or have been newly released on the market. Every dosage schedule or every form of application used is entirely at the user's own risk and responsibility. The authors and publishers request every user to report to the publishers any discrepancies or inaccuracies noticed. If errors in this work are found after publication, errata will be posted at www.thieme.com on the product description page.

Some of the product names, patents, and registered designs referred to in this book are in fact registered trademarks or proprietary names even though specific reference to this fact is not always made in the text. Therefore, the appearance of a name without designation as proprietary is not to be construed as a representation by the publisher that it is in the public domain.

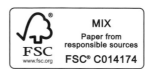

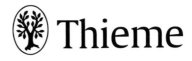

To Ronald W. Isele, MA, who first introduced me to the
International Phonetic Alphabet and whose enthusiasm for clinical teaching
and our profession influenced me throughout my career.

To Barbara W. Hodson, PhD, whose work in applying theory
to clinical practice enabled me and my students to make a difference
in the lives of countless children with severe speech sound disorders.

CONTENTS

FOREWORD FOR THE INSTRUCTOR ix

FOREWORD FOR STUDENTS. xi

PREFACE xiii

CHAPTER 1   INTRODUCTION. 1

CHAPTER 2   THE SPEECH PRODUCTION MECHANISM
            AND PROCESSES 11

CHAPTER 3   VOWELS AND DIPHTHONGS 26

CHAPTER 4   AMERICAN-ENGLISH CONSONANTS. 56

CHAPTER 5   CONNECTED SPEECH: SEGMENTAL
            AND SUPRASEGMENTAL EFFECTS. 86

CHAPTER 6   MULTICULTURAL VARIATIONS: DIALECTS 115

CHAPTER 7   APPLIED PHONETICS. 135

GLOSSARY 149

APPENDIX A. CHAPTER EXERCISES 163

APPENDIX B. ANSWER KEY: CHAPTER CONCEPT QUESTIONS 196

APPENDIX C. ANSWER KEY: CHAPTER EXERCISES 205

APPENDIX D. REFERENCES. 227

INDEX 235

FOREWORD FOR THE INSTRUCTOR

This edition has been designed for college-level students as an introductory text. No previous knowledge of phonetics is required—only a rudimentary knowledge of anatomy, physiology, and physics. Each chapter begins with an outline. New terms are highlighted when they are introduced and are also found in the glossary at the end of the text. Exercises designed to help the student learn and understand chapter content as well as to master International Phonetic Alphabet transcription are provided in Appendix A. Even with this "reader-friendly" text, there is no substitute for a course that includes lecture, examples, and multiple opportunities for transcription practice. Instructors may find that they wish to use all or only parts of this book, depending on the course's focus and content. In cases where more than one transcription or symbol use is possible, students are directed to ask for their instructor's teaching preference.

This book is intended to enable students to accomplish the following:

1. Develop listening and analytic skills

2. Gain knowledge and understanding of speech

3. Recognize and identify some of the specialty areas of phonetics

4. Gain access to resource materials that may be helpful in applying this knowledge

The following list shows these objectives matched with chapter designations:

1. Develop Listening and Analytic Skills: Chapters 1 to 6
   - Broad and narrow transcription, International Phonetic Alphabet: Chapters 1 to 5
   - Analysis of how speech units are produced: Chapters 3 to 5
   - Indication of speech rhythm features: Chapter 5
   - Word sets contrasting similar or often confused phonemes (minimal pair differences): Chapters 3 and 4

2. Gain knowledge and understanding of speech: Chapters 1 to 7
   - Nature of orthographic systems: Chapter 1
   - Anatomy and physiologic processes of speech production: Chapter 2
   - Categorization of vowels and consonants according to traditional and distinctive feature classifications: Chapter 3
   - Categorization of vowels by placement and height of tongue elevation: Chapter 3
   - Categorization of consonants by place, manner, and voicing: Chapter 4
   - Influences of phonetic context and coarticulation: Chapter 5
   - Relation of speech rhythm and pronunciation: Chapter 5

3. Recognize and identify some of the specialty areas of phonetics
   - Dialectic variations: Chapter 6
   - Relation of acoustic parameters to oral positions: Chapters 3 to 5
   - Vocabulary associated with phonetics: Chapters 1 to 7
   - Physiologic phonetics: Chapters 2 to 5
   - Mainstream American English pronunciations: Chapters 1 and 3 to 7
   - Multicultural considerations and dialectic variations: Chapters 3, 4, 6, and 7
   - Acoustic phonetics: Chapters 3 to 5
   - Applications of phonetics: Chapter 7
4. Access resource material for reference
   - Word examples of phonemes in all positions: Chapters 3 and 4
   - Formation of primary American English phonemes: Chapters 2 to 4
   - Spellings for primary phonemes: Chapters 1, 3, and 4
   - General American symbol system for reading and spelling: Chapter 1

You will notice that most objectives are not confined to just one chapter. Even in Chapter 1 students are introduced to International Phonetic Alphabet consonant and vowel symbols. The book returns to these symbols repeatedly, especially in Chapters 3, 4, and 5. Basic knowledge underlying physiologic phonetics is found in Chapter 2 and reiterated in later chapters as consonant and vowel symbols are introduced. After basic transcription skills are developed, students can learn about advanced narrow transcription in Chapter 5, followed by dialectic variations and applied phonetics in Chapters 6 and 7. The expanded workbook exercises included in this book are designed to accompany the text material and reinforce the development of cumulative skill in International Phonetic Alphabet transcription. An instructional recording covering introductory, vowel, and consonant workbook exercises is also available. Whether you use this textbook by itself or in conjunction with the recording, I hope that you find it a helpful teaching and learning tool.

Pamela Garn-Nunn, PhD

FOREWORD FOR STUDENTS

Many years ago, I, like you, enrolled in my first class in phonetics. I "took" to it immediately, finding the International Phonetic Alphabet interesting and sometimes even fun to use, and I'm sure you will, too. It can be useful in your other classes, because if you take your class notes (or doodle) in the International Phonetic Alphabet, no teachers or students will be able to read them. It's a bit like using your own secret code.

More importantly, I was soon to learn that phonetics would be a lifelong professional tool that allowed me to make a tremendous difference in the lives of children with speech sound disorders, especially those whose speech was unintelligible. All that hard-learned knowledge about how consonants and vowels were formed later enabled me to analyze children's speech and then help them hear and produce the contrasts that distinguish speech sounds from each other. New research findings, built on my basic knowledge of phonetics, allowed me to become a much more effective clinician and supervisor.

My first phonetics instructor was young and enthusiastic and enhanced his teaching with real professional examples. I later followed in his footsteps, teaching courses in phonetics and speech sound disorders myself. This book gives you many practical examples to make phonetics come "alive" for you. Make no mistake: learning the International Phonetic Alphabet and its varied applications takes time and patience. If you learned to read with any type of phonics instruction (if you can remember that far back), you will probably find that phonetics comes more easily to you than to your classmates who learned by a non–phonics-based method. Nevertheless, my students who applied themselves and quickly learned to focus on phonemes, rather than on alphabetic letters, always succeeded.

As you complete the readings and transcription exercises, keep reminding yourself of how much you have learned and that the International Phonetic Alphabet is a tool that could prove useful to you throughout your professional life. I wish all of you success in your career, with many opportunities to make a difference in the lives of others!

Pamela Garn-Nunn, PhD

PREFACE

This fourth edition of *Calvert's Descriptive Phonetics* follows Dr. Donald Calvert's original lead in writing a high-quality text that would be useful to a wide variety of readers, especially students in speech production who intend to become speech-language pathologists, teachers of children who are hearing impaired or deaf, auditory-verbal therapists, teachers of English as a second language (ESL), or coaches of dramatics and diction. I hope that students and instructors in these specialties will find the text informative, comprehensive, and useful in learning the International Phonetic Alphabet.

This edition differs from its predecessors in that it consists of one, rather than two, volumes. The previous phonetic workbook exercises and keys have been incorporated as appendices in the text. Students now have only one book to work with and to pay for! Although the content areas covered remain much the same as in previous editions, there are organizational changes, new information, and lots of additional practice examples for students. In particular, Chapter 2 and the chapters on dialectic variations (Chapter 6) and applied phonetics (Chapter 7) have been extensively rewritten. Information about acoustic phonetics is included in Chapter 2 as well as throughout the text; however, there is no chapter devoted exclusively to acoustic phonetics. Chapter 3's content from the third edition is now distributed in the chapters on vowels, consonants, connected speech, and applied phonetics. The presentation of vowels (the new Chapter 3) precedes that of consonants, based on the author's teaching experience with a large number of undergraduate students over the years. Otherwise, the emphases of this text remain much the same.

This book is designed primarily as a text for students beginning the study of phonetics. The exercises in Appendix A are intended to help the student understand and learn the information. Concept questions have been added at the end of each chapter to help students master the text information.

The pronunciations in this book are those most commonly associated with what has previously been referred to as standard American English or mainstream American English (MAE). In this text, we discuss MAE and its dialectic variations. In Chapter 6, MAE serves as the reference for discussing a number of dialectic variations. Students should realize that no single dialectic variation of English has an inherent value in and of itself. Based on the most recent studies by linguists, a variety of dialects can be found within our borders. Thus, both background information and characteristics of dialectic variations are included.

Chapter 7, covering applied phonetics, has been expanded and especially emphasizes analysis of speech sound disorders and differentiating dialectic variation and disorders. Depending on the orientation of the student, for example speech-language pathology or voice and diction, this chapter may vary in its applicability. Nevertheless, it can introduce the student to the correspondence between International Phonetic Alphabet knowledge and its applicability to a variety of differences and disorders.

1

INTRODUCTION

SYMBOL SYSTEMS
DIFFERENCES BETWEEN SPELLING AND PHONEMES
BASIC TERMS AND DEFINITIONS
CONCEPT QUESTIONS

SYMBOL SYSTEMS

Imagine that you are from the American Midwest and are now a student at a university in Massachusetts. Your suitemates are from a variety of places, including Boston. When your roommate from Georgia says, "Hi," for the first time, you realize that the way you both pronounce English is not always the same. It sounds to you as if she said "Hah" rather than "Hi." She also talks about losing her *pen* except you think that she said *pin*. Then there's your roommate from Maine who wonders why you pronounce *hawk* and *hock, Dawn* and *Don* with the same vowel sound, *ah*. She uses two different vowel sounds for those words, *aw* for *hawk* and *Dawn*, and ah for *hock* and *Don*. All three of you have noticed that your suitemate from Boston doesn't use the *r* sound after vowels so that "park the car" sounds like "*pahk* the *cah*," like many other speakers in eastern Massachusetts.

So whose speech is correct? The answer is that none of you is correct or incorrect. You simply speak different dialects of American English (American Speech-Language-Hearing Association, 2003; Wolfram, 1991; Wolfram, Adger, & Christian, 1999). So how can you figure out the differences in your pronunciation to communicate more easily? Well, you could use the Roman alphabet that you learned in kindergarten, as shown in the examples in the first paragraph. But in trying to figure out the difference in your two pronunciations of *i* in *hi,* you first have to realize that you're discussing the *i* in *height* and *buy,* not the *i* in *inch* and *sit.* Then, you think that your roommate's production of *i* sounded like the letter *a* instead of *i.* But do you mean the *a* in *calm,* the *a* in *add,* or even the other *a* in *base?* Then there's your confusion over her pronunciation of *pen.* "You're using *i* instead of *e,*" you tell her. "Which *e?*" she replies. "The one in *each* or the one in *red?*"

Obviously, even when we have a common orthographic system, communication can be a problem. Each of us learned **orthography** (the accurate or accepted spelling of words using alphabet symbols) very early in our education. And we've been using it ever since, so we're very used to it. But some languages use symbol systems different from that of English; for example, Russian uses the Cyrillic alphabet. We would pronounce the Russian word for *no* as *nyet* (Roman alphabet symbols), but in Cyrillic it would be written as *нет*. To further complicate matters, some sounds occur in one language but not in others. For example, German doesn't have *th* sounds (*thorn* and *them*), but English lacks the pharyngeal sounds of other languages.

We can bypass these problems by using a common symbol system, the **International Phonetic Alphabet (IPA)** (**Tables 1.1** and **1.2**). In the IPA, each symbol corresponds to one and only one speech sound or **phoneme.** For example, the *i* in *hi* is transcribed as /aɪ/, but the *i* in *inch* is transcribed as /ɪ/. Your roommate from Georgia pronounces *hi* as *hah*, transcribed as /hɑ/. That /ɑ/ is different from the /æ/ in *apple*. Your roommate who uses different vowels for *Don* and *Dawn* notes that the words are spelled differently, but you're using the same vowel sound. In orthographics, *o* can represent a number of different vowel sounds, for example *hot*, *done*, and *hold*. The spelling of words can be (and often is) variable (**Tables 1.1** and **1.2**), but IPA transcription is consistent in its sound–symbol relationships. Notice that **Tables 1.1** and **1.2** show "primary" orthographic symbols in the first column but also give alternative spelling examples in the "Key Words" column. **Table 1.3** shows you just how often spelling does (or doesn't) correspond to specific orthographic symbols for vowels. In some cases, e.g., "a-e" and "u-e" spelling and phonetic

TABLE 1.1 INTERNATIONAL PHONETIC ALPHABET: VOWEL AND DIPHTHONG SYMBOLS FOR MAINSTREAM AMERICAN ENGLISH

Primary Orthographic Symbols	IPA Symbol	Spelling Examples
ee, ea	/i/	Lee, eat, beet, hobby, seize
i	/ɪ/	it, kiss, sick, fill, busy
e	/ɛ/	etch, bet, less, said, lead
a	/æ/	add, bat, pass, cabin, laugh
oo	/u/	ooze, pool, too, news, super
oo	/ʊ/	book, good, would, push, full
aw	/ɔ/	saw, yawn, off, caught, laud
o	/ɑ/	odd, bond, pot, palm, calm
ur, er	/ɝ/	turn, verse, earth, bird, search (stressed)
	/ɚ/	hammer, under, scenery, over (unstressed)
u	/ʌ/	up, come, must, flood, other (stressed)
u	/ə/	elephant, sofa, about, tuba (unstressed)
a-e	/eɪ/	late, made, able, may, reign (stressed)
a-e	/e/	vibrate, rotate, rebate, vacate (unstressed)
oa	/oʊ/	boat, load, code, bowl, show (stressed)
oa	/o/	rotation, donation, location (unstressed)
i-e	/aɪ/	kite, ideal, I've, my, heist
ou	/aʊ/	out, couch, our, now, town
oi	/ɔɪ/	oil, coin, boy, royal, soy

Source: Garn-Nunn, & Lynn, 2004

TABLE 1.2 INTERNATIONAL PHONETIC ALPHABET SYMBOLS: CONSONANT SYMBOLS FOR
MAINSTREAM AMERICAN ENGLISH

Primary Orthographic Symbols	IPA Symbol	Spelling Examples
p	/p/	pie, stopped, cup, camp, ape
b	/b/	boy, baby, robot, crab, herb
t	/t/	top, later, seat, city, trust
d	/d/	down, ladder, red, jade, lady
k, c	/k/	kite, bake, book, cub, ache
g	/g/	go, bug, log, bigger, vague
f, ph	/f/	four, offer, if, prophet, rough
v	/v/	vine, over, believe, live, of
th	/θ/	thin, Athens, earth, teeth
th	/ð/	this, they, other, breathe
s	/s/	see, missing, bus, bicycle, ice
z	/z/	zoo, buzzer, eyes, rose, miser
sh	/ʃ/	shoe, washer, fish, ocean
zh	/ʒ/	measure, beige, vision, rouge
h	/h/	he, hoe, hair, ahead, behind
ch	/ʧ/	chin, matches, such, watch
j, dg	/ʤ/	jump, angel, fudge, magic
w	/w/	we, awake, away, twin, sway
y	/j/	yes, bayou, yell, use, cute
l	/l/	listen, low, hollow, fill, sled
r	/ɹ/	rain, arrange, very, car, tray
m	/m/	me, omen, among, home, am
n	/n/	new, owner, pan, snail, pint
ng	/ŋ/	sing, singer, linger, longer

Source: Garn-Nunn & Lynn, 2004.
PLEASE NOTE: the correct *phonetic* symbol for the letter g is /g/; it has to be inserted from the IPA chart. Substituting g for /g/ is incorrect.

symbols always agree. However, in others, e.g., a (bad and able), or e (bet and be) several different phonemes may be represented by the same letter.

As a beginning student in the study of phonetics, you have spent many years using the orthographic system for reading and writing in your language. Whether you realize it or not, you tend to view words in terms of *alphabet letters* rather than the *phonemes* perceived. Consequently, you will need to disregard what you know about spelling in order to master phonetics. The next section of this chapter discusses the differences between phonemes and alphabet letters. In addition, there are exercises throughout this book that will help you develop your phoneme listening skills.

DIFFERENCES BETWEEN SPELLING AND PHONEMES

The difference between the spelling of words and their pronunciation results from a variety of factors. Spoken language tends to change more quickly than written

TABLE 1.3 PERCENTAGE OF TIMES EACH OF 19 ALPHABET SPELLINGS REPRESENTS THE DESIGNATED VOWEL SOUNDS IN 7,500 COMMON WORDS

Orthographic Symbol	Word	Alphabet-Sound Agreement	Orthographic Symbol	Word	Alphabet-Sound Agreement
a-e	gave	100%	-a-	cat	81%
				table	13%
u-e	cute	100%	-u-	cup	73%
				unite	24%
aw	law	100%	-ea-	meat	74%
				head	24%
i-e	kite	99%	-e-	bet	70%
				be	30%
oi	boil	99%	ee	beet	96%
oa	boat	98%			
ou	out	60%	oo	boot	59%
	rough	35%		cook	41%
-i-	pin	91%	-o-	top	53%
	child	9%		told	40%
			ow	low	52%
ai	bait	90%		cow	48%
au	caught	88%	o-e	home	34%
				come	66%

language. The English language originated from a variety of sources across Europe. These include Germanic dialects, Scandinavian languages (northern Europe), French, and Romance languages from southern Europe, as well as classic Greek and Latin (Graddol, Leith, & Swann, 1996; Merriam-Webster, 2012). Thus, two words can contain the same speech sound/phoneme but vary in their spelling as a result of their origin. For example, the first phonemes in the words *fan* and *phone* (IPA transcription: /f/) are the same, but the spelling (*ph* or *f*) differs. The *ph* spelling is most likely indicative of the word's Greek origin, whereas the *f* spelling is indicative Middle English and Latin origins.

A major problem of orthography is that the Roman alphabet used in English does not contain enough symbols to represent all the different English phonemes that you will learn to listen for. We have only 26 alphabet letters to represent 43 basic phonemes. In elementary school you learned that there are five vowels: *a, e, i, o,* and *u* (and sometimes *y*). In reality, English uses 18 different vowel and diphthong phonemes and 25 different consonant phonemes (as opposed to the 21 orthographic letters). Some phonemes have no specific letter to represent them, for example the middle consonant in *leisure* and *pleasure*. Still other speech sounds require a combination of letters to stand for the single phoneme they represent (e.g., the initial sound in *shoe* and *share* or those in *chin* and *chair*). These letter combinations are known as **digraphs**.

Another difference between spelling and phonemes is that the same spelling does not always equate to the same phoneme in different words. For example, the words *chorus* and *chair* both begin with the same orthographic symbol, *ch*. However, the initial phonemes in these words are different (IPA: /k/ and /ʧ/, respectively). Similar examples are found in words such as *measure* and *raisin*. The middle consonant phoneme is spelled as *s* in each word, but it represents two different phonemes, *zh* (IPA: /ʒ/ in *measure*) and *z* (IPA: /z/ in *raisin*).

On the other hand, words can differ in spelling even if the same phoneme is contained in each word. An example of this can be found in the words *sugar* and *short*. Both words start with the phoneme /ʃ/, but their spelling of that speech sound differs (*s* and *sh*, respectively). Similarly the sound of *f* (IPA: /f/) can be spelled in several different ways (e.g., *file, phone, differ, trough)*.

The orthographic system for vowels provides additional (and often frustrating!) examples of how the same orthographic letter does not necessarily represent the same phoneme. Consider the orthographic symbol *o*. We use this letter to represent a number of different vowel phonemes, for example *ton, top, told, tomb,* and *woman* (IPA symbols: /ʌ ɑ o u ʊ/, respectively).

In case you're not yet convinced about the unreliability of spelling, here is another example. English spelling also includes letters that have no corresponding phoneme. In the word *knave*, there are really only three phonemes (IPA: /n e v/), but the spelling consists of five letters. In the word *honest*, there are six orthographic letters but only five phonemes (IPA: /ɑ n ə s t/) because the letter *h* is silent. The same principle applies to the word *house*, but a different letter is involved. The five letters correspond to only three phonemes: /h aʊ s/. This time the *h* does symbolize a phoneme, but there is only one vowel (symbolized by two orthographic letters), and the *e* is silent. This will make more sense as you complete **Exercise 1.5** in Appendix A.

A similar example is found in words in which *two* orthographic letters correspond to only *one* speech sound/phoneme. In the word *running*, there is only one middle consonant phoneme (IPA: /n/), even though there are two letters (*nn*) in spelling. Another example, using vowels, can be found in the word *troupe* in which two letters, *ou*, stand for only one phoneme (IPA: /u/).

For most American English speakers, these inconsistencies and irregularities are ultimately manageable obstacles to be overcome in learning to read and spell. This is not necessarily the case for children with reading disabilities or communication disorders (Anthony et al, 2011; Apel & Lawrence, 2011; Pascoe, Stackhouse, & Wells, 2006). Furthermore, nonnative English speakers' mispronunciations are often related to the irregularities between orthographic spelling and the pronunciation of a word. Again, your key task in learning phonetics will be to listen for each phoneme and associate it with its IPA symbol. Thinking about how the word is spelled will not help, and more likely will hinder, your growth in this process.

Listening Exercises: Appendix A. To help you develop your listening skills, you should turn to Appendix A and complete Exercises 1.1–1.7. These will help you to become more aware of the frequent contrasts between spelling and actual phonemes.

BASIC TERMS AND DEFINITIONS

Phonetics, the focus of this textbook is defined most simply as the study of speech sounds of a spoken language. Within this broad definition, a number of subtypes or branches are important to the student of phonetics. In particular, this book empha-sizes **physiologic phonetics** to build understanding of the English language sound system. Researchers in physiologic phonetics analyze speech sounds in terms of the anatomic and physiologic concepts involved. Thus, studies in physiologic phonetics would focus on the interaction of physical structures, muscles, and movements in-volved in producing speech sounds. In **acoustic phonetics**, the researcher is fo-cused on the acoustic properties of speech sounds, that is, the frequency (heard as pitch) and intensity (heard as loudness) of the sounds heard. These topics, especially physiologic phonetics, are addressed in more detail in Chapter 2.

Although phoneticians focus on the study of phonemes, the definition of *phoneme* is more complex than "speech sound." In fact, each phoneme is a group of sounds, or **allophones.** You see, each time we produce a speech sound, we produce it in a slightly different way. As long as the physiologic formation and its acoustic result are consistent enough, we still hear each allophone as a member of the same phoneme class. For example, try saying the word *cap* in these two different ways. First, open your lips as you finish the word so that lip closure for /p/ is followed by a small puff of air. Now, say the word again, but keep your lips closed (no puff of air released). You just produced two allophones of the phoneme /p/, the audibly aspirated (puff of air) and unaspirated (no air released). Despite that small difference in air release, you still hear the last sound in both words as /p/; the word meaning—something you wear on your head—remains the same.

You will perceive allophonic variations of a particular phoneme as being the same phoneme as long as certain requirements are met. For example, if you say *cap* and then *cat*, you hear two different phonemes at the end of the words. It does not matter whether you release the air or not; the *places* where the sounds are made are differ-ent. /p/ is produced with the lips, and /t/ is made with the tongue tip and alveolar ridge. Requirements to hear an allophone as /p/ include lip closure; tongue tip–alveolar ridge closure produces a different phoneme, /t/. Finally, a word that varies only by allophones will still be heard as two versions of the same word. Changing the phoneme /p/ to /t/ in *cap* and *cat*, however, results in a difference in meaning; that is, the phoneme change means that you hear two different words.

The IPA transcription of words may or may not reflect allophonic variation. **Broad transcription** (also known as **phonemic transcription**) does not reflect allo-phonic variation. It is contained in virgules or slashes (/ /). If you wish to reflect the difference between our two allophones of /p/ (previous example), you have to use **narrow transcription**, also known as **phonetic transcription**. Phonetic tran-scription, enclosed in brackets ([ ]), includes **diacritic markings** to reflect allo-phonic differences. So, a phonemic transcription of *cap* would be /k æ p/. A phonetic, or narrow transcription, would have to represent each word separately and use dia-critical markings indicative of audible aspiration/air released ([k ^{h} æ p ^{h}] or [k ^{h} æ p ˀ]) for the production without audible air release.

Although phoneticians focus on formation and acoustic characteristics of pho-nemes and allophones, **phonologists** have a related, but different focus. They are interested in **phonology,** the study of how phonemes can be *combined* to transmit meaning. **Developmental phonology** is the study of how children acquire the sound system of their language. In early development, English-speaking children often omit final consonants in words (e.g., ca for cat and ro for rose). Because final consonants are important in signaling meaning in English, the child must eventually learn to "finish" or "close" words. If a child fails to do so in a timely manner, he or she is said to have a **phonological disorder**.

Another aspect of phonology is **phonotactics**, the rules for how sounds can be combined to form syllables and words. This is not as simple as it might sound. In English, some phoneme combinations are not possible or typical. For example, the phoneme /ŋ/ (as in si*ng*) cannot begin words in English. English allows word-beginning consonant clusters or blends of up to three sounds (e.g., *str*eet) but does not permit four-consonant blends to begin words. The Russian word for hello (transliterated as *sdrastvweetyeh*) seems hard to pronounce for English speakers because the *stvwee* combination is not found in English.

Phonemes signal their meaning within the context of **morphemes.** Morphemes are the smallest meaningful units of language. A morpheme can consist of one or more phonemes or of an entire word. And a word can contain more than one morpheme. The word *view* is composed of one morpheme; it cannot be broken down further and still retain its meaning of "look at." But if we add the phoneme /s/ to the end of the word, we change the meaning: *views* means "more than one view" and contains two morphemes (*view* + *s*). Next, if we add the prefix *pre-*, we have created a word with three morphemes (*pre* + *view* + *s*) (meaning to look at in advance or ahead of time).

The meaningful words (one morpheme each) *cap* and *cat* show us how phonemes differentiate meaning within the context of morphemes. *Cat* and *cap* differ in their final phonemes, /t/ and /p/. It is that simple difference in phonemes that tells us whether someone is talking about a furry feline or a hat. One-morpheme words like *cat* and *cap* are also called **minimal pairs**: two words that differ by only one phoneme. Other examples of minimal pairs are *seat* and *seal*, *rush* and *rash*, and *see* and *she*. Later, in Chapter 7, you will learn how minimal pairs may be used in therapy to treat children with speech sound disorders.

As you use this book, you will learn to recognize and transcribe the phonemes of English primarily within the context of words. This puts these physiological and acoustic units into their language role: to signify differences in meaning. And it will help you to disregard alphabetic symbols and learn to listen for phonemes.

CONCEPT QUESTIONS

The following exercises are designed to help you expand both your conceptual knowledge and your phonological awareness skills. In the first section, true–false questions are designed to help you integrate the different concepts covered in this chapter. The second section will help you to better hear all the consonant and vowel phonemes. After you have completed the exercises, you can check your answers in Appendix B, Chapter 1 Key.

PART I: CONCEPT INTEGRATION

Are the following statements true or false?

_____ 1. A phoneme is composed of a group of allophones.

_____ 2. In the words *side* and *site*, /t/ and /d/ are different allophones.

_____ 3. A child who has not learned all age-appropriate rules governing phonology is said to have a phonological disorder.

_____ 4. The vowel phonemes in English are *a*, *e*, *i o*, *u*, and sometimes *y*.

_____ 5. In English, there are more alphabet letters than phonemes.

_____ 6. The letter *e* can correspond to more than one vowel phoneme.

_____ 7. In English, two words can be spelled differently but have the same phoneme.

_____ 8. In orthography, there is a one-to-one relationship between letters and sounds.

_____ 9. The word *listeners* has 4 morphemes.

_____ 10. Phonetic transcription is sensitive to allophonic variation and uses / /.

Part II: Supplemental Exercises—Listening for Phonemes

As you learned in this chapter, the relationship between phonemes and their orthographic representation can be highly variable. The following exercises are designed to help you further develop your listening skills and decrease your reliance on visual orthographic symbols. In each exercise, remember to focus on *phonemes*, not letters. Answers for all these exercises are in Appendix B.

Consonant Exercises

1. Underline all the words that contain the same *beginning* phoneme in each line, regardless of spelling/letters. For each list, there are four words beginning with the same consonant phoneme. Then, using **Table 1.2**, enter the phoneme symbol in the slashes at the end. The first line is completed for you.

a.	chorus	chime	<u>cobra</u>	<u>Canada</u>	<u>Kyle</u>	<u>chord</u>	/ k /
b.	first	phony	fairy	phase	pair	pan	/ /
c.	hope	who	honest	hill	heather	those	/ /
d.	think	tone	Thomas	tie	thumb	table	/ /
e.	them	Thames	third	three	thirteen	thick	/ /
f.	this	Thomas	there	that	them	thicket	/ /
g.	write	rain	who	wrought	rest	web	/ /
h.	science	skirt	school	sci-fi	show	shall	/ /

2. Underline all the words that contain the same *ending* phoneme in each line, regardless of spelling/letters. For each list, there are four words ending with the same consonant phoneme. Then, using **Table 1.2**, enter the phoneme symbol in the slashes at the end of the line. The first line is completed for you.

a.	<u>back</u>	<u>ache</u>	watch	<u>sac</u>	cache	<u>work</u>	/ k /
b.	cope	graph	rope	leaf	hop	map	/ /
c.	with	bathe	boot	sight	eight	last	/ /
d.	less	mash	bats	dogs	ice	box	/ /
e.	reach	Bach	ache	such	patch	fetch	/ /
f.	mines	rose	razz	books	ease	boss	/ /
g.	rash	crèche	batch	such	clash	seiche	/ /
h.	Harry	far	pore	hair	dare	curl	/ /

3. Underline all the words that contain the same *middle* phoneme in each line, regardless of spelling/letters. For each list, there are four words with the same
consonant phoneme in the middle of the word. Then, using **Table 1.2**, enter the
phoneme symbol in the slash marks at the end of the line. The first line is completed for you.

a.	danger	Roger	budgie	regal	manager	angle	/dʒ/
b.	banner	singer	ranger	hanger	ringing	manganese	/ /
c.	hugger	finger	region	hunger	range	ugly	/ /
d.	pressure	measure	lessen	assure	Bashir	cashier	/ /
e.	whistle	washer	rashly	listener	dancing	relaxing	/ /
f.	razor	reason	reserve	azure	lessen	observe	/ /
g.	measure	leisure	laser	treasure	casual	Caesar	/ /
h.	backache	record	acre	bacon	racing	nicer	/ /

VOWEL EXERCISES

1. For this word list, underline the four words in each row that have the same beginning *vowel* sound, regardless of spelling. Then, using **Table 1.1**, enter the symbol
for the common phoneme in the slash marks at the end of each line. The first line
is completed for you.

a.	able	at	and	atrium	eight	aim	/e/
b.	evil	every	ending	ember	emu	etch	/ /
c.	one	on	over	old	Oprah	ogee	/ /
d.	on	offer	aardvark	obelisk	oath	ostrich	/ /
e.	eel	east	even	ever	eerie	elevator	/ /
f.	inner	Irish	iPad	if	is	Iliad	/ /
g.	apart	after	axe	upon	afghan	aspirin	/ /
h.	eyelid	Ivan	I'll	aisle	insect	air	/ /

2. For this word list, underline the four words in each row that have the same vowel
sound, regardless of position. Then, using **Table 1.1**, enter the IPA symbol for the
common phoneme in the slash marks at the end of the line. The first line is completed for you.

a.	turn	fair	birch	work	earth	part	/ɝ/
b.	seam	pear	measure	least	reach	eagle	/ /
c.	fried	shriek	pie	bind	license	mystery	/ /
d.	bait	age	lady	mane	match	atom	/ /
e.	apple	cater	fact	patch	fate	pasture	/ /
f.	bend	lean	edit	mellow	rein	session	/ /
g.	I'm	itch	sign	singe	list	fill	/ /
h.	done	fuss	gone	bush	upper	wonder	/ /

CHALLENGE EXERCISES

To further develop your listening skills before beginning to learn the IPA, try the
next two exercises.

1. Count the number of phonemes in each word and enter the number in the space
next to the word. For example, the number of sounds in the word *maker* is 4:

m/a/k/er or /mekɚ/, the same as the number of phonemes in *fix: f/i/k/s* or /f ɪ k s/. Remember to listen for *sounds* and ignore letters as much as possible! Sometimes the number of phonemes and letters will be the same, but more often that will not be the case. The first one is completed for you.

ax	_3_	baker	___	knot	___	squeeze	___	sure	___	first	___
panda	___	afghan	___	karate	___	received	___	peachy	___	wreath	___
boxer	___	slope	___	coupe	___	quest	___	bonding	___	honest	___

2. Reverse the sounds in the word to create a new, real word. For example, if you reverse the sounds in *aisle*, you get *lie* because *ai* is one vowel, and the *s* and *e* are silent: /l aɪ/→/aɪ l/. Another example would be *peach,* which becomes *cheap* when reversed: /p i ʧ/→/ʧ i p/. But be careful; the reversed word may not contain the same letters as the original word, but the phonemes will be the same. The first one is done for you.

Luke	_c oo l_	bag	_____	dumb	_____	rots	_____
stun	_____	niece	_____	knife	_____	licks	_____
Mack	_____	ouch	_____	caught	_____	zoo	_____
lean	_____	gnome	_____	sigh	_____	bats	_____

THE SPEECH PRODUCTION MECHANISM AND PROCESSES

THE SPEECH MECHANISM: SUPRAGLOTTAL STRUCTURES
THE LARYNX AND SUBGLOTTAL STRUCTURES
SPEECH PROCESSES AND ASSOCIATED STRUCTURES
CONCLUSION
CONCEPT QUESTIONS

Among the creatures on Earth, only *Homo sapiens* has achieved oral language. All species of animals communicate, many through vocalizations as well as physical signals. No species, however, has approached the complexity and sophistication of our oral language. In fact, current research continues to support the uniqueness of humans to support this function (Spiteri et al, 2007). The body parts we use to produce speech do not appear to be vastly different from those of other animals, which also have teeth, tongues, and palates. Like other species, we also use these oral structures regularly for basic biological functions such as breathing and eating. However, we know that a healthy human infant has an innate *potential* to communicate orally. Research tells us that humans have some unique neurological and structural characteristics that allow us to use these body parts for speech production in addition to their basic, vegetative function. More recent research has also indicated that the muscle range and movement for speech are qualitatively and quantitatively different from those used for vegetative functions, such as breathing, chewing, and swallowing (Bunton, 2008; Connaghan, Moore, & Higashakawa, 2004; Green, Moore, & Reilly, 2002; Lof, 2008; Moore, Caulfield, & Green, 2001; Parham, Buder, Oller, & Boliek, 2011; Reilly & Moore, 2009; Wilson, Green, Yunusova, & Moore, 2008).

Speech is the result of four processes or actions that occur simultaneously and cooperatively: **respiration**, **phonation**, **resonation**, and **articulation**. **Audition**, which involves the auditory mechanism, is an additional crucial feedback loop in speech. It is very important to understand the implications of the terms *simultaneously* and *cooperatively*. Speaking is not a linear sequence of events that starts with the lungs and ends with the listener's ear. The act of speaking requires continuous, overlapping action as well as feedback adjustments across all the systems involved. To understand the speech processes, you need to begin with a description of the basic structures involved in speech production. If you're wondering why you need to learn this information, rest assured that it will be important in distinguishing and learning the characteristics of consonants and vowels in the following chapters.

THE SPEECH MECHANISM: SUPRAGLOTTAL STRUCTURES

Information for each structure of the speech mechanism includes location, speech function, and terms commonly associated with each structure. In particular, the associated terms are important as you learn about vowel and consonant formation in Chapters 3 and 4. Even though the speech mechanism structures are covered separately, you should remember that all these structures function *synergistically* in order to produce speech. That is, all the parts working together produce something that could not be produced by each individual part alone. To emphasize the interaction, the text sections are grouped according to location and function of the structures.

SUPRALARYNGEAL STRUCTURES

The supralaryngeal structures refer to those parts of the speech mechanism located above the level of the larynx. Each of these structures is contained in one of three cavities or spaces: **oral, nasal,** or **pharyngeal**. The pharyngeal cavity, or **pharynx,** extends from the opening of the larynx to the posterior boundaries of the **oral cavity** (mouth) and **nasal cavity** (nose) (**Fig. 2.1**). Positioning and movements of the structures in these cavities shape the outgoing airstream into the vowels and consonants we recognize as speech.

LIPS

The lips are the external boundary of the oral cavity. They are a complex of numerous internal and external muscles and other tissues. In speech, they perform a variety of actions. For vowels, lip position can range from rounded to neutral to spread. These changes in shape also contribute to the resonant patterns that characterize different vowels. Several consonants are classified as **labial** (involving the lips). Some of these consonants are **bilabial** (using both lips) such as /b/, and others **labiodental** (using upper lip and lower teeth), such as /v/. In most speakers, the lower lip is more mobile in rapid connected speech.

TEETH

The role that teeth play in speech is primarily passive but still important. In English, two consonants are classified as **dental** or **interdental** (involving the teeth): the /θ/ in **th***orn* and the /ð/ in **th***em*. However, production of a number of consonants, such as /s/ and /z/, also requires the use of the posterior sides of the tongue. For several consonants, including /s/ and /z/, the tongue sides must touch against the back teeth (molars) to direct the airstream appropriately. Otherwise, air may escape laterally, resulting in a distortion of the sound(s). Loss of the central **incisors** (front teeth) between ages 5 and 7 results in many children having a **lisp** (/s/) problem (**Fig. 2.2**). The lisp usually disappears when the permanent incisors grow in fully.

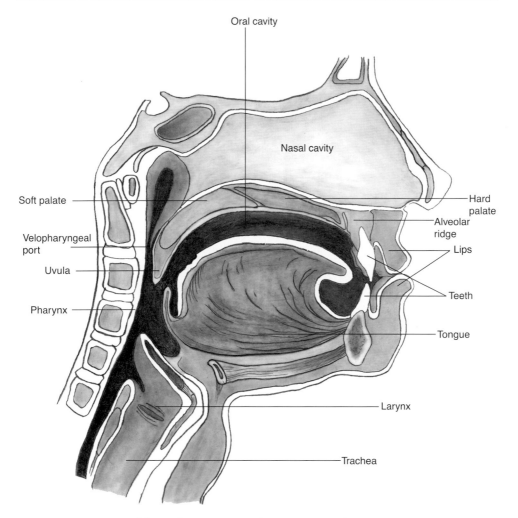

Figure 2.1 *Structures of the vocal tract. (From Van de Water, T., & Staecker, H. Otolaryngology. New York: Thieme, 2005. Reprinted with permission.)*

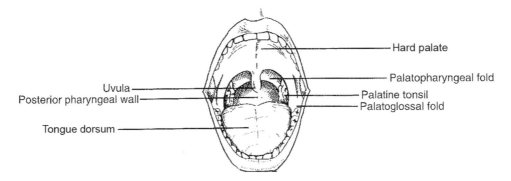

Figure 2.2 *Structures of the oral cavity. (From Van de Water, T., & Staecker, H. Otolaryngology. New York: Thieme, 2005. Reprinted with permission.) Modified from Beasley, P. Anatomy of the pharynx and esophagus. In: Gleeson, M., ed. Scott-Brown's Otolaryngology. Bath, England: University of Bath Press, 1997. Reprinted with permission).*

ALVEOLAR RIDGE

In both the **maxilla** (upper jaw) and **mandible** (lower jaw), the teeth are contained in the **alveolar ridge** (alveolar processes, more commonly known as the gum ridges). In speech, many consonants involve tongue contact with, or placement near, the upper alveolar ridge (found behind the maxillary incisors.) **Alveolar** consonants such as /t/, /s/, and /l/, to name just a few, involve the maxillary alveolar ridge. In addition, the alveolar ridge, along with the anterior palate, serves as a reference point for the tongue in front vowel formation.

HARD PALATE

The hard palate is composed of bony tissue and covered by mucous membrane. It divides the oral and nasal cavities, forming the roof of the oral cavity and the floor of the nasal cavity. It is involved in both vowel and consonant production for speech. For vowels, it plays a role in oral cavity shaping. Several consonants are considered **palatal**: /ʃ/ (as in *sh*oe), /ʒ/ (as in *measure*), /ʧ/ (as in *ch*air), /ʤ/ (as in *jump*), /ɹ/ (as in *r*un and *dr*ink), and /j/ (as in *yes* and *youth*). All these consonants require the tongue to be positioned near, or to move in relation to, the hard palate.

SOFT PALATE (VELUM)

Posterior to the hard palate (behind it), the **velum** or **soft palate** forms the remainder of the roof of the mouth and the floor of the nasal cavity. It is composed of muscle and connective tissue and is covered by a continuation of the mucous membrane of the hard palate. Opening and closing of the **velopharyngeal port** (aperture/opening that connects the nasal and oral cavities) requires participation of the velum (**Fig. 2.1**). Composed of a complex of muscles, the velum is highly flexible and important for speech function. By helping to close the velopharyngeal port, the velum helps direct the breath stream to the oral cavity for articulation of oral resonant phonemes (especially vowels). Relaxation of the velum opens the velopharyngeal port and is necessary to produce the three **nasal** consonant phonemes: /m/, /n/, and /ŋ/. Consonants involving tongue contact with the velum (/k/ /g/ /ŋ/) are referred to as **velar** consonants.

TONGUE

The tongue, composed of muscle and connective tissue and covered by mucous membrane, is extremely important for production of many consonants and all vowels. Highly flexible and mobile, the tongue can shape the oral cavity almost infinitely. It arises from the floor of the oral cavity and is dually controlled by both intrinsic (within the tongue) and extrinsic (connecting the tongue to other structures) muscles. To understand the specific role of the tongue in vowel and consonant production, you need to be familiar with various tongue landmarks. The tongue itself has a root, apex, dorsum, septum, and frenum (**Fig. 2.2**). The root is the posterior portion, connecting to the hyoid bone and epiglottis. The anterior end of the tongue is its **apex**, and the superior (upper) surface, the **dorsum**. The **lingual septum** is a midline structure of connective tissue. The front tongue undersurface is connected to the mandible by the **lingual frenum**. In describing speech articulation, we refer to various landmarks on the tongue surface (**Fig. 2.2**): **back, middle, front/blade,** and **tip**. Consonants such as /s/ and /t/ involve the tongue tip (**alveolar** consonants), whereas /k/ and /g/ production (**velar** consonants) involve the back of the tongue. In producing consonants and vowels, the tongue shape can vary from broad to narrow, flat to curled, and whole tongue positioning to differential positioning of tongue segments. All the vowels and most of the consonants require tongue movement; only /m/, /p/, /b/, /f/, and /v/ do not.

Mandible

The mandible or lower jaw plays both an active and passive role in articulation of speech sounds. It forms the base for the tongue and houses the mandibular teeth. For speech, the mandible can be raised or lowered by varying degrees, contributing to changes in vowel articulation.

Nasal Cavity

The nasal cavity lies directly superior to the oral cavity (**Fig. 2.1**). Horizontally, it extends from the external nares (nostrils) to the posterior pharyngeal wall. Vertically, it is bounded by the base of the skull and the palate and velum. With its soft, moist lining, it contributes to the distinctive resonance characteristics of the cavity. The nasal cavity participates in speech resonance with either closure or opening of the velopharyngeal port. It is always open anteriorly, at the nostrils, unless you have a cold or other infection. Even if the velopharyngeal port is closed, the nasal cavity resonates the vibrating airstream from the larynx. In this case, the resonation of oral and nasal air combines to help produce an individual speaker's distinctive voice quality. Unlike all the other consonants, production of /m/, /n/, and /ŋ/ require *closure* somewhere in the oral cavity combined with *opening* of the velopharyngeal port (lowering the velum). This allows the nasal cavity to serve as the primary resonator. Consequently, these three phonemes are referred to as **nasal** consonants.

Pharyngeal Cavity

Anatomically, the **pharynx** (pharyngeal cavity) extends from the posterior portion of the nasal cavity downward past the back of the oral cavity to (but not including) the larynx (**Fig. 2.1**). A vertical tube, the pharynx can be subdivided into three parts: **nasopharynx** (continuation of nasal cavity), **oropharynx** (continuation of oral cavity), and **laryngopharynx** (just above larynx). For American English speech production, the pharynx acts as a resonating chamber. (Although some languages use the pharynx for consonant articulation, English is not one of them.) The primary pharyngeal alteration occurs in velopharyngeal closure. This closure both directs voice into the oral cavity and reduces the length of the pharyngeal tube (by closing off the nasopharynx). Pharyngeal circumference (diameter) can also be changed by constriction or relaxation of the muscular pharyngeal walls. Such changes alter the resonating characteristics of the pharynx, and, consequently, the sound of the human voice as well as contributing to vowel resonance.

THE LARYNX AND SUBGLOTTAL STRUCTURES

The larynx is composed of cartilage and muscle. It sits on top of, and is connected to, the trachea (**Fig. 2.3**). It is suspended from the **hyoid bone** by a complex of muscles and ligaments and lies posterior and slightly inferior to the tongue root. It contains the **vocal folds** necessary for **phonation** (vocal fold vibration). The vocal folds are shelves of muscles and connective tissue, lined with mucous membrane. The space between the vocal folds is referred to as the **glottis**. Sometimes laryngeal structures are referred to as **subglottal** (below) or **supraglottal** (above), depending on their spatial relationship with the vocal fold opening. The vocal folds are anchored to the inner surface of the large **thyroid cartilage** anteriorly. Posteriorly, the folds attach to the movable **arytenoid cartilages**. These cartilages allow the vocal folds to be **abducted** (positioned apart) or **adducted** (positioned together, or approximated). Inferiorly, the **cricoid cartilage** forms the base of the larynx and rests atop the trachea (**Figs. 2.3, 2.4, 2.5, 2.6**). In summary, the structures important to laryngeal function in speech are the cricoid cartilage, paired arytenoid cartilages, thyroid cartilage, hyoid bone, and vocal folds.

Phonemes that are produced with vocal fold vibration (vocal folds adducted) are referred to as **voiced** sounds; those produced with the vocal folds abducted are **voiceless**. All American-English vowels as well as the majority of consonants are voiced.

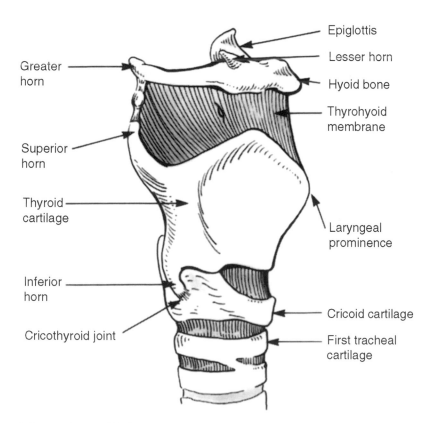

Figure 2.3 *Lateral view of the larynx. (From Blitzer, A., Brin, M., & Ramig, L. Neurologic Disorders of the Larynx. New York: Thieme, 2009. Reprinted with permission.)*

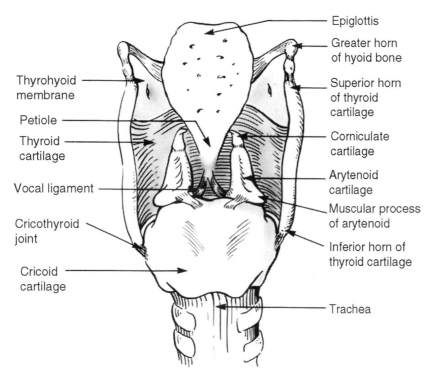

Figure 2.4 *Posterior view of the larynx. (From Blitzer, A., Brin, M., & Ramig, L. Neurologic Disorders of the Larynx. New York: Thieme, 2009. Reprinted with permission.)*

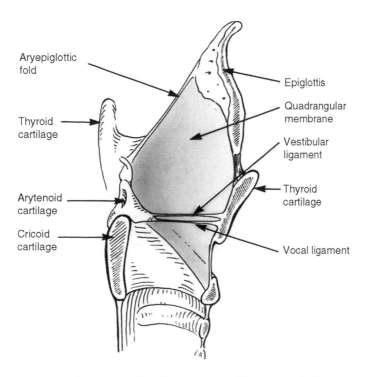

Figure 2.5 *Sagittal view of the larynx. (From Blitzer, A., Brin, M., & Ramig, L. Neurologic Disorders of the Larynx. New York: Thieme, 2009. Reprinted with permission.)*

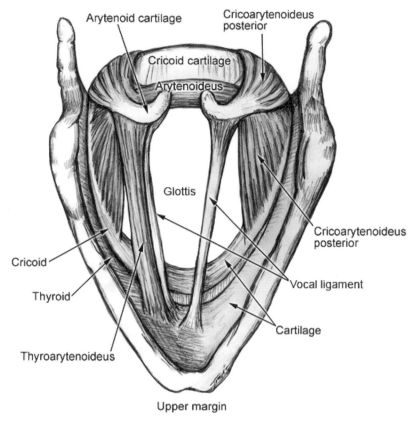

Figure 2.6 *Superior view of the vocal folds. (From Medscape, 2014. http://emedicine.medscape.com/ article/867575-overview. Reprinted with permission.)*

Sublaryngeal structures are the organs of respiration that provide the breath stream necessary for speech production (**Fig. 2.7**). The **trachea** is immediately below the larynx and is attached to the cricoid cartilage. It is a tube of cartilaginous rings and other connective tissue that descends in front of the esophagus and bifurcates (divides in half) into two **primary bronchi.** The paired bronchi enter the lungs and continue to bifurcate into smaller **bronchioles**. Ultimately, the bronchioles terminate in **alveolar ducts,** which lead to the **alveolar sacs**. The **alveoli** are contained in the walls of the alveolar sacs and serve as the site for exchange of oxygen and carbon dioxide in speech and for life support. Other sublaryngeal structures necessary for speech include the **rib cage**, **diaphragm**, and other muscles of respiration, including the **internal** and **external intercostal** muscles.

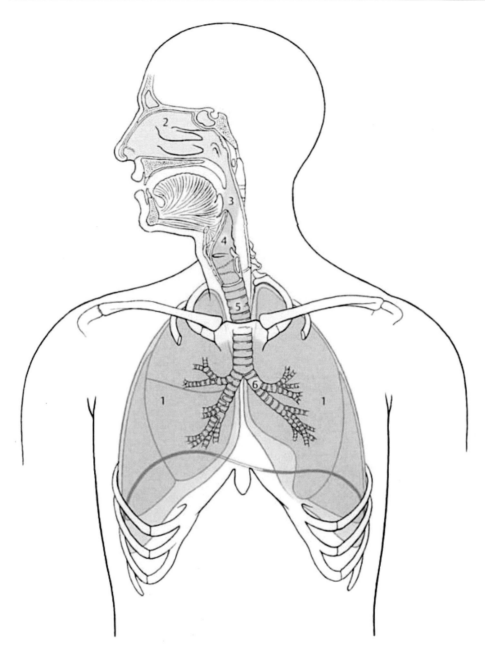

Figure 2.7 *Respiratory tract. Key: 1, lungs; 2, nasal cavity; 3, oropharynx; 4, epiglottis; 5, trachea; 6, primary bronchus. (From Fritsch, H., & Kuehnel,W. Color Atlas of Human Anatomy: Internal Organs, vol. 2. NewYork:Thieme, 2008. Reprinted with permission.)*

SPEECH PROCESSES AND ASSOCIATED STRUCTURES

Now that you are familiar with the individual structures involved in the speech process, it is time to discuss their integrated roles in speech production. The resulting, overlapping processes of respiration, phonation, resonation, and articulation together are responsible for the variety of sounds we use to transmit oral language. Coordination of these processes requires complex interaction, feedback, and adjustments, mediated by the nervous system (brain, cranial nerves, and spinal cord).

RESPIRATION

Human oral communication requires some type of air source for its occurrence. That source is provided by the process of respiration. Respiration is accomplished by a complex interaction of respiratory structures and muscles. The structures involved in respiration, as we noted earlier, include the lungs, bronchi, bronchioles, alveoli, and trachea. The muscles involved in respiration primarily include the **diaphragm** and the **external** and **internal intercostals.** However, respiration for speech requires more than just structures and muscle activity, as you will discover in the next section.

Whether breathing for speech or simply breathing quietly (life support), you inhale (bring air into the lungs) and exhale (release air from the lungs). Oxygen and carbon dioxide exchange occurs in the lungs each time you inhale and exhale, whether you speak or not. The exhalation phase of respiration provides the flow of breath for speech in pulmonic languages like English. **Inhalation** consists of taking air into the lungs. Contraction of the diaphragm causes the thoracic cavity space to expand. Co-occurring upward and outward rib cage movement due to the action of thoracic and neck muscles also expands this space. The elastic properties of the lungs allow them to expand as well. **Exhalation** (which provides the **egressive** or outgoing airstream for speech) is achieved by a combination of these factors: (1) gravity, (2) elastic properties of cartilage and lung tissue, and (3) relaxation of the muscles of inhalation. In addition, for speech and heavy breathing, there is progressive contraction of the muscles of exhalation.

In **vegetative breathing** (for life support), the relative duration of inhalation and exhalation is about the same. You can see this for yourself as you sit quietly reading this book or listening in class. But in **speech breathing**, the duration of exhalation in a single respiratory cycle is usually about 10 times longer than that of inhalation. Notice that when you speak, you inhale quickly and then exhale slowly to produce as much speech as possible. Practiced speakers may have their exhalation phase last 50 times longer than inhalation! Despite differences in the inhalatory and exhalatory cycle length for life support and speech, the *amount* of air exchanged is about the same, regardless of purpose. The extended duration of exhalation for speech reflects extremely efficient control of the breath stream. This efficiency results from the synergistic functioning of the respiratory muscles, larynx, and articulatory mechanisms. Changes in the larynx and articulatory system cause adjustments in the exhalation process. This degree of control takes time to master. Researchers have noted differences in control of breathing for vegetative function and vocalization (prespeech) even in infants (Moore et al, 2001; Reilly and Moore, 2009). Additional studies have found that a child's development of adult-like control of the airstream for speech requires a period of years (Boliek, Hixon, Watson, & Jones, 2009; Connagham et al, 2004; Parham et al 2011). Consider how babies may cry and run out of breath but how a trained adult speaker can easily sustain voice for long periods!

PHONATION

Phonation (vocal fold vibration) or voicing is accomplished by the interruption of the outgoing airstream by rapid rhythmic closing and opening of the glottis with the vocal folds. At rest and for quiet breathing, the vocal folds are **abducted** (apart) posteriorly. For phonation, the vocal folds are steadily but lightly approximated (together) when the arytenoid cartilages are **adducted** (brought together in midline) by muscle action. This degree of closing allows the folds to be parted by accumulated subglottal air pressure coming from the lungs. After the air escape, the folds then reapproximate (return to the central position) from the combined effects of muscular tension and aerodynamic effect. For phonation to occur, subglottal pressure must be sufficient to overcome both supraglottal air pressure and the glottal resistance or tension of the vocal folds. The process follows this rhythmic cycle:

1. Closing of the glottis (vocal folds adducted)
2. Increasing of air pressure beneath the glottis
3. Bursting apart of the folds from air pressure with release of a puff of compressed breath
4. Reclosing of the folds under constant muscle tension, with temporarily decreased subglottal air pressure drawing or sucking the folds back together

Air pressure beneath the glottis builds again as air continues to flow from the lungs and trachea. Consequently, the cycle is repeated many times per second.

The opening and closing of the folds is not a simple open and shut process. As we noted before, the vocal folds are muscular tissue shelves with vertical depth (**Fig. 2.6**). Consequently, in each phonatory cycle the folds open from bottom to top and posterior to anterior. In closing, the inferior part of the folds closes before the superior part, and horizontal closure proceeds from anterior to posterior. When seen through high-speed photography, the motion of the folds appears wavelike. Each complete opening and closing of the glottis constitutes one **cycle**.

The rate of release of these puffs of air determines the **fundamental frequency** or F_o of a speaker's voice. Fundamental frequency varies, affected by age, sex, and voluntary control. For men, the average fundamental frequency of vocal fold vibration is 125 **hertz** (Hz, or cycles per second). The average fundamental frequency for women is faster, about 220 Hz. Not surprisingly, the fundamental frequency of infants' and children's voices is even faster! A faster F_o is heard as a higher **pitch,** whereas a slower F_o characterizes a lower pitch.

Changes in fundamental frequency require interaction of the lungs and larynx. In addition, the size and mass of the vocal folds determine the range of frequencies possible for a given speaker. You can change your F_o through a combination of alterations of (1) vocal fold tension and (2) subglottal air pressure. Higher or rising F_o is associated with greater vocal fold tension and higher subglottal air pressure. A drop in F_o, conversely, is associated with a reduction in vocal fold tension, and, especially, lower subglottal pressure. When you are conversing (rapid connected speech), your fundamental frequency will vary constantly according to these two factors of vocal fold tension and subglottal air pressure. That variation is perceived as changes in **intonation** of your voice. (See Chapter 5 for details about the prosody of speech.)

Not just fundamental frequency is produced by the rapid opening and closing of the glottis. Remember, the movement of the folds is complex, and the folds open more slowly than they close. Consequently, a *complex* harmonic sound is produced by the opening and closing of the vocal folds. This secondary complex harmonic signal is composed of **harmonics** or **overtones** of the fundamental frequency. Thus, the sound that emerges is complex, more of a buzz. It is not recognizable as the human voice. Instead, it must pass through the resonatory system to develop those characteristics (see the following section).

Intensity of voice, heard by listeners as **loudness**, results from an interaction of vocal fold characteristics, subglottal and supraglottal pressure. Greater loudness results from (1) increased subglottal pressure; (2) vocal fold control that allows rapid, firm, longer closure of the folds; and (3) expansion of the vocal tract to reduce supraglottal pressure. The opposite adjustments produce a quieter voice intensity. Thus, a speaker whose voice is too soft can learn how to change respiration, phonation, and resonation to develop a louder voice.

In summary, vocal fold vibration is affected not only by the function of laryngeal structures but also by respiration (subglottal pressure) and resonation (supraglottal shaping and pressure). Feedback between and among these systems causes changes in their actions, resulting in the complex sound waveform that serves as the basis for speech.

Resonation

Resonation occurs as the vibrating air stream passes through the pharyngeal, oral, and nasal cavities. These cavities can be altered in size, shape, and coupling or connections. The resonating cavities selectively amplify parts of the complex sound produced by phonation. The result is what you perceive as the distinctive sound of an individual's voice, also known as **voice quality**.

It may help to understand a little more about resonation in general before learning more about the resonation process in speech. A simple example of a resonating chamber is a bottle partially filled with liquid. If you blow into the air space in the bottle, you hear a tone. The tone will vary depending on how much liquid is in the bottle. If the bottle is almost full, the sound will seem higher than when the bottle is almost empty. (Feel free to try this yourself.) The level of the liquid determines the amount of air space in the bottle. Less liquid means more air space, which emphasizes lower resonating frequencies. Higher frequencies are amplified when the bottle is almost full and the air space is minimal. The bottle is a fairly simple space, but the vocal tract is not. That makes for an even more complex result in speech resonation.

Resonation requires a vibrating source as well as an air space through which the vibration can move. For the human voice, the vibrating source is the larynx, as discussed previously. The air space is composed of pharynx, oral, and nasal cavities. Those cavities are very complex in shape as well as being composed of variable soft tissue surfaces. In addition, you can change your vocal tract shape in a large number of ways, depending on velopharyngeal coupling and movements of the articulators. The quality of a person's voice is produced primarily by a combination of the person's habitual F_o range, blended with the overtones that are amplified (made louder) or subdued by resonation. The influences of resonation on voice quality include the following:

1. The overall length of the vocal tract

2. The relative length of the oral, nasal, and pharyngeal cavities

3. Habitual muscle tensing, which can raise the larynx and change the size and shape of the pharynx

4. The size of the tongue in relation to the oral cavity

5. The moistness and softness of the cavity walls (greater moistness and soft-ness is associated with a lower, more "hollow"-sounding voice)

6. The relative opening of the jaw and lips during speaking (wider openings cor-respond to amplification of higher frequencies)

7. Relative openness of the velopharyngeal port during production of vowels and oral resonant consonants (a greater opening is associated with a nasal quality to the voice)

The low-resonance pattern characteristic of the voice of the Disney cartoon char-acter Goofy exemplifies the interaction of these factors. The low, hollow-sounding voice of this character is produced by a tongue posture that is low and toward the back (greater cavity space), small openings (lips, between resonating cavities), and soft, moist cavity walls. These adjustments amplify lower harmonics and are associ-ated with the character's distinctive voice.

Overall, the process of resonation shapes and amplifies selected frequencies of the laryngeal tone. It does not occur in isolation but is affected by the nature of respira-tion, phonation, and articulation processes. It also plays a role in articulation, as you will see in the next section.

ARTICULATION

Articulation is defined as the shaping of the voiced or unvoiced breath stream to form the sounds of speech. The vowels and resonant consonants (/m/, /n/, /ŋ/, /l/, /ɹ/, /w/, /j/) are articulated primarily by adjustments in resonance. For ex-ample, the nasal consonants /m/, /n/, and /ŋ/ are all articulated with the velopha-ryngeal port open, or *coupled* to the pharynx. For /m/, the lips are closed (bilabial), for /n/, the tongue tip touches the alveolar ridge (lingua-alveolar). The fairly fixed position of the oral articulators, combined with the open velopharyngeal port, pro-duces the distinctive resonance characteristics of nasal consonants. For /l/ and /ɹ/ production, the voiced airstream flows through relatively fixed oral articulators, and the velopharyngeal port is closed. Different frequencies are amplified, and different consonants are heard. Most of all, the characteristic resonances of different vowels are produced by adjustments in the oral cavity.

In contrast, the remaining consonants are shaped by action of the tongue, jaw, and lips. The velopharyngeal port is closed for articulation of these consonants. If airflow is constricted between the maxillary incisors and the lower lip, a /f/ (unvoiced air-stream) or /v/ (voiced airstream) results. This friction-like quality is also characteristic of nonresonant consonants produced with constriction in other parts of the oral cavity, for example the alveolar ridge (/s/) and palate (/ʃ/). Another type of non-resonant consonant is produced when the outgoing airstream is suddenly stopped and (sometimes) released. Such closure with the lips produces the bilabial /p/ (un-voiced) and /b/ (voiced). Similarly, air is stopped between the tongue tip and the alveolar ridge for /t/ and /d/. Detailed descriptions of the articulatory processes for vowels and consonants are found in Chapters 3 and 4.

CONCLUSION

Even this short discussion should make it clear that speech production is not a sim-ple, one-step-at-a-time process, beginning with the lungs and ending with a stream of articulated speech sounds. The breath stream for speech, provided by the respira-tory system, is constantly adjusting in response to the activity of the vocal folds, resonators, and articulators. Laryngeal changes in frequency of vibration character-ize connected speech and also require reciprocal adjustments across systems. Precise timing between articulation and phonation is necessary to produce appropriate voic-ing for consonants. Upper airway pressure changes, resulting from movement of the articulators, require changes in the glottis and respiratory system. If each process operated independently of each other, fluent speech would be impossible. It is the simultaneous and cooperative functioning of these systems and their structures that allow us to produce speech.

CONCEPT QUESTIONS

PART I: STRUCTURAL TERMS

1. List the structure(s) associated with the following terms:
   - a. Bilabial _____
   - b. Glottal _____
   - c. Dental _____
   - d. Velar _____
   - e. Pharyngeal _____
   - f. Nasal _____
   - g. Alveolar _____
   - h. Palatal _____

2. List the supralaryngeal structures.

3. List the sublaryngeal structures.

4. Name the structure associated with the following functions or locations:
   - a. Larynx suspended from it _____
   - b. Protects larynx in swallowing _____
   - c. Anterior attachment for vocal folds _____
   - d. Space between vocal folds _____
   - e. Responsible for vocal fold abduction _____
   - f. Most inferior laryngeal cartilage, attached to trachea _____
   - g. Muscular tissue shelves in larynx _____

PART II: CONCEPT INTEGRATION

1. Trace the pathway for a respiratory cycle. List the structures involved and their actions. _____
   _____

2. Explain frequency and intensity of vocal fold vibration in phonation. Name the acoustic products associated with each of them. _____

_____

PART III: DIAGRAM OF THE VOCAL TRACT

From memory, label the structures indicated on this diagram:

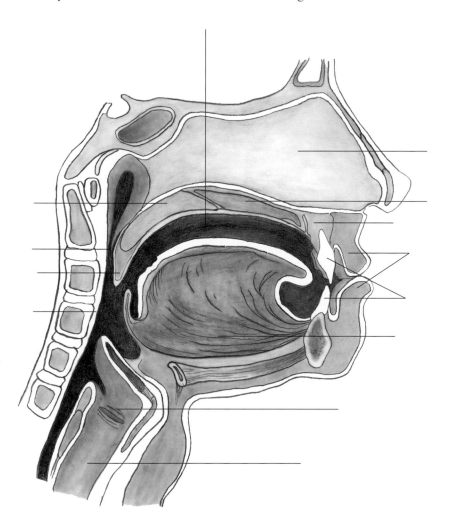

VOWELS AND DIPHTHONGS

OVERVIEW: VOWELS AND CONSONANTS
TRADITIONAL ANALYSIS OF VOWELS
CONCEPT QUESTIONS

OVERVIEW: VOWELS AND CONSONANTS

Speech sounds, or phonemes, traditionally have been divided into two categories, consonants and vowels, with vowels further subdivided into monophthongs and diphthongs. Although this book uses this classification system as a reference for this chapter and Chapter 4, many phoneticians have disagreed over the definitions and identities of these two categories. You might find that hard to understand because in many cases the differences between consonants and vowels seem very obvious. For example, the consonant /t/ is short in duration and does not require vocal fold vibration. Unlike consonants, the vowels are usually longer in duration and are all voiced. But in contrast to the example with /t/, many consonants resemble vowels in characteristics such as voicing and oral resonance. Some consonants are very similar to vowels, for example /w/ (*wing*, *web*) and /j/ (*yes*, *yoyo*). Both /w/ and /j/ are voiced, both have oral resonance, and both are initiated from a high vowel position. The /j/ begins in a position very similar to /i/ and the /w/ begins in a position similar to /u/. (See Chapter 4, section Approximants/Oral Resonant Consonants, for a full explanation.) Nevertheless, there are several ways that phoneticians have typically distinguished vowels from consonants: (1) their role in syllable formation, (2) the degree of vocal tract constriction, and (3) classification schemes.

ROLE IN SYLLABLE FORMATION

One of the most commonly used and agreed upon ways to distinguish between vowels and consonants has been their different roles in syllable formation. With very few exceptions (see Chapter 5), only a vowel can be a syllable nucleus. Thus, a single vowel can constitute a full syllable, for example /aɪ/ (*eye*, *I*). Consonants may be added to a vowel, for example /haɪ/, /laɪ/ (*high*, *lie*), but they are not required for syllable formation. It is the vowel, not the consonant, that is necessary to make a syllable. If a word contains two vowels, then it also consists of two syllables. Examples include words like *higher* (/haɪɚ/) and *liar* (/laɪɚ/).

DEGREE OF VOCAL TRACT CONSTRICTION

A second, generally accepted way to distinguish between vowels and consonants is based on the degree of closure, or constriction, in the vocal tract. Vowels are produced with a relatively open or unconstricted vocal tract that does not change during production. Consonants, however, are all produced with constriction in the vocal tract. To help illustrate this, try the following sound production exercise while looking in a mirror. Pay close attention to your tongue and jaw position, the tongue movement (or lack of it), and the closeness of your tongue to your hard palate and alveolar ridge. Now, produce the vowel /ɑ/ as in *hop*. Next, try to produce /s/ for several seconds. What you should notice is that your jaw is much lower and your mouth is much more open for production of the /ɑ/. Also, your tongue tip is very close to your alveolar ridge for the /s/ but not for the vowel. Not all vowels are as "open" as /ɑ/, nor are all consonants as constricted as /s/. However, they do demonstrate the principle that, relatively speaking, the vocal tract is much more open (less constricted) for vowel production than for consonant production.

CLASSIFICATION SCHEMES

TRADITIONAL CLASSIFICATION: TWO SEPARATE SYSTEMS

Within the traditional vowel and consonant classification system, the two sound types have separate classification schemes (**Fig. 3.1** and **Table 3.1**). Vowels are classified on the basis of tongue placement (**front, central,** or **back**) and degree of tongue

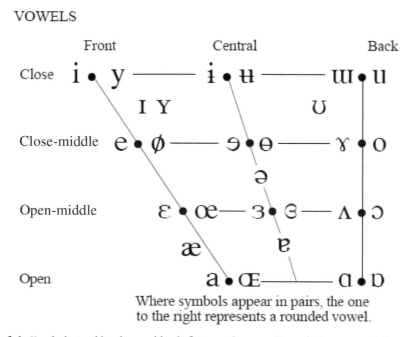

Figure 3.1 Vowels depicted by place and level of tongue elevation. (From the International Phonetic Association (http://www.langsci.ucl.ac.uk/ipa/). Copyright 2005 by International Phonetic Association. Reprinted with permission.)

TABLE 3.1 AMERICAN-ENGLISH CONSONANT SOUNDS BY PLACE AND MANNER OF ARTICULATION

Manner of articulation	Place of Articulation						
	Bilabial	Labio-dental	Lingua-dental	Lingua-alveolar	Lingua-palatal	Lingua-velar	Glottal
Stops	p b			t d		k g	
Fricatives	ʍ	f v	θ ð	s z	ʃ ʒ	(ʍ)	h
Affricates					ʧ ʤ		
Nasals	m			n		ŋ	
Liquids				l	ɹ		
Glides	w				j	(w)	

elevation (**high**, **mid**, or **low**) with some supplemental notation for lip rounding. (Further details about vowel classification appear later in this chapter.) Using a traditional scheme, you will learn to classify consonants in a different way than vowels by using these characteristics: place, manner, and voicing. **Place of articulation** refers to the location of the articulators involved (e.g., alveolar, palatal) in consonant production. **Manner of articulation** is the way in which the airstream is modified (e.g., narrowing for /s/ versus air blockage for /t/). Finally, consonants will be either **voiced** or **voiceless**, depending on whether or not there is vocal fold vibration.

These traditional categorization systems (vowels vs consonants) will be a primary focus as you progress through this book. There is another system, however, that you should also know about that is used to classify and distinguish phonemes. This is known as *distinctive feature classification.*

DISTINCTIVE FEATURE CLASSIFICATION

Distinctive feature classification was described in detail by Noam Chomsky and Morris Halle in 1968 and has been widely studied and applied since that time (Bernhardt & Stemberger, 1998; Blache, 1978; Elbert & Gierut, 1986; Gierut, 1992; Grunwell, 1982; Lowe, Knutson, & Monsen, 1985). Unlike the older, separate vowel and consonant classes of the traditional system, distinctive features allow classification of all consonants and vowels using one system. Chomsky and Halle (1968) proposed and described distinctive feature characteristics as both articulatory and acoustic. In contrast, traditional vowel and consonant classifications depend only on the articulatory/physiologic characteristics. These distinctive features share many characteristics with the traditional vowel and classification systems discussed previously. A key difference lies in the ability to distinguish vowels from consonants using one system (distinctive features) rather than two (traditional system).

With distinctive feature systems, each phoneme is viewed as a "bundle" of acoustic and articulatory features. The features themselves are binary, which means that each phoneme will possess (indicated by +) or will not possess (indicated by −) a particular feature. For example, look for the feature *nasal* in **Table 3.2**. As you go across that row, you will find only three phonemes that are + nasal: /m/, /n/, and /ŋ/; thus,

TABLE 3.2 SELECTED PHONEMES DISTRIBUTED ACCORDING TO 11 DISTINCTIVE FEATURE PROPERTIES FROM CHOMSKY AND HALLE (1968)

Feature	p	d	k	f	v	θ	ð	s	z	ʃ	dʒ	h	m	n	ŋ	ɹ	l	w	j	i	æ	u	ɑ
Sonorant	−	−	−	−	−	−	−	−	−	−	−	−	+	+	+	+	+	+	+	+	+	+	+
Consonantal	+	+	+	+	+	+	+	+	+	+	+	+	+	+	+	+	+	−	−	−	−	−	−
Vocalic	−	−	−	−	−	−	−	−	−	−	−	−	−	−	−	+	+	−	−	+	+	+	+
Coronal	−	+	−	−	−	+	+	+	+	+	+	−	−	+	−	+	+	−	−	−	−	−	−
Anterior	+	+	−	+	+	+	+	+	+	−	−	−	+	+	−	−	+	−	−	−	−	−	−
Nasal	−	−	−	−	−	−	−	−	−	−	−	−	+	+	+	−	−	−	−	−	−	−	−
High	−	−	+	−	−	−	−	−	−	+	+	−	−	−	+	−	−	+	+	+	−	+	−
Back	−	−	+	−	−	−	−	−	−	−	−	−	−	−	+	−	−	+	−	−	−	+	+
Continuant	−	−	−	+	+	+	+	+	+	+	−	+	−	−	−	+	+	+	+	+	+	+	+
Voiced	−	+	−	−	+	−	+	−	+	−	+	−	+	+	+	+	+	+	+	+	+	+	+
Strident	−	−	−	+	+	−	−	+	+	+	+	−	−	−	−	−	−	−	−	−	−	−	−

the feature + *nasal* corresponds to the traditional manner of articulation referred to as nasal (as opposed to nonnasal consonants). Notice that with this one classification system, the vowels are also – *nasal* like the remaining consonants.

For another example, look at the *consonantal* distinctive feature in **Table 3.2**. Almost all consonants share the + *consonantal* feature. But look at the consonants /w/ (*we, were*) and /j/ (*young, yes*): they are considered – *consonantal,* even though they are classified as consonants in traditional classification schemes. Phonemes that are + *consonantal* have either *total closure* or *extreme narrowing* (producing friction) in the oral cavity. The consonants /w/ and /j/, along with the vowels, are produced with a more open vocal tract than the typical consonant. That difference makes /w/ and /j/-*consonantal*, just like vowels. (Recall that we noted similarities between the vowels and /w/ and /j/ earlier.)

Distinctive features, then, allow us to classify all phonemes with one system rather than having separate methods for vowels and consonants. Distinctive features have been applied to treatment schemes for patients with speech sound disorders. Use of this system to analyze phoneme confusions and contrasts can also be helpful for speakers of English as a second language when they are trying to learn new, unfamiliar American-English phonemes (see Chapter 6). Nevertheless, the traditional system introduced first in this chapter remains more frequently used. For the remainder of this chapter and the next, we will introduce the phonemes according to the traditional classification systems.

TRADITIONAL ANALYSIS OF VOWELS

NATURE OF VOWELS

American-English vowels are all formed with essentially the same manner of production. They are all produced with oral resonance (velopharyngeal closure/velopharyngeal port closed), and they are all voiced (vocal fold vibration). Each vowel's identity is primarily a product of shaping of the oral cavity. That shaping is affected primarily by tongue movements, but jaw opening/closing and lip rounding also play a role. Consequently, American-English vowel categorization has been based on the height and the placement of tongue elevation, with supplemental notation for lip rounding and tenseness.

We measure tongue height in tongue-to-palate or tongue-to-velum distance. In articulating American-English vowels from high to low, your jaw movement and tongue position will change vertically because the tongue follows the vertical movement of the mandible. Thus, vowels can be classified as **high**, **mid**, or **low**, depending on the degree of tongue elevation. Within each high and mid vowel category, vowels may be distinguished as **close** or **open,** referring to the relative closeness of the tongue to the palate. For example, there are two high front vowels /i/ and /ɪ/. /i/ is described as *close high*, as opposed to the *open high* classification of /ɪ/ because the tongue is closer to the palate in /i/ production. Similarly, for the mid back vowels, /o/ (*location*) is classified as *close high* and /ɔ/ (bought) as *open high*.

Placement or area of tongue elevation refers to that part of the tongue and oral cavity in which elevation occurs. Using this scheme, the vowels fall into three primary classes: **front**, **back**, and **central**. In the descriptions that follow, the vowels are presented in groups according to this classification. Study of front, back, and central monophthong vowels will be followed by coverage of diphthongs. Again, these dimensions can be seen in **Fig. 3.1**.

Lip position also serves as a supplemental way of classifying vowels. In particular, it is noted especially for rounded vowels such as /u ʊ o ɔ ɝ/ and the highly retracted vowels such as /i/. Another characteristic, *tenseness* (and its opposite characteristic, *laxness*) refers to the degree of muscular effort as well as the duration involved in articulating a particular vowel. The tense vowels are /i e u o ɝ/. These characteristics are also included in the discussion and descriptions of vowels in the following pages, in addition to the primary placement and height categories.

MONOPHTHONGS VS. DIPHTHONGS

Vowels can also be classified as monophthongs or diphthongs. The front, back, and central vowels are **monophthong** vowels; that is, they are produced with one, unchanged (mono-) position. **Diphthongs** involve a transition from one vowel position (**on-glide/nucleus**) to another vowel position (**off-glide**). There are two vowels that can be monophthongal or diphthongal in mainstream American English: the close mid front monophthong vowel /e/ (diphthong /eɪ/)and the close mid back vowel /o/ (diphthong /oʊ/). The diphthong forms are found in stressed syllables and at the end of words. The monophthong forms occur only in syllables not marked by primary accent.

On the following pages each monophthong and diphthong vowel is described individually. Monophthong vowels are presented in order for front, back, and central vowels, followed by the diphthong descriptions. Each vowel is described in terms of tongue height, placement, lip shape (when applicable), and tenseness/laxness, followed by a step-by-step analysis of production. The appropriate International Phonetic Alphabet (IPA) symbol, key words, and examples are supplied for each vowel. You will also find additional information about some of the vowels, especially those that are more often affected by dialectic variation.

FRONT VOWELS

The front vowels of English, from high to low, are /i ɪ e ɛ æ/. The tongue tip lies just behind and usually touches the inner surface of the mandibular incisors. At the same time, the front or blade of the tongue is raised toward the palate but not closely enough to touch or to cause air turbulence or friction (**Fig. 3.2**). The necessary tongue-to-palate difference can be achieved in several ways: by differential elevation of the front tongue in relationship to the (stationary) mandible, by holding the front tongue in a high steady position and raising/lowering the mandible, or by some combination of both. Sound confusing? Try this exercise. You will need a mirror so that you can watch your lips and jaw. First, keep your mandible in one position by putting a pencil eraser or tongue depressor between your upper and lower front teeth. Now, say the front vowels from high to low: /i ɪ e ɛ æ/. Then, begin again with the same amount of jaw opening and tongue position as before but without the pencil. Try to hold your tongue in a steady position and again say these vowels from high to low by dropping your jaw in progressive steps. Did you see your jaw move? You were able

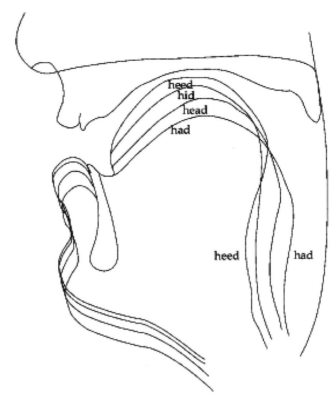

Figure 3.2 Front tongue vowel position: high to low. (From Ladefoged, P. Vowels and Consonants: An Introduction to the Sound of Languages, 3rd ed. New York: Wiley-Blackwell, 2012. Reprinted with permission.)

to produce the front vowels either way; you simply changed from tongue motion to jaw motion to make it happen. Don't be surprised if you find that one way feels easier or more natural than the other. Either way is appropriate, however. In connected speech, the tongue height for front vowels may be achieved by a combination of both types of adjustments.

/i/

IPA Symbol:	/i/
Description:	close high, front, retracted, tense
Key Words:	eat, seed, be
Common Spellings:	e, ee, ea, -y

/i/ Production

The velopharyngeal port is closed, and the sides of the back of the tongue are closed against the upper molars. The middle to front portion of the tongue is raised high, nearly touching the palate and maxillary alveolar ridge. Simultaneously, the tongue tip touches lightly behind the lower front teeth and voicing occurs. The upper and lower front teeth are slightly open with lips often retracted at the corners.

/i/ Words

Initial		Medial		Final	
eat	either	seed	reed	be	trustee
eve	east	leave	feet	he	free
eel	equal	beech	green	key	tea
even	eager	teach	bead	three	sea
each	enough	these	chief	plea	money
eagle	email	lease	sheep	knee	candy

/i/ Contrasts/Minimal Pairs

/i/–/ɪ/		/i/–/ɛ/		/i/–/æ/	
deep	dip	meat	met	beat	bat
deed	did	bead	bed	beak	back
beat	bit	neat	net	seem	Sam
peak	pick	seat	set	leak	lack
bean	bin	mean	men	keep	cap
peach	pitch	teen	ten	teen	tan

Additional Notes

/i/ has the highest tongue position of the front vowels. It is sometimes modified to /ɪ/, depending on phonetic context and conventions of transcription. For example, the high vowel in *hear* may be produced as [ɪɹ], [h ɪ ɹ]. If /i/ is in an unstressed syllable in a word such as *rehearse*, it may also be produced as /ɪ/, [ɹ ɪ h ɝ s]. It is the third most frequently occurring American-English vowel, following only /ə/ and /ɪ/ in its occurrence in adult speech (Mines, Hanson, & Shoup, 1978, referenced by Shriberg & Kent, 2013).

/ɪ/

IPA Symbol:	/ɪ/
Description:	open high, front, slightly retracted, lax
Key Words:	if, sit, middle
Common Spellings:	i, y

/ɪ/ Production

The velopharyngeal port is closed, and the sides of the back of the tongue are closed against the upper molars. The middle to front portion of the tongue is raised toward the palate and alveolar ridge, slightly lower and farther back than for the /i/. Simultaneously, the tongue tip touches lightly behind the lower front teeth and voicing occurs. The tongue musculature is less tense than for /i/, and the lips are not as retracted.

/ɪ/ Words

Initial		Medial	
in	into	his	pill
it	ignore	busy	quill
if	interest	limb	sit
itch	insect	mitt	tin
ill	idiom	Nick	victor
imp	Ithaca	wit	whisper

/ɪ/ Contrasts/Minimal Pairs

/ɪ/–/i/		/ɪ/–/ɛ/		/ɪ/–/æ/	
fist	feast	lit	let	list	last
wit	wheat	kin	ken	lick	lack
sip	seep	pin	pen	in	an
lid	lead	bids	beds	pitch	patch
rid	reed	tin	ten	tin	tan
fill	feel	lift	left	lift	laughed

Additional Notes

/ɪ/ is one of the most frequently occurring vowels in American English (Mines et al, 1978, referenced by Shriberg & Kent, 2013). It is not produced in the final position of words except for unstressed final *y* by some speakers of New England and Southern American English dialects.

/e/ (monophthong) and /eɪ/ (diphthong)

IPA Symbol:	/e/
Description:	close mid, front, tense
Key Words:	/e/ fatality, vacation, chaotic
	/eɪ/ able, base, away
Common Spelling:	a (in syllables not receiving primary stress)

/e/ Production

The velopharyngeal port is closed, and the sides of the back of the tongue are closed against the upper molars. The middle to front portion of the tongue is raised toward the palate and alveolar ridge, slightly lower and farther back than for the /ɪ/. Simultaneously, the tongue tip touches lightly behind the lower front teeth and voicing occurs. The upper and lower front teeth are open. If the lips move from this position to the /ɪ/ position, then the diphthong /eɪ/ results. (See Additional Notes and the section Diphthongs, later in this chapter, for further details and clarification.)

/e/ Words

This symbol is used to transcribe only the vowel of syllables that do not receive primary stress or occur at the beginning or end of words. Its diphthong form, /eɪ/ occurs much more often in mainstream American English.

/e/			/eɪ/	
crybaby	fatality	acre	major	today
operate	chaotic	atrium	Mayflower	may
cavalcade	vacation	age	vacation	Parkay
excavate	creativity	ailing	remain	neigh
imitate	radiate	April	stage	delay
appreciate	evaluate	aim	male	ray

Additional Notes

The diphthong form of this vowel occurs much more frequently than the monophthong form. Phoneticians vary in their views and transcription of these forms, which are allophones of each other. Check with your instructor to see if one or the other symbol will be used more frequently in your class. As with other vowels, there will be variation between these two forms depending on speech context and dialectic variation.

/ɛ/

IPA Symbol:	/ɛ/
Description:	open mid, front, slightly retracted, lax
Key Words:	end, bet
Common Spellings:	e

/ɛ/ Production

The velopharyngeal port is closed, and the sides of the back of the tongue are closed against the upper molars. The middle to front portion of the tongue is raised slightly toward the palate and alveolar ridge but lower and farther back than for the /ɪ/ or /e/. At the same time, the tongue tip touches lightly behind the lower front teeth and voicing occurs. The upper and lower front teeth are open slightly wider than for /ɪ/.

/ɛ/ Words

Note that /ɛ/ does not occur in the final position of words.

Initial		Medial	
edge	extra	men	head
end	elephant	red	said
egg	else	get	many
elm	engine	them	friend
ever	excel	beg	guest
any	effort	neck	best

/ɛ/ Contrasts/Minimal Pairs

/ɛ/–/i/		/ɛ/–/ɪ/		/ɛ/–/eɪ/		/ɛ/–/æ/	
Nell	kneel	send	sinned	test	taste	send	sand
guess	geese	bet	bit	bell	bail	vet	vat
wreck	reek	met	mitt	led	laid	met	mat
fend	fiend	neck	nick	Ben	bane	neck	knack
ken	keen	mess	miss	when	wane	mess	mass
lest	least	rest	wrist	fell	fail	lest	last

Additional Notes

Like /ɪ/, /ɛ/ is one of the most frequently occurring vowels occurring in mainstream American English (Mines et al, referenced by Shriberg & Kent, 2013). It may be produced as /ɪ/ before nasal consonants in Southern English, for example *pin* and *pen* both produced as [p ɪ n] (see Chapter 5 for further details). In addition, it is one of the American-English vowels that has been affected in the Northern American cities shift (Labov, Ash, and Boberg, 2006).

/æ/

IPA Symbol:	/æ/
Description:	low, front, lax
Key Words:	at, has, ham
Common Spellings:	a

/æ/ Production

The velopharyngeal port is closed, and the mouth is open wider than for the other front vowels. The middle to front portion of the tongue is raised slightly lower and farther back than for the other front vowels. The sides of the back of the tongue may move away from the upper molars, and the tongue tip may move slightly behind the lower front teeth.

/æ/ Words

Note that /æ/ does not occur at the ends of words in English.

Initial		Medial	
ax	add	cat	camera
album	Adam	sand	sag
after	absolute	laugh	rather
atom	answer	that	grab
ask	agony	dance	salmon
actor	aster	radical	pad

/æ/ Contrasts/Minimal Pairs

See examples under previous sections.

Additional Notes

The /æ/ is usually in an accented syllable of a multisyllabic word. It may sound closer to /eɪ/ when it occurs before a nasal consonant (e.g., <u>ka</u>ngaroo, <u>ra</u>ng). Like other vowels, /ae/ can vary as a product of context and dialect. In particular, the New England *a* (/ɒ/) is a common alternate pronunciation for /ae/ in the northeastern United States (see Chapter 6).

Transcription

Now that you have been introduced to the front vowels, you should practice listening for and transcribing them. Before you begin, you need to know some guidelines for the format and spacing relationships of transcription symbols. First, notice that the vowels /i/ and /e/ resemble the lower case letters *i* and *e*, respectively. The symbol for /ɪ/ closely resembles a capital *I*, but in lower case size. Transcription of /ɛ/ should resemble a backwards *3*, but again, lower case in proportion. Finally, /æ/ looks like a combination of the letters *a* and *e*; be sure that the two symbols touch each other for accurate transcription.

Exercises 3.1 and 3.2 in Appendix A require you to listen to the recording or to your instructor's live-voice presentation of word lists to identify or discriminate front vowels. Exercises 3.3 and 3.4 require transcription of the words dictated.

BACK VOWELS

The back vowels of mainstream American English, in order of tongue height, are /u/, /ʊ/, /o/, /ɔ/, /ɑ/. For back vowels, the back of the tongue is raised toward the velum near its junction with the soft palate (**Fig. 3.3**). At its highest point, the tongue does not touch the velum, nor does it come close enough to cause air turbulence or audible friction. The tongue tip rests behind and slightly below the mandibular incisors or lightly touches the lower gum ridge.

Like the front vowels, the tongue-to-velum distance needed for each back vowel results from a combination of lingual and mandibular adjustments. With decreasing tongue elevation, the point of back tongue elevation also becomes slightly farther forward in the mouth. The higher the tongue, the more rounded the lips. As the highest back vowel, /u/ has the most lip rounding and the smallest lip opening. Conversely, /ɑ/, the low back vowel, is unrounded (but not retracted like the front vowels). The /ɑ/ has the greatest jaw opening of all the mainstream American-English vowel sounds. Look at your mouth in a mirror as you produce the back vowels from high /u/ to low /ɑ/; notice the changes in degree of mouth opening and lip rounding.

/u/

IPA Symbol:	/u/
Description:	close high, back, rounded, tense
Key Words:	ooze, boot, too/to/two
Common Spellings:	oo

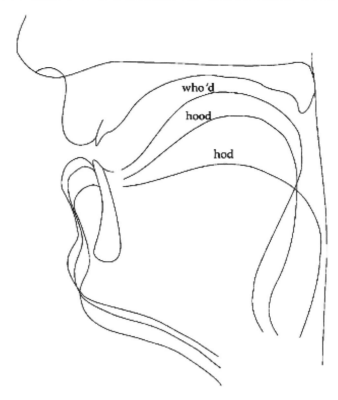

Figure 3.3 *Back tongue vowel positions: high to low. (From Ladefoged, P. Vowels and Consonants: An Introduction to the Sound of Languages, 3rd ed. New York: Wiley-Blackwell, 2012. Reprinted with permission.)*

/u/ Production

With the velopharyngeal port closed, the sides of the back of the tongue are closed against the molars. The back of the tongue is raised high and tense, nearly touching the palate. The lips are rounded and might be slightly protruded, producing a small opening. Voice is given. The tongue tip is just behind the lower front teeth, and the upper and lower teeth are slightly open.

/u/ Words

Initial	Medial		Final	
oodles	boot	moon	too	do
ooze	crew	move	who	drew
oolong	doom	rude	Q	blew
oops	fruit	tomb	shoe	through
	group	school	you	flu
	lose	whom	true	canoe

/u/ Contrasts/Minimal Pairs

/u/–/ʊ/		/u/–/ɔ/		/u/–/ɑ/	
pool	pull	pool	Paul	pool	pall
fool	full	fool	fall	loot	lot
stewed	stood	boot	bought	ooze	Oz
shooed	should	toot	taught	toot	tot
Luke	look	loose	loss	Luke	lock
cooed	could	cool	call	coop	cop

Additional Notes

A few words may vary in the pronunciation of either /u/ or /ʊ/, depending on the speaker's dialect (e.g., *roof*, *hoof*, *root*). The /u/ pronunciation is more common in mainstream American English. (See Chapter 6 for further details on American English dialects.)

/ʊ/

IPA Symbol:	/ʊ/
Description:	open high, back, rounded, lax
Key Words:	cook, pull, should
Common Spellings:	oo, u

/ʊ/ Production

With the velopharyngeal port closed, the sides of the back of the tongue are closed against the molars. The back of the tongue is raised high but lower and with less tension than for /u/, nearly touching the palate. The lips are rounded and might be slightly protruded, producing an opening larger than for /u/. Voice is given. The tongue tip is just behind the lower front teeth, and the upper and lower teeth are slightly open.

/ʊ/ Words

Note that /ʊ/ only occurs in the medial position of words in American English

cook	hood	pull
look	woolen	bush
hook	wooden	could
shook	full	should
good	put	would
stood	push	wolf

/ʊ/ Contrasts/Minimal Word Pairs

/ʊ/–/ɔ/		/ʊ/–/o/		/ʊ/–/ɑ/	
cook	caulk	cook	coke	cook	cock
soot	sought	should	showed	soot	sot
could	cawed	could	code	could	cod
hood	hawed	hood	hoed	hood	hod
full	fall	full	foal	look	lock
pull	Paul	good	goad	good	god

Additional Notes

As previously noted, /ʊ/ occurs only in the medial position of words. It can vary with /u/ in production of some words, depending on the speaker's dialect.

/o/ (monophthong) and /oʊ/ (diphthong)

IPA Symbol:	/o/
Description:	close mid, back, tense, rounded
Key Words:	/o/ donation, location
	/oʊ/ know, over, slow
Common Spellings:	o (in syllables not receiving primary stress)

/o/ Production

With the velopharyngeal port closed, the back and middle portions of the tongue are slightly raised, with elevation slightly lower and more forward than for /ʊ/. The tongue tip touches behind the lower front teeth, and voice is given. The upper and lower front teeth are open. The lips are rounded and might be slightly protruded, producing an opening larger than for /ʊ/. (If the lips and tongue move from this /o/ position and briefly assume the position for /ʊ/, then the diphthong /oʊ/ is produced.) The relationship between /o/ and /oʊ/ is similar to that of /e/ and /eɪ/. (See Additional Notes, below, and the section Diphthongs for further details and clarification.)

/o/ Words

This symbol is only used to transcribe the vowel that occurs in syllables that do not receive primary stress or occur at the beginning or ends of words. Its diphthong form, /oʊ/ occurs much more often, in stressed syllables and in initiating and ending words.

/o/		/oʊ/		
innovation	utmost	open	most	low
momentous	cooperate	own	soap	window
proliferate	nobility	Oprah	dole	beau
Cochise	professional	ocean	load	doe
renovate	bodacious	over	pose	sew
innovate	renovation	odor	roast	dough

/o/ Contrasts/Minimal Pairs

See the subsection on /oʊ/ in the Diphthongs section.

Additional Notes

The diphthong form of this vowel occurs much more frequently than the monophthong form. Phoneticians vary in their views and transcription of these forms, which are allophones of each other. Check with your instructor to see if one or the other symbol will be used more frequently in your class. As with other vowels, there will be variation between these two forms depending on speech context and dialectic variation.

/ɔ/

IPA Symbol:	/ɔ/
Description:	open mid, back, rounded, tense
Key Words:	awed, caught, law
Common Spellings:	au, aw

/ɔ/ Production

The velopharyngeal port is closed, and the back and middle portions of the tongue are slightly raised, with elevation just below that for /o/. The mouth is open wider than for /o/ production, and the lips are rounded and slightly protruded. Voice is given and the tongue tip touches the lower front teeth.

/ɔ/ Words

Use of the /ɔ/ vowel is very much affected by a speaker's dialect; see Additional Notes, below, for more information.

Initial		Medial		Final	
always	awesome	taut	gaudy	saw	straw
off	awning	pawed	caught	raw	craw
audio	awestruck	vault	thought	paw	thaw
often	auction	talk	haughty	caw	gnaw
auto	audience	walk	wrong	jaw	slaw
auger	almost	yawn	bought	law	raw

/ɔ/ Contrasts/Minimal Word Pairs

/ɔ/–/u/		/ɔ/–/o/–/oʊ/	
caught	coot	saw	so
bought	boot	bought	boat
taught	toot	taught	tote
lawn	loon	lawn	loan
dawn	dune	fawn	phone
loss	loose	law	low

Additional Notes

The /ɔ/ is one of the most inconsistently used sounds in American-English speech. Compared with /ɑ/, /ɔ/ differs only by having a slightly higher tongue elevation and lip rounding. /ɔ/ is consistently differentiated from /ɑ/ in only a few regional American-English dialects but is almost always replaced by /ɑ/ in all others (Labov et al, 2006) (see Chapter 6 for more information). The presence or lack of differentiation of /ɔ/ from /ɑ/ does not appear to have a significant effect on a speaker's understandability.

/ɑ/

IPA Symbol:	/ɑ/
Description:	low, back, open, tense
Key Words:	top, cotton bother
Common Spellings:	o

/ɑ/ Production

With the velopharyngeal port closed, the tongue is slightly raised in the back, with the tongue tip touching behind the lower front teeth. The mouth is open wider than for any other vowel as voicing is given. The lips are not rounded or protruded but may be described as slightly retracted. /ɑ/ differs primarily from the neutral vowel /ʌ/ in having a wider mouth opening and lower back of tongue elevation.

/ɑ/ Words

Initial		Medial		Final
on	honest	father	Tom	la
onset	Olive	copper	beyond	baa
honor	ominous	bomb	Bob	Pa
odder	oxen	calm	doll	cha-cha
Oz	onyx	Don	palm	ha
opera	October	mom	stop	rah

/ɑ/ Contrasts/Minimal Word Pairs

/ɑ/–/o/		/ɑ/–/ɔ/		/ɑ/–/ʊ/		/ɑ/–/æ/	
cot	coat	cot	caught	Bach	book	hot	hat
rot	rote	rot	wrought	lock	look	rot	rat
Bonn	bone	hock	hawk	wad	would	Bonn	ban
hocks	hoax	mod	Maude	rock	rook	mod	mad
got	goat	odd	awed	god	good	Tom	tam
socks	soaks	knot	naught	knock	nook	not	gnat

Additional Notes

The /ɑ/ is quite variable in American English, often interchanged with /ɔ/ and /æ/. The "broad a" of some eastern New England speakers makes words like *aunt* and *bath* be pronounced as [ɒ n t] and [b ɒ θ]. Actually, the word *aunt* is an excellent example of how vowels may vary across dialects. The pronunciation can vary from [æ n t] (most regional dialects) to [ɒ n t] (see above) to [eɪ n t] (some Southern English speakers). See Chapter 6 for more information on dialectic variations for vowels.

Transcription

Now that you have been introduced to the back vowels, it's time for you to combine them with your transcription of front vowels. Like the front vowels, there are some guidelines for the format of transcription of back vowels. First, notice that the vowels /u/ and /o/ resemble the lower case letters *u* and *o*, respectively. The symbol for /ʊ/, however, looks like an upside-down Greek omega. Some of the author's students have remembered the form for this vowel by calling it "handlebar U." Transcription of /ɔ/ should resemble a backwards *C*, but in lower case in proportion. Finally, /ɑ/ looks like the lower case *a,* which you were taught to use in elementary school, not the typeset letter a. Remember that the proportions for all the vowels are like those of lower case letters.

Exercises 3.6 and 3.7 in Appendix A are designed to further develop your listening skills. Word transcription of only back vowels will appear in Exercise 3.8, but transcription of both front and back vowels will be required for Exercise 3.9.

CENTRAL VOWELS

There are four central vowels in American English: /ɝ/ and /ɚ/ (stressed and unstressed vowel *-er*) and /ʌ/ and /ə/ (stressed and unstressed vowel *–uh*). They are produced with more central tongue elevation, hence the term *central vowels*. The /ʌ/ is the vowel heard in monosyllabic words such as *mud* and *up* and in stressed syllables of multisyllabic words (e.g., *r<u>u</u>nning, b<u>u</u>tter*). The /ə/ occurs in unstressed syllables and is the first vowel in words like *<u>a</u>round* and *<u>u</u>nhappy*. The /ɝ/ and /ɚ/ are also referred to as *r-colored* or *rhotacized* vowels.

/ɝ/ is the vowel heard in monosyllabic words such as *h<u>ur</u>t*, *<u>ear</u>th,* and *b<u>ir</u>d*. It is also the vowel heard in the stressed syllable of multisyllabic words (e.g., *c<u>er</u>tain, p<u>ur</u>chase, l<u>ear</u>ning*). The unstressed counterpart, /ɚ/, occurs in the unstressed syllable of multisyllabic words such as *hamm<u>er</u>, ov<u>er</u>,* and *teach<u>er</u>*. Because of their r-coloring, these vowels may be confused with postvocalic /ɹ/ or /ɚ/ diphthongs (e.g., purr [p ɝ] vs pear [p ɛɹ]). You will find further explanations and examples below.

Learning the central vowels adds several layers of complexity to your listening and transcription tasks. First, you must distinguish these vowels as distinct from the identities of the front and back vowels. Then, having decided whether the vowel is *-er* or *-uh*, you must determine whether it is contained in a stressed or unstressed syllable to determine the correct symbol.

/ʌ/

IPA Symbol:	/ʌ/
Description:	close mid, central, lax, stressed
Key Words:	cup, done, rough
Common Spellings:	u

/ʌ/ Production

With the velopharyngeal port closed, the tongue is slightly elevated in the middle to back portion. The upper and lower front teeth are separated about the same distance as for /ɛ/. The tongue tip touches lightly behind the lower front teeth. The airstream is voiced. Because the tongue is in a somewhat relaxed position, /ʌ/ has also been called a "neutral" vowel. This vowel occurs in stressed syllables only.

/ʌ/ Words

Initial		**Medial**	
upper	upward	cup	flood
under	ugly	tub	blood
up	ultimate	hunt	rough
other	oven	some	nothing
uncle	usher	done	mother

/ʌ/ Contrasts/Minimal Pairs

/ʌ/–/ɑ/		/ʌ/–/ʊ/		/ʌ/–/ɛ/	
bum	bomb	luck	look	bun	Ben
come	calm	tuck	took	nut	net
cub	cob	stud	stood	but	bet
nut	not	shuck	shook	hull	hell
putt	pot	putt	put	lug	leg
duck	dock	buck	book	mutt	met
cut	cot	cud	could	pun	pen
rub	rob	crux	crooks	money	many

Additional Notes

This vowel is used only for the stressed vowel *uh* in one-syllable words and in the stressed syllable of words of more than one syllable.

/ə/

IPA Symbol:	/ə/
Description:	open-mid central, lax, unstressed
Key Words:	elephant, lemon, sofa
Common Spellings:	highly variable

/ə/ Production

The velopharyngeal port is closed with tongue placement in the mid-central part of the oral cavity. The tongue is more relaxed than for /ʌ/ production, and duration is shorter than for /ʌ/. The airstream is voiced.

/ə/ Words

Initial		Medial		Final	
about	appeal	alphabet	relative	sofa	Alabama
above	arouse	chocolate	syllable	soda	camera
away	attach	company	emphasis	tuba	gorilla
allow	abate	buffalo	accident	quota	arena
awhile	alive	elephant	parasol	zebra	cinema
amaze	another	parachute	cinnamon	drama	stamina
across	obscene	minimum	aluminum	vanilla	Brenda
adore	awry	comedy	Canada	Anna	manna

Additional Notes

The /ə/ is also commonly referred to as the **schwa** vowel. In casual or rapid speech, it is not uncommon for vowels to become /ə/. For example, formal speech would include full pronunciation of all the vowels in *indigo* [ɪ n d ɪ g oʊ]. In rapid, casual speech, the second vowel is most likely to be replaced by /ə/ [ɪ n d ə g oʊ]. Because of this tendency, /ə/ (like /ɪ/ and /ɛ/) is one of the most commonly occurring vowels in English.

/ɝ/

IPA Symbol:	/ɝ/
Description:	close-mid, central, rounded, tense
Key Words:	bird, furnace, prefer
Common Spellings:	er

/ɝ/ Production

The velopharyngeal port is closed, and the sides of the tongue are closed against the upper molars, with the tongue slightly retracted, in a mid-central position. Production is often accompanied by some lip rounding. There are several ways of producing this vowel. The tongue tip may be elevated and curled back toward the alveolar ridge, or the tip may be lowered while the body is bunched near the palate. The airstream is voiced. Duration is longer, and there is more muscular tension than for production of /ɚ/. The /ɝ/ differs from the consonant /ɹ/ in several ways: (1) /ɝ/ has greater duration; (2) /ɝ/ constitutes a syllable; (3) it has tongue movement toward, rather than away from, the consonant /ɹ/ position; and (4) it is never voiceless following voiceless consonants, as /ɹ/ can be.

/ɝ/ Words

Initial		Medial		Final	
earth	earn	pearl	courage	her	stir
early	urchin	sturdy	learn	burr	aver
earl	urn	herd	pertinent	fur	her
Earl	Irving	heard	furnish	purr	sir
irked	earnest	kernel	stern	were	occur
Ernie	urged	work	bird	infer	spur
Urdu	erst	worm	person	recur	assure
herb	erg	curry	learning	whirr	cur

/ɝ/ Contrasts / Minimal Pairs

/ɝ/–/ʊ/		/ɝ/–/ʌ/		/ɝ/ /ɚ/ or /ɹ/ blend	
shirk	shook	hurt	hut	terrain	train
stirred	stood	lurk	luck	beret	bray
curd	could	shirk	shuck	duress	dress
lurk	luck	shirt	shut	curried	creed
furl	full	burn	bun	stirring	string
gird	good	curt	cut	burrow	bro
Turk	took	burrs	buzz	furrow	fro
birch	butch	Turk	tuck		

Additional Notes

The /ɝ/ is subject to dialectic variation in eastern New England (Labov et al, 2006). It may also be confused with **rhotic** (r-colored) diphthongs or when consonant /ɹ/ follows a vowel as in *card* /k ɑɹd/ (as opposed to *curd* /k ɝd/) or *bear* /b ɛ ɹ/ (as opposed to *burr* /b ɝ/). You will find further instruction about these differences in the section Diphthongs, as well as in the section Approximants/Oral Resonant Consonants in Chapter 4. Those sections have a more intense drill on /ɝ/–/ɚ/ as opposed to consonant /ɹ/ discrimination skills.

/ɚ/

IPA Symbol:	/ɚ/
Description:	open-mid, central, lax
Key Words:	brother, Saturday
Common Spellings:	er (unstressed syllables)

/ɚ/ Production

The velopharyngeal port is closed, and the tongue position is similar to that for /ɝ/. However, /ɚ/ is produced with less muscular tension and is shorter in duration than /ɝ/. The airstream is voiced. Lip rounding is variable. This vowel occurs only in unstressed syllables.

/ɚ/ Words

urbane	labor
terrain	mother
percent	martyr
centered	improper
understand	anger
refrigerator	sister
researcher	pewter
gingerbread	hammer
gathered	matter
intern	mortar

Additional Notes

The /ɚ/ symbol is similar in appearance to the /ə/. It is sometimes referred to as "schwar." It may be affected by dialectic variation, particularly by speakers in eastern New England and in some parts of the southern United States (Labov et al, 2006).

TRANSCRIPTION

Now that you have been introduced to the central vowels, it is time to work on listening for them and adding them to the vowels you have already learned to recognize and transcribe. Turn to Exercises 3.9 to 3.12 in Appendix A. As in previous exercises, the first two are designed to improve your recognition of, and discrimination among, the back vowels. The remaining two exercises focus on further developing both discrimination and transcription skills.

Before you begin, here are some reminders about transcription. First, all these symbols should be the size of lower case letters. The stressed /ʌ/ symbol looks like a caret or an inverted *v*. For unstressed /ə/, your transcription should resemble a backwards inverted *e*. The form for the stressed /ɝ/ is sometimes described as the numeral *3* with a "wing" added to it, again in lower case proportion. Finally, the /ə/ symbol can serve as a reference in transcribing /ɚ/. Like /ɝ/, it looks like a "wing" has been added to it.

DIPHTHONGS

Like monophthong vowels, diphthongs serve as syllable nuclei. They are considered single phonemes even though they are composed of a sequence of two vowel positions. The first position is always the dominant nucleus or **on-glide,** which has greater duration and stress than its successor, the **off-glide** portion. Both positions, however, are taken in a single syllable.

The traditional, or **rising diphthongs** of mainstream American English are /eɪ/ (*aim, may*), /oʊ/ (*low, over*), /aɪ/ (*ice, mine*), /ɔɪ/ (*boy, joy*), and /aʊ/ (*out, town*). Another set of diphthongs, **centering diphthongs**, have /ɚ/ as their off-glide. Some phoneticians transcribe postvocalic *r*s as centering diphthongs, but more frequently they use consonant /ɹ/, for example [kɑɚ] as opposed to [k ɑ ɹ] to transcribe *car*. Both types of diphthongs are presented in this chapter. Ultimately, however, the more common /ɹ/ will be used to follow the vowel in transcription. This will

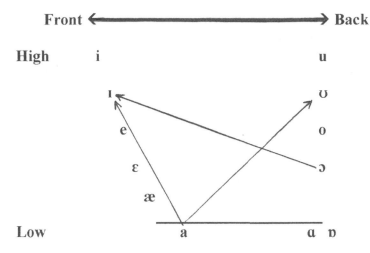

Figure 3.4 *Movements for rising diphthongs. (Adapted from the International Phonetic Association (http://www.langsci.ucl.ac.uk/ipa/). Copyright 2005 by International Phonetic Association. Reprinted with permission.)*

be more understandable when you learn about the liquid consonants /ɹ/ and /l/ in Chapter 4. Because diphthongs are characterized by change in production, they need to be depicted by tongue movement, as in **Figs. 3.4.** and **3.5**. These figures use the now-familiar vowel diagram to indicate direction of movement from the nucleus/ on-glide to the off-glide position. For traditional diphthongs, movement is from a lower tongue elevation to a higher elevation, ending in either the /ɪ/ or /ʊ/ position

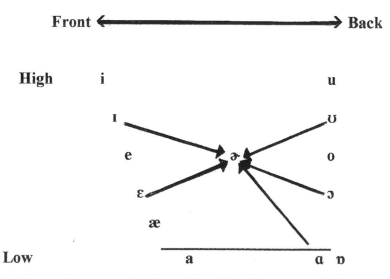

Figure 3.5 *Movements for centering diphthongs. (Adapted from the International Phonetic Association (http://www.langsci.ucl.ac.uk/ipa/). Copyright 2005 by International Phonetic Association. Reprinted with permission.)*

to complete the diphthong. For /ɚ/ diphthongs, movement is toward the central vowel position so that the off-glide is transcribed as /ɚ/. For both types of diphthongs, transcription requires that the two symbols used touch each other. If you separate the symbols, you must use this symbol over them [‿]. Otherwise, you will be transcribing two separate vowels rather than one coarticulated diphthong.

RISING DIPHTHONGS

IPA Symbol:	/eɪ/	/oʊ/	/aʊ/	/aɪ/	/ɔɪ/
Description:	Front, rising diphthongs (3)				
	Back, rising diphthongs (2)				
Key Words:	/eɪ/	hay, safer			
	/oʊ/	old, mow			
	/aɪ/	eye, high			
	/aʊ/	out, tower			
	/ɔɪ/	oil, oyster			

/eɪ/

IPA Symbol:	/eɪ/
Description:	Front, rising diphthong
Key Words:	able, maze, say
Common Spellings:	a-e

/eɪ/ Production

With the velopharyngeal port closed and the sides of the back of the tongue against the upper molars, the middle and front portions of the tongue are raised toward the palate and the alveolar ridge, slightly lower and farther back than for /ɪ/; then the tongue briefly rises toward the /ɪ/ height. The airstream is voiced throughout production. The tongue tip touches lightly behind the lower front teeth. The upper and lower front teeth are open and the lips may move from the /e/ to the /ɪ/ opening. The /e/ portion is the longer nucleus or on-glide, and the /ɪ/ portion is the shorter off-glide. For many speakers, the off-glide portion may have a tongue position close to /i/ but of short duration.

/eɪ/ Words

Initial		Medial		Final	
age	apex	bale	label	may	neigh
ache	eight	came	baby	bay	weigh
aim	alien	dale	making	say	decay
aid	aviary	face	place	spray	away
able	apron	stale	taper	they	matinee
ape	acre	gain	relation	prey	ballet

/eɪ/ Contrasts/Minimal Pair Word Lists

/eɪ/–/ɛ/		/eɪ/–/ɪ/		/eɪ/–/æ/	
mate	met	mate	mitt	made	mad
date	debt	late	lit	sate	sat
bait	bet	tame	Tim	tape	tap
rake	wreck	wait	wit	ale	Al
main	men	bait	bit	fate	fat
gate	get	chain	chin	lace	lass
laid	led	laid	lid	laid	lad
fade	fed	hate	hit	fade	fad
bane	Ben	male	mill	shame	sham

Additional Notes

In words like *air* and *care* (vowel followed by postvocalic /ɚ/), the vowel may be heard and transcribed as /eɪ/, /e/, or /ɛ/. The /ɛ/ is the most common variant, particularly if you transcribe with centering diphthongs (e.g., [ɛɚ], [k ɛɚ]). In American English, the /eɪ/ usually occurs in a syllable with a primary accent. It can also occur with a secondary accent if it is in a final, open syllable (e.g., *Monday*, *Saturday*, transcribed as [m ʌ n d eɪ], [sæ t ɚ d eɪ], respectively). Use of /e/ tends to be restricted to unaccented syllables that occur next to the accented syllable, as noted in the section on front vowels.

/oʊ/

IPA Symbol:	/oʊ/
Description:	Back, rising diphthong
Key Words:	own, bowl, no
Common Spellings:	-o-e, -oa

/oʊ/ Production

With the velopharyngeal port closed, the middle and back portions of the tongue are raised toward the palate, slightly lower than for /ʊ/. The lips are rounded and may be slightly protruded, with the opening slightly larger than for /ʊ/. The airstream is voiced. The tongue rises briefly to the /ʊ/ height, and the rounded lip opening decreases in size. The tip of the tongue touches lightly behind the lower front teeth. The /o/ portion is the longer nucleus, and the /ʊ/ portion is the shorter off-glide.

/oʊ/ Words

Initial		Medial		Final	
oak	ocean	bone	toes	go	toe
oats	over	pole	thrown	no	hoe
only	oaf	code	both	so	woe
opal	odor	rose	sewed	row	sew
own	omen	broke	hope	low	dough
open	oval	road	showed	beau	though

/oʊ/ Contrasts/Minimal Pairs

/oʊ/–/ʊ/		/oʊ/–/ɔ/	
pole	pull	phone	fawn
bowl	bull	boat	bought
code	could	coat	caught
stowed	stood	pose	pause
goad	good	bowl	bawl
broke	brook	coal	call
coke	cook	foal	fall
hoed	hood	tote	taut

Additional Notes

When *o*, *ao-*, and *o-e* or other spellings associated with /oʊ/ are followed by postvocalic /ɹ/, the vowel is more often transcribed as /ɔ/ or /o/, for example *for* as [f ɔɹ] or [f oɹ]. In mainstream American English, the /o/ occurs in syllables with a primary accent (e.g., *only*, *emotion*). /oʊ/ is also used for open (no final consonant), final, unaccented syllables (e.g., *window*, *yellow*). As noted previously in the section on /o/, the /oʊ/ diphthong occurs much more often than the monophthong /o/. Most often, an unaccented vowel is transcribed as the monophthong /o/ when the sound is in the syllable next to the accented syllable. See the examples in the section on back vowels earlier in this chapter.

/aɪ/

IPA Symbol:	/aɪ/
Description:	Back, rising diphthong
Key Words:	ice, mine, high
Common Spellings:	i, y, ie, igh

/aɪ/ Production

The velopharyngeal port is closed and the mouth is open as for /æ/, with the middle and front portions of the tongue raised more than for /ʌ/ but less than for /æ/. The tongue rises briefly in front toward the /ɪ/ height, and the mouth opening is slightly decreased. The tongue tip touches lightly behind the lower front teeth, and the airstream is voiced throughout production. The [a] portion is the longer nucleus, and the [ɪ] portion is the shorter off-glide. For some speakers, the nucleus may be closer to the /ɑ/ position and the off-glide close to /i/ but of short duration.

/aɪ/ Words

Initial		Medial		Final	
ice	item	find	light	by	die
ivy	idea	child	psyche	my	lie
idle	icicle	wild	shine	guy	sigh
iris	eyes	kind	fright	deny	bye
aisle	eyed	pine	type	thigh	buy
ivory	island	hide	height	sky	rye

/aɪ/ Contrasts/Minimal Pair Words

/aɪ/−/ɑ/		/aɪ/−/ɪ/		/aɪ/−/aʊ/	
type	top	ride	rid	dine	down
ride	rod	fine	fin	mice	mouse
pipe	pop	like	lick	nine	noun
like	lock	type	tip	lied	loud
light	lot	sign	sin	by	bow
fire	far	hide	hid	high	how
side	sod	light	lit	file	fowl
hide	hod	bite	bit	spite	spout

/aʊ/

IPA Symbol:	/aʊ/
Description:	Back, rising diphthong
Key Words:	out, loud, now
Common Spellings:	ou, ow

/aʊ/ Production

The velopharyngeal port is closed, and the mouth is opened as for /æ/. The middle and front tongue portions are raised more than for /ʌ/ but less than for /æ/. The tongue briefly rises in the back toward the /ʊ/ height, the mouth opening is slightly decreased, and the lips are round as for /ʊ/. The tip of the tongue touches lightly behind the lower front teeth and may move back slightly for the /ʊ/ portion. The airstream is voiced throughout production. The /a/ portion is the longer nucleus, and the /ʊ/ portion is the shorter off-glide. For some speakers, the nucleus may be closer to the /ɑ/ position and the off-glide close to /u/ but of short duration.

/aʊ/ Words

Initial		Medial		Final	
out	outlaw	count	town	now	vow
ouch	outline	found	foul	cow	endow
ounce	outfit	mouse	gown	sow	allow
oust	output	doubt	dowel	prow	somehow
ours	outlet	noun	towel	how	eyebrow
owl	hour	about	brown	bough	thou

/aʊ/ Contrasts/Minimal Pair Words

/aʊ/ – /ɑ/		/aʊ/ – /ʌ/		/aʊ/ – /aɪ/	
shout	shot	town	ton	down	dine
spout	spot	down	done	mouse	mice
down	Don	gown	gun	noun	nine
cowed	cod	bout	butt	loud	lied
scout	Scott	found	fund	bow	buy
gout	got	cowl	cull	how	high
pout	pot	noun	nun	fowl	file

/ɔɪ/

IPA Symbol:	/ɔɪ/
Description:	Back, rising diphthong
Key Words:	oil, coin, boy
Common Spellings:	oi, oy

/ɔɪ/ Production

The velopharyngeal port is closed, and the back and middle portions of the tongue are slightly raised with elevation as for /ɔ/ with the lips rounded and slightly protruded. The lip rounding then relaxes, and the tongue briefly rises toward the /ɪ/ height. The /ɔ/ is the longer nucleus, and the /ɪ/ portion is the shorter off-glide. The airstream is voiced throughout production. For many speakers, the off-glide portion may have a tongue-mouth position close to /i/ but of short duration.

/ɔɪ/ Words

Initial	**Medial**		**Final**	
oil	foil	boycott	boy	toy
oiler	coin	royal	soy	deploy
ointment	voice	mastoid	cloy	coy
oyster	join	appoint	joy	enjoy
oily	soil	goiter	Roy	destroy
	loin	thyroid	poi	Troy

/ɔɪ/ Contrasts/Minimal Pair Words

/ɔɪ/ – /aɪ/		/ɔɪ/ – /ɔ/		/ɔɪ/ – /ɝ/	
toil	tile	coil	call	oil	earl
poise	pies	foil	fall	loin	learn
toys	ties	toil	tall	voice	verse
loin	line	boil	bawl	boil	burl
foil	file	joy	jaw	poise	purrs
boy	buy	cloy	claw	boys	burrs
voice	vice	soy	saw	coil	curl

Additional Notes

Some dialects may substitute /ɔɪ/ and /ɝ/ in different words; for example, [g ɔɪ l] for *girl* but [ɝl] for *oil*.

CENTERING DIPHTHONGS

IPA Symbol: /ɪɚ/   /ɛɚ/   /ʊɚ/   /ɔɚ/   /ɑɚ/
Description: Front, centering diphthongs
            Back, centering diphthongs
Key Words: /ɪɚ/   ear, hear
            /ɛɚ/   air, care
            /ʊɚ/   pure, cure
            /ɔɚ/   soar, pore
            /ɑɚ/   car, jar

Additional Notes

Listening and transcription for /ɚ/ diphthongs/postvocalic /ɹ/ will be covered in Chapter 4 in the Approximants/Oral Resonant Consonants section. **Figure 3.3** depicts the movements involved in formation of centering diphthongs.

  Now that you have been introduced to all the diphthongs, you can complete the corresponding exercises in Appendix A. They are designed to help you learn to accurately recognize, discriminate among, and transcribe all the rising diphthongs. For the form of rising diphthongs, there are several important points to remember. First, remember that the symbols for the two portions of each diphthong must either touch or be tied by [͡]. If not, they symbolize two different vowels, not a single diphthong. Also notice that for /aɪ/ and /aʊ/, the correct form for the on-glide is /a/, not /ɑ/. And, for the back rising diphthongs, the off-glide symbol is /ʊ/, not [u]. Exercises for listening for /ɚ/-diphthongs are included in this chapter, but transcription will be saved for Chapter 4.

CONCEPT QUESTIONS
PART I

Are the following statements true or false?

_____   1. A vowel is necessary to have a syllable.

_____   2. Vowels are characterized by constriction in the vocal tract.

_____   3. Traditional consonant classification is based on place, manner, and voicing.

_____   4. All the front vowels are unrounded.

_____   5. All the back vowels are rounded.

_____   6. The vowel phonemes in *banana* are /ɑ æ ɑ/.

_____   7. A word that contains two syllables must have at least two consonants.

_____   8. The words *pat* and *pet* are minimal pair words.

_____   9. The most commonly occurring American-English vowels are /ɛ ɪ ə/.

_____ 10. The high vowels include /i u ɝ ɚ/.

PART II

1. Use **Fig. 3.1** and text information to complete these questions:
    a. List all the back vowels from high to low. _____
    b. List all the front vowels from low to high. _____
    c. List all the central vowels. _____
    d. For the following vowels, list the characteristic(s) they share in common:
        (1) /u o ɔ ʊ/ _____
        (2) /e ɛ o ɔ/ _____
        (3) /æ ɑ/   _____
        (4) /i e u o/ _____
        (5) /ɪ ɛ ə ʊ/ _____
        (6) /i e ɛ æ/ _____
        (7) /e ɚ o ʌ/ _____

2. Using **Table 3.2**, list the phonemes that are classified as:
    (a) + coronal   _____
    (b) − anterior _____
    (c) + strident _____
    (d) + back   _____
    (e) + nasal   _____
    (f) + high   _____

AMERICAN-ENGLISH CONSONANTS

OVERVIEW OF CONSONANTS: PLACE, MANNER, VOICING
CONSONANT SINGLETONS, SEQUENCES, AND SYLLABLE PLACEMENT
CONSONANT ANALYSIS BY MANNER OF ARTICULATION
CONCEPT QUESTIONS

OVERVIEW OF CONSONANTS: PLACE, MANNER, VOICING

As discussed in Chapter 3, consonants have traditionally been classified according to three characteristics: place of articulation, manner of articulation, and voicing. Place of articulation refers to the location (e.g., labial, alveolar) of airstream modification or to those parts of the speech mechanism used most prominently in consonant production. You learned the terms to describe **place of articulation** in Chapter 2. For example, /p/ and /b/ share a *bilabial* place of articulation, whereas /h/ has a *glottal* place of articulation. **Manner of articulation** refers to the way the airstream is modified. In this chapter the consonants are presented according to their manner of articulation: **stop, fricative, affricate, nasal,** and **approximant/oral resonant** (**liquids** and **glides**). The third classification category, **voicing,** refers to vocal fold vibration, as you also learned in Chapter 2. Consonants such as /b/ and /z/, which involve phonation, are **voiced,** and consonants such as /p/ and /s/, made without phonation, are **voiceless.** Many of the consonants occur in **cognate pairs.** Cognates are phonemes which share the same place and manner but differ in voicing. Thus, /p/ and /b/ are cognates, as are /s/ and /z/.

CONSONANT SINGLETONS, SEQUENCES, AND SYLLABLE PLACEMENT

It is also important to understand the terminology that refers to the role of consonants in relation to vowels. We can refer to consonants as **singletons** (one consonant with no consonants adjacent to it) or **sequences** (two or more consonants in succession in the same syllable or word). We can also refer to consonant singletons or sequences as **prevocalic, intervocalic,** or **postvocalic** (or **initial, medial,** and **final,** respectively). Prevocalic refers to consonant(s) occurring before a vowel, at the beginning of a word, and postvocalic refers to consonant(s) occurring after a vowel, at the end of a word. If a consonant is intervocalic, then it occurs between two vowels in a multisyllabic word. Thus, /p/ is a prevocalic consonant singleton in the word /paɪ/ (*pie*), and /sp/ is a prevocalic consonant sequence in the word /spaɪ/ (*spy*). The word /paɪp/ (*pipe*) ends with a postvocalic /p/, and the word /paɪps/ (*pipes*) ends with a postvocalic consonant sequence. In the word /baɪsɪkəl/ (*bicycle*), /s/ and /k/ are intervocalic consonant singletons. Correspondingly, the /sk/ is an intervocalic consonant sequence in the word /bæskɪt/ (*basket*).

There are also two kinds of consonant sequences: **blends** and **abutting** consonants. Blends consist of two or more adjacent consonants occurring within the same syllable, for example /bl/ in /blu/ (*blue*). Abutting consonants consist of two or more adjacent consonants that cross a syllable boundary, for example /t p/ in /patpaɪ/ (*pot pie*). Both blends and abutting consonants are examples of consonant sequences, but they are just two different kinds of sequence. (For more examples of these terms, see **Table 4.1**.)

The consonant phonemes of American-English speech are described individually in this chapter. Their symbols, as used in the International Phonetic Alphabet (IPA), key words, and most common spellings are listed for each phoneme. Each consonant production is described in simple place and manner terms and also step by step. These descriptions are followed by examples of words (organized by position), and discrimination lists for each consonant. These lists contain **minimal pairs,** which are two words that differ by only one phoneme. Notes are also added about some phonemes with regard to frequency of occurrence, age of acquisition, and possible dialectic variations.

Although these production descriptions may sound absolute or "cut-and-dried," this is not really the case, particularly in connected speech! Each description is more

TABLE 4.1 EXAMPLES OF CONSONANT SINGLETONS AND SEQUENCES IN RELATIONSHIP TO VOWELS

Word	Phonemes	Singleton/Sequence	Position
house	/h/	Singleton	Prevocalic
	/s/	Singleton	Postvocalic
telephone	/t/	Singleton	Prevocalic
	/l/	Singleton	Intervocalic
	/f/	Singleton	Intervocalic
	/n/	Singleton	Postvocalic
girl	/g/	Singleton	Prevocalic
	/l/	Singleton	Postvocalic
orange	/ɹ/	Singleton	Intervocalic
	/n ʤ/	Sequence	Postvocalic
stars	/s t/	Sequence	Prevocalic
	/ɹ z/	Sequence	Postvocalic
spoon	/s p/	Sequence	Prevocalic
	/n/	Singleton	Prevocalic
toothbrush	/t/	Singleton	Prevocalic
	/θ b ɹ/	Sequence	Intervocalic
	/ʃ/	Singleton	Postvocalic

a generalization of how most people produce speech sounds. We all make accommodations for our unique anatomy and for our skill in moving the speech mechanism rapidly about. Most of us did not learn speech through detailed instruction, carefully watching and copying someone else's tongue or lip movements. Instead, we learned speech by listening, and, by trial and error, moving our speech mechanism until we produced a sound that sounded similar to that of more mature speakers. There is more than one possible way to produce the same sound, and there are individual differences in the particular way people habitually produce speech. Nevertheless, there are enough common characteristics to devise "typical" descriptions. Such descriptions serve as excellent reference points for teaching someone who has not acquired a particular consonant or consonants. (See Chapter 7)

CONSONANT ANALYSIS BY MANNER OF ARTICULATION

STOP CONSONANTS

There are six stop consonants in American English: /p/, /t/, /k/, /b/, /d/, and /g/. All are produced with the velopharyngeal port closed. This manner of articulation requires that the voiced or voiceless airstream be interrupted by closure within the oral cavity. The airstream interruption has two possible phases. The **stop** (or necessary) **phase** requires rapid closure within the oral cavity. The second, more variable phase, is the **aspiration** (**plosive**) phase, in which the impounded or blocked airstream is released. These two phases have led some phoneticians to refer to this manner of articulation as stop-plosives. Some allophones (variants) of stops are made with or without aspiration. Try saying the word *hop* in these two ways: first, release the air (puff of air, stop + aspiration phase) as you produce the /p/ in the word. Next, say *hop*, but keep your lips closed (no air release, stop phase only). Both productions sound like the intended word, but the aspiration phase was not required for meaning. Stops may or may not be released with aspiration in connected speech. We discuss the different conditions for aspiration in Chapter 5.

As a phoneme class, the stops are all acquired early in speech development and seldom pose production difficulties for children (Bleile, 2006; Smit, 2003a,b; Smit, Hand, Freilinger, Bernthal, & Bird, 1990). In this section each stop is introduced individually and linked to cognate and to place of articulation. At the end of the section you will find exercises to help you practice listening for, and transcribing, the stop consonants in Appendix A.

/p/

Cognate:	/b/
Description:	Voiceless bilabial stop
Key Words:	pie, happy, top
Common Spellings:	p, pp

/p/ Production

The /p/ is made with the velopharyngeal port closed and without voicing. For the necessary stop phase, the lips close and the breath is held and compressed in the oral cavity. Lip closure for /p/ is made with more tension and greater duration than for /b/. In the variable aspiration, or plosive phase, the compressed air is released suddenly as an audible explosion of air between the lips. In connected speech the /p/ may or may not be released with aspiration.

/p/ Words

Prevocalic		Intervocalic		Postvocalic		Sequences	
pack	pool	upon	paper	up	shop	pry	prey
pie	pun	apple	rapid	cap	cape	plot	press
peas	peak	tapping	appeal	chop	deep	raspy	whisper
pill	pot	happy	stopping	ape	mope	laptop	popcorn
pine	paint	stupid	oppose	reap	hoop	grasps	hopped
port	peace	upper	repay	soap	sleep	wept	camp

/p/ Contrasts/Minimal Pair Words

/p/–/b/		/p/–/t/		/p/–/k/	
pack	back	pie	tie	pear	care
pill	bill	pan	tan	pan	can
peas	bees	pin	tin	peep	keep
pear	bear	pile	tile	pill	kill
rope	robe	pop	pot	lap	lack
cup	cub	peep	Pete	nip	nick
tap	tab	rap	rat	seep	seek
mop	mob	hop	hot	mop	mock

Additional Notes

The /p/ is developed early by children and is seldom misarticulated. It occurs less frequently than all the other stops except for /g/ in mainstream American English.

/b/

Cognate:	/p/
Description:	Voiced bilabial stop
Key Words:	be, cab, elbow
Common Spellings:	b, bb

/b/ Production

The /b/ is made with the velopharyngeal port closed and with voicing. In the necessary stop or closure phase, the lips close as voicing begins or continues, and air is held briefly in the oral cavity. Closure for /b/ is less tense and of shorter duration than for /p/. If the optional release phase then follows, the lips are opened as voicing continues.

/b/ Words

Prevocalic		Intervocalic		Postvocalic		Sequences	
be	boot	baby	maybe	tub	orb	blue	brew
by	bad	robot	nobody	crab	curb	bread	bless
bed	boy	about	labor	globe	herb	number	rainbow
book	boom	ribbon	sober	cube	knob	amber	fumbles
bait	bead	pebble	October	bib	lab	rubbed	fibbed
born	base	robin	rubble	mob	rub	mobs	pubs

/b/ Contrasts / Minimal Pair Words

/b/–/p/		/b/–/v/		/b/–/m/		/b/–/d/	
bend	penned	berry	very	bee	me	bore	door
ban	pan	best	vest	best	messed	Ben	den
beat	peat	boat	vote	by	my	bid	did
bar	par	bee	vee	bear	mare	bill	dill
tab	tap	given	gibbon	hub	hum	cab	cad
robe	rope	bow	vow	lab	lamb	lab	lad
cob	cop	buy	vie	lobe	loam	lobe	load
nab	nap	bane	vane	rub	rum	tab	tad

Additional Notes

The /b/ is mastered early by children and seldom misarticulated. It occurs more frequently in American English than its cognate, /p/. Speakers of English as a second language may show some alterations of /b/. (See Chapter 6 for more information.)

/t/

Cognate:	/d/
Description:	Voiceless (lingua-) alveolar stop
Key Words:	tie, sit, later
Common Spellings:	t, tt, -ed

/t/ Production

The /t/ is made with the velopharyngeal port closed and without voicing. In the first, (necessary) stop phase, the tip of the tongue closes against the alveolar ridge with the sides of the tongue against the molars. The breath is held and compressed in the oral cavity at this point. Closure is more tense and of greater duration than for the cognate /d/. In the (optional) aspiration phase, the compressed air behind the tongue is released suddenly as an audible explosion between the alveolar ridge and the tip of the tongue through slightly open teeth and lips.

/t/ Words

Prevocalic		Intervocalic		Postvocalic		Sequences	
too	tie	otter	potato	at	eat	trust	stretch
take	tone	pretty	city	cut	wait	treat	twin
tube	teak	letter	shouted	gate	goat	winter	fainted
toe	time	rotate	batted	seat	shut	Bantu	into
team	tip	meter	gator	plate	pleat	waked	guests
time	tower	attack	eating	wrote	hurt	paints	dropped

/t/ Contrasts/Minimal Pair Words

/t/–/d/		/t/–/θ/		/t/ Singleton-Sequence	
tie	dye	tin	thin	tee	tree
ton	done	tick	thick	two	true
tier	deer	torn	thorn	bay	bray
metal	medal	tinker	thinker	slip	slipped
mat	mad	bat	bath	pass	past
coat	code	boat	both	wash	washed
bat	bad	heat	heath	guess	guest
bite	bide	bet	Beth	can	can't

Additional Notes

The /t/ is one of the most frequently occurring sounds in American English. It is mastered early by children in the prevocalic and postvocalic positions. Intervocalic /t/, especially in unstressed syllables, is sometimes produced as a brief, voiced "flap" (/ɾ/) of the tongue, rather than a voiceless stop, for example *better, butter, pity, waiting, beautiful*. See Chapter 5 for further information on this topic.

/d/

Cognate:	/t/
Description:	Voiced (lingua-) alveolar stop
Key Words:	day, mud, fading
Common Spellings:	d, dd, ed

/d/ Production

The /d/ is made with the velopharyngeal port closed and vocal fold vibration. In the necessary stop phase, the tip of the tongue closes against the alveolar ridge with the sides of the tongue against the molars. Air is held briefly in the oral cavity at this closure. Closure is usually less tense and of shorter duration than for /t/. In the optional release phase, the closure of the tongue tip to the alveolar ridge is released while voicing continues.

/d/ Words

Initial		Medial		Final		Sequences	
do	date	somebody	model	bad	code	dwell	drain
day	dyne	ladder	jaded	did	used	drop	drink
dog	dine	lady	madder	read	made	under	wander
dish	deep	lowdown	reader	bird	bead	undo	boulder
down	deal	nobody	adore	load	amid	razed	bond
dust	door	body	aiding	bride	lad	roads	hands

/d/ Contrasts/Minimal Pair Words

/d/–/t/		/d/–/ð/		/d/–/n/	
dying	tying	dine	thine	done	nun
dean	teen	den	then	do	new
dare	tear	doze	those	door	nor
medal	metal	fodder	father	madder	manner
riding	writing	udder	other	raiding	raining
hide	height	seed	seethe	seed	seen
cod	cot	breed	breathe	dud	done
bode	boat	ride	writhe	mad	man

Additional Notes

Like /p/ and /b/, /d/ is mastered fairly early by children and is among the "Early Eight." It is misarticulated more often than /p/ and /b/, however. Like /t/, it is one of the most frequently occurring consonants in American English.

/k/

Cognate:	/g/
Description:	Voiceless (lingua-) velar stop
Key Words:	key, become, back
Common Spellings:	k, c, ck

/k/ Production

The velopharyngeal port is closed and there is no vocal fold vibration throughout /k/ production. In the necessary stop phase, the back of the tongue closes against the front of the velum or back portion of the palate, and the breath is held and compressed in the oral cavity and oropharynx. Closure is usually more tense and of longer duration than for /g/. If the optional aspiration phase follows, the compressed air is released suddenly between the tongue and roof of the mouth.

/k/ Words

Prevocalic		Intervocalic		Postvocalic		Sequences	
key	chord	jacket	stocking	hook	oak	cry	clown
cat	cold	acre	okay	rock	stick	creed	crow
could	count	bucket	bacon	wake	tick	biscuit	picture
coal	caught	become	backache	cake	duck	anchor	banker
kite	camp	baker	beacon	peek	rake	silk	looked
ketch	kind	weaker	beckon	lake	stock	thinks	asks

/k/ Contrasts/Minimal Pair Words

/k/–/g/		/k/–/t/		/k/–/p/	
cap	gap	cone	tone	care	pear
coal	goal	came	tame	cool	pool
cab	gab	carry	terry	calm	palm
bicker	bigger	backer	batter	sicker	sipper
backer	bagger	scare	stare	seek	seep
rack	rag	peek	Pete	coke	cope
stack	stag	ache	ate	leak	leap
buck	bug	Luke	lute	ax	apps

Additional Notes

The /k/ is acquired fairly early by children, but later than /p/ and /b/. It is not usually misarticulated unless a child has a hearing loss or a phonological disorder. When it is misarticulated, it is most often replaced by /t/ so that *cake* becomes [t eɪ t]. The /k/ is one of the most frequently occurring American-English consonants, but not as frequent as /t/.

/g/

Description	Voiced (lingua-) velar stop
Cognate:	/k/
Key Words:	go, foggy, log
Common Spellings:	g, gg

/g/ Production

The /g/ is made with the velopharyngeal port closed and with voicing. In the necessary stop phase, the back of the tongue closes against the front of the velum or the back portion of the palate, and air is held briefly in the back of the oral cavity and oropharynx. Closure is less tense and of shorter duration than for /k/. In the variable release phase, the closure of the back of the tongue and the velum or palate is released as voicing continues.

/g/ Words

Prevocalic		Intervocalic		Postvocalic		Sequences	
go	guest	again	buggy	egg	vague	glass	green
gate	give	begin	bigger	dog	rogue	Gwen	grow
gun	geese	ago	logger	tug	intrigue	single	giggling
good	ghost	ego	bagger	bag	tag	finger	mingle
gap	gasp	beggar	sagging	dig	big	sags	nagged
gourd	gain	bagel	wiggle	nag	bug	eggs	bugs

/g/ Contrasts/Minimal Pairs

/g/–/k/		/g/–/d/		/g/–/ŋ/	
gain	cane	guy	dye	sag	sang
goal	coal	gale	dale	bag	bang
guile	Kyle	get	debt	rig	ring
bigger	bicker	bigger	bidder	dig	ding
tag	tack	buggy	buddy	hag	hang
hag	hack	bug	bud	hug	hung
bag	back	rig	rid	wig	wing
bug	buck	rogue	road	dig	ding

Additional Notes

The /g/ is mastered at about the same time as /k/ and is seldom misarticulated. Children who have difficulty acquiring /g/ usually substitute /d/ instead. For example, *dog* may be produced as [d ɔ d] by a very young child (before age 3). The /g/ is the least frequently occurring stop in American English. All the stop consonant symbols look very much like the lower case alphabetic letters you learned to print when you began school. However, note that the symbol for the velar /g/ appears like a hand-printed *g* rather than the typeset *g*.

Transcription

Now that you have been introduced to all the stops, you can begin listening and transcription exercises. Remember that all the stops resemble their lower case alphabetic counterparts. You will find the exercises for stops in Appendix A.

FRICATIVES

Consonants classified as fricatives are the largest category of all the consonants. They are all characterized by audible friction. This air turbulence results from the passage of the voiced or voiceless airstream through a narrow opening, usually in the oral cavity. For example, if the narrow opening is between the upper incisors and the lower lip, the fricative /f/ or /v/ will be produced. /s/ and /z/ result from constriction between the tongue tip and the alveolar ridge. If the constriction is between the vocal folds, the consonant /h/ results. There are 10 fricative consonants in American English, eight of which occur in cognate pairs: /f/ and /v/, /θ/ and /ð/, /s/ and/z/, and /ʃ/ and /ʒ/. The glottal /h/ is the only fricative without a cognate.

The tenth fricative, /ʍ/, is seldom used in mainstream American English. It will be covered in the section Approximants/Oral Resonant Consonants, later in this chapter. The fricatives are presented in cognate pairs (when applicable), in order of place of articulation, from most anterior to most posterior.

/f/

Cognate:	/v/
Description	Voiceless labiodental fricative
Key Words:	fan, offer, leaf
Common Spellings:	f, ff, ph

/f/ Production: Voiceless Labiodental Fricative

With the velopharyngeal port closed, the lower lip approximates the upper front teeth. Breath is continuously emitted between the teeth and lower lip as audible friction. There is no vocal fold vibration. The /f/ is usually of greater duration and produced with more force than /v/.

/f/ Words

Prevocalic		Intervocalic		Postvocalic		Sequences	
fun	fair	offer	refer	if	beef	fly	float
feet	fight	before	effort	off	cough	free	frost
fast	four	coffee	office	wife	tough	softly	lifted
five	fine	prophet	coughing	puff	staff	rafted	breakfast
follow	fort	laughing	prefer	laugh	safe	raft	laughs
face	phone	loafers	defer	rough	scuff	sifts	surfed

/f/ Contrasts/Minimal Pairs

/f/–/v/		/f/–/θ/		/f/–/p/	
fan	van	Fred	thread	fast	past
fine	vine	fin	thin	fool	pool
fest	vest	free	three	fry	pry
surface	service	first	thirst	flee	plea
feel	veal	offer	author	leaf	leap
proof	prove	oaf	oath	hoof	hoop
belief	believe	reef	wreath	Jif	gyp
half	halve	roof	Ruth	calf	cap

Additional Notes

The /f/ is not a frequently occurring consonant. It is acquired fairly early in development and is seldom misarticulated.

/v/

Cognate:	/f/
Description	Voiced labiodental fricative
Key Words:	vote, ever, have
Common Spellings:	v

/v/ Production

/v/ is produced in the same way as /f/ except that the airstream is voiced.

/v/ Words

Prevocalic		Intervocalic		Postvocalic		Sequences	
vine	voice	ever	servant	have	believe	advent	obvious
very	vowel	over	fever	gave	weave	envy	advantage
vote	vane	server	diver	live	twelve	velvet	advice
visit	value	lover	oven	serve	groove	lived	saves
van	vague	aver	proving	move	carve	served	carved
vest	verse	hover	every	rave	love	craved	raves

/v/ Contrasts/Minimal Pairs

/v/–/f/		/v/–/θ/		/v/–/b/		/v/–/w/	
very	fairy	vine	thine	van	ban	vine	wine
veal	feel	van	than	very	berry	vent	went
vest	fest	clover	clothier	vest	best	vet	wet
waver	wafer	veil	they'll	vent	bent	vee	we
calve	calf	lever	leather	Vic	Bic	vest	west
halve	half	vie	thy	savor	saber	very	wary
prove	proof			serve	Serb	Vic	wick

Additional Notes

The /v/ is mastered fairly late by children, somewhat later than /f/. It is misarticulated with moderate frequency, more often than /f/ but less than fricatives such as /s/. Hispanic English speakers may substitute /b/ for /v/ and substitute the voiced bilabial fricative /β/ (a Spanish phoneme) for /v/ in the medial position of words.

/θ/

Cognate:	/ð/
Description	Voiceless (lingua-) dental fricative
	Voiceless (inter) dental fricative
Key Words:	thumb, nothing, tooth
Common Spellings:	th

/θ/ Production

The velopharyngeal port is closed, and the sides of the tongue are against the molars. The tip of the tongue, spread wide and thin, approximates the edge of inner surface of the upper front teeth. The voiceless breath stream is continuously emitted between the front teeth and tongue to create audible friction. The /θ/ is of greater duration and is produced with more force than its cognate, /ð/.

/θ/ Words

Prevocalic		Intervocalic		Postvocalic		Sequences	
thin	thaw	anything	nothing	cloth	booth	three	threw
thank	thud	cathedral	ethics	teeth	growth	threat	thrive
theft	thigh	everything	pathetic	breath	path	wealthy	earthquake
third	theater	Athens	ether	oath	mouth	filthy	earthly
think	thorn	author	Ethel	south	bath	width	fifth
theme	thermal	within	ethos	faith	lath	month	length

/θ/ Contrasts/Minimal Pairs

/θ/–/ð/		/θ/–/t/		/θ/–/f/		/θ/–/s/	
ether	either	thigh	tie	thin	fin	thumb	some
wreath	wreathe	thin	tin	Thor	four	think	sink
thigh	thy	thick	tick	three	free	thaw	saw
teeth	teethe	bath	bat	wreath	reef	bath	bass
loath	loathe	both	boat	Ruth	roof	faith	face
		Beth	bet	frothed	frost	north	Norse

Additional Notes

The /θ/ is one of the weakest phonemes acoustically. It is mastered later than many other phonemes and is frequently misarticulated. It is one of the phonemes found among residual errors, those phonemes that continue to cause difficulty even for some school-aged children (Smit, 2003b). Substitutions for /θ/ typically are /f/, /t/, or /s/. Thus, **thumb** might be produced as [f ʌ m], [t ʌ m], or [s ʌ m]. The /θ/ often creates difficulty for speakers of English as a second language because /θ/ occurs in so few world languages.

/ð/

Cognate:	/θ/
Description	Voiced (lingua-) dental fricative
	Voiced (inter) dental fricative
Key Words:	this, weather, breathe
Common Spellings:	th

/ð/ Production

The /ð/ is produced like the /θ/ except that the airstream is voiced. It is of slightly shorter duration and produced with less force than /θ/.

/ð/ Words

Prevocalic		Medial		Postvocalic	
the	these	bother	other	soothe	smooth
this	though	weather	lather	bathe	breathe
that	those	rather	feather	writhe	loathe
they	their	either	soothing	tithe	seethe
them	thus	father	mother	teethe	clothe
there	thine	brother	southern		

/ð/ Contrasts / Minimal Pairs

/ð/–/θ/		/ð/–/d/		/ð/–/v/	
either	ether	then	den	than	van
teethe	teeth	those	doze	that	vat
mouth (verb)	mouth (noun)	they	day	they'll	veil
this	thin	though	dough	thee	vee
these	theme	their	dare	thou	vow
		father	fodder	thy	vie
		teethe	teed		
		lathe	laid		

Additional Notes

Like its cognate /θ/, /ð/ is acquired later in development and is likely to be a residual error in children. Misarticulations may be particularly noticeable because /ð/ occurs in a number of important words such as *the*, *this*, *that*, *then*, *there* (*their*), *them*, *these*, and *those*. /ð/ also causes difficulty for many speakers of English as a second language because /ð/ does not occur in many languages. Frequent substitutions for /ð/ include /v/, /d/, and /z/. *Them* could be misarticulated as [v ɛ m], [d ɛ m], or [z ɛ m].

Transcription

Now that you have been introduced to some of the fricative consonants, you can begin to learn to listen for them and transcribe them. Because there are so many fricatives, listening and transcription exercises are divided into two groups: /f v θ ð/ and then /s z ʃ ʒ h/, followed by additional exercises for all the fricatives. The IPA symbols for /f v h s z/ look very much like the lower case alphabetic letters you learned to print when you began school. However, the remaining symbols do not resemble English alphabetic letters. The /θ/ looks like a 0 (zero) with a line drawn through the middle or somewhat like the Greek letter *theta*. For its voiced cognate, /ð/, the symbol resembles a backwards 6, slightly tilted, with a cross on the stem. You will find the exercises for /f v θ ð/ in Appendix A.

/s/

Cognate:	/z/
Description	Voiceless (lingua-) alveolar fricative
Key Words:	sun, missing, moss
Common Spellings:	s, ss, c, x (/k/ + /s/)

/s/ Production

There are two positions commonly used by American English speakers to produce /s/: with tongue tip up and with tongue tip down. You can use a mirror to see for yourself: try producing /s/ and noting where your tongue tip is. For most people, the tongue tip is raised, but a sizable minority produce /s/ with the tongue tip lowered. Either position is acceptable as long as a clear /s/ is produced. Both positions, of course, require velopharyngeal closure and a voiceless airstream. In addition, the sides of the tongue rest against the molars for both types. Duration of /s/ is generally longer, and breath pressure is greater than for its cognate /z/.

Alveolar /s/: tongue-tip up position. This is the more commonly occurring position for production of /s/. The tongue tip is narrowly grooved and approximates the alveolar ridge just behind the upper incisors. Air flows through the narrow opening created by the tongue tip, alveolar ridge, and closely approximated teeth, producing an audible friction or hissing sound.

Dental /s/: tongue-tip down position. For this position, the tongue tip approximates the lower incisors near the gum ridge. The front of the tongue is slightly grooved and raised toward the alveolar ridge. Airflow through the narrow opening created by tongue front, alveolar ridge, and teeth results in the friction or hissing quality of /s/.

/s/ Words

Prevocalic		Intervocalic		Postvocalic		Sequences	
see	sun	fasten	missile	us	boss	splash	skin
sign	sick	lesson	possible	miss	this	spring	straw
sour	sip	basin	recent	horse	peace	basket	history
soup	soap	lasso	gasoline	yes	mice	asking	whisker
suit	send	hustle	passing	ice	loss	jokes	tax
cell	cider	passer	facing	trace	gross	mists	wasps

/s/ Contrasts/Minimal Pairs

/s/–/z/		/s/–/θ/		/s/–/ʃ/	
sip	zip	some	thumb	sore	shore
see	z	sin	thin	sue	shoe
sue	zoo	sank	thank	sign	shine
racer	razor	seem	theme	fasten	fashion
bus	buzz	gross	growth	mass	mash
fuss	fuzz	face	faith	Swiss	swish
fleece	flees	pass	path	lass	lash
loose	lose	moss	moth	Gus	gush

Additional Notes

The /s/ is one of the most frequently occurring American-English consonant sounds as well as being a common residual error in children. Consequently, a problem with /s/ (**lisp**) can be quite disruptive to speech understandability. The /θ/ is a frequent substitution for /s/, making words such as *sun* become [θ ʌ n]. Dentition issues can play a role in poor /s/ production; for example, dentures in an older adult may lend a whistling quality to /s/. The loss of central incisors by children between ages 5 and 7 also frequently results in a temporary lisp. High-frequency hearing loss may also be associated with misarticulation of /s/.

/z/

Cognate:	/s/
Description	Voiced (lingua) alveolar fricative
Key Words:	zoo, razor, size
Common Spellings:	z, zz

/z/ Production

Like /s/, there are two prevalent formations for /z/ production, with the tongue-tip up position more often used. These formations are exactly like those for /s/ with one exception: the airstream is voiced. Duration and breath pressure for /z/ are usually less than for its cognate /s/.

/z/ Words

Prevocalic		Intervocalic		Postvocalic		Sequences	
zoo	zebra	easy	visit	buzz	is	songs	buds
zipper	zinc	dozen	nozzle	jazz	was	webs	wrongs
zone	Zen	music	dizzy	these	breeze	gives	arrives
zero	zodiac	puzzle	raisin	use	those	raised	breezed
zest	xylophone	busy	weasel	nose	lose	buzzed	amazed
zip	zest	rosy	measles	wise	awes	frowns	greens

/z/ Contrasts/Minimal Pairs

/z/–/s/		/z/–/ð/		/z/–/ʒ/	
zeal	seal	bays	bathe	bays	beige
Zack	sack	breeze	breathe	lows	loge
zing	sing	lows	loathe	rues	rouge
zone	sewn	close	clothe	Caesar	seizure
zip	sip	seas	seethe	glazer	glazier
fleas	fleece	tease	teethe		
eyes	ice	rise	writhe		
lose	loose				

Additional Notes

The /z/, like its cognate /s/, often continues to cause difficulty for children. Speakers who have difficulty with /z/ often substitute /ð/. Thus, *zoo* and *buzz* would be produced as [ð u] and [b ʌ ð].

/ʃ/

Cognate:	/ʒ/
Description	Voiceless (lingua-) palatal fricative
Key Words:	shoe, wishing, wash
Common Spellings:	sh, s

/ʃ/ Production

The velopharyngeal port is closed and a voiceless airstream is used throughout production. The sides of the tongue are against the upper molars, and the broad front surface of the tongue is raised toward the palate just behind the alveolar ridge. This forms a central opening that is slightly broader and farther back than for /s/ production. The voiceless airstream is directed continuously through and against the slightly open front teeth to produce audible friction. The lips are usually slightly rounded and protruded, similar to the position for /ʊ/.

/ʃ/ Words

Prevocalic		Intervocalic		Postvocalic		Sequences	
sheep	shine	wishes	fashion	mash	radish	shrimp	shrink
chic	shut	bushel	fishing	mesh	English	shred	shrew
shall	shake	rushing	ashamed	wish	splash	action	insurance
shield	show	ocean	fuchsia	fresh	crush	ensure	banshee
ship	shade	assure	nation	relish	push	fished	washed
show	sham	ashes	machine	leash	rush	wished	meshed

/ʃ/ Contrasts/Minimal Pairs

/ʃ/–/ʒ/		/ʃ/–/s/		/ʃ/–/tʃ/	
glacier	glazier	sheet	seat	shad	chad
Aleutian	allusion	shoe	sue	chic	cheek
assure	azure	she	see	ship	chip
leash	liege	lashes	lasses	lashes	latches
dilution	delusion	mush	muss	leashes	leeches
		gash	gas	bush	butch
		cash	Cass	cash	catch
		dished	dissed	crush	crutch

Additional Notes

The /ʃ/ is also one of the consonants found among residual error sounds. The /s/ is a common substitution for /ʃ/ so that **sh**oe becomes [s u]. The /ʃ/ may also be affected if English is a speaker's second language; for example, Hispanic English speakers may substitute /tʃ/ for /ʃ/. Further details regarding dialectic variation may be found in Chapter 6.

/ʒ/

Cognate:	/ʃ/
Description	Voiced (lingua-) palatal fricative
Key Words:	measure, corsage
Common Spellings:	variable (see Additional Notes)

/ʒ/ Production

The velopharyngeal port is closed and the airstream is voiced throughout production. Formation of /ʒ/ is just like that for /ʃ/ except that the airstream is voiced.

/ʒ/ Words

Note that /ʒ/ occurs only in the medial and final positions of words in English.

/ʒ/ Words

Intervocalic		Postvocalic	
vision	aphasia	beige	corsage
usual	treasure	loge	garage
casual	occasion	rouge	prestige
measure	seizure	montage	camouflage
lesion	regime	collage	triage
Asian	collision		

/ʒ/ Contrasts

/ʒ/–/ʃ/		/ʒ/–/ʤ/	
glazier	glacier	pleasure	pledger
vision	vicious	lesion	legion
measure	pressure	vision	pigeon
occasion	vacation	rouge	huge
azure	assure	prestige	vestige

Additional Notes

The /ʒ/ is one of the last consonants to be developed and mastered by children. It is also one of the least frequently occurring consonants in English. In some American-English dialects, /ʒ/ may be replaced by /ʤ/ in certain words. For example, *garage* might be pronounced as [gəraʒ] or [gəraʤ].

/h/

Cognate:	None
Description	Voiceless glottal fricative
Key Words:	he, ahead
Common Spellings:	h, wh

/h/ Production

The velopharyngeal port is closed. The vocal folds are partially abducted, creating a constriction through which the voiceless airstream is forced. This results in the friction sound recognized as /h/. Because /h/ is formed at the glottis, the oral cavity structures are free to assume any of the vowel positions that follow it.

/h/ Words

Note that /h/ occurs only in the prevocalic and intervocalic positions in English.

Prevocalic		Intervocalic	
he	high	ahead	unhook
his	how	behind	mahogany
her	hat	rehire	perhaps
hoe	home	behold	rehearse
who	hook	mohair	Mojave

/h/ Contrasts/Minimal Pairs Words

//–/h/		/h/–/θ/	
eat	heat	hatch	thatch
it	hit	high	thigh
ate	hate	hum	thumb
air	hair	heard	third
Ed	head	hug	thug
ugh	hug	had	Thad
ear	hear	hump	thump
eye	high	horn	thorn

Additional Notes

The /h/ is one of the earliest sounds mastered by children and has been noted to occur in the first 50 vocabulary words of toddlers. Consequently, complete omission of /h/ in words, even in young children, may indicate a problem with speech development. The /h/ is subject to some voicing when it occurs between voiced phonemes. We will discuss this further in Chapter 5.

Transcription of Fricatives

Exercises 4.7–4.10 are designed to help you listen for, and transcribe the remaining fricatives as well as all the phonemes you have learned previously. Remember to follow the conventions for correct IPA form that appeared earlier in this chapter.

AFFRICATES

There are only two affricates in American English, the cognates /ʧ/ and /ʤ/ (as in *chair* and *jump*, respectively). Affricates share characteristics of both stops and fricatives in their manner of formation. Consequently, their symbols are a combination of those you already know. Each is still one phoneme, however, because of the coarticulation involved. The single phoneme is also indicated by the touching of the component symbols in transcription for each affricate.

For both American-English affricates, the oral airflow is briefly interrupted or stopped (like a stop) and then released with friction (like a fricative). The stop and the fricative sound are smoothly blended as one phoneme.

/ʧ/

Cognate:	ʤ
Description	Voiceless (lingua-) palatal affricate
Key Words:	chair, teacher, watch
Common Spellings:	ch, tch

/ʧ/ Production

The velopharyngeal port is closed, and the sides of the tongue approximate the upper molars. The tongue tip closes on or just behind the alveolar ridge, and the voiceless air-stream is held and compressed in the oral cavity. Following this air compression, the air is forced through a narrow constriction formed by the tongue and palate to complete the /ʃ/ phase of /ʧ/. The entire phoneme is produced on a single impulse of breath.

/ʧ/ Words

Prevocalic		Intervocalic		Postvocalic	
chain	chair	kitchen	bachelor	watch	each
choose	cheese	nature	natural	much	such
change	chase	virtue	capture	birch	reach
chin	children	matches	preacher	coach	which
chilled	chapter	richest	patches	beach	latch
chant	chore	watching	catcher	hutch	Dutch

/ʧ/ Contrasts/Minimal Pairs Words

/ʧ/–/ʤ/		/ʧ/–/ʃ/		/ʧ/–/t/	
chain	Jane	cherry	sherry	chime	time
cheap	jeep	chair	share	chew	two
batch	badge	chin	shin	chin	tin
chunk	junk	cheer	sheer	which	wit
char	jar	much	mush	beach	beat
chess	Jess	match	mash	hatch	hat
lunch	lunge	hutch	hush	batch	bat
rich	ridge	witch	wish	cherry	Terry

Additional Notes

The /ʧ/ also is one of the residual error sounds that may be difficult for young children. In general, affricates are mastered later than stops, nasals, and glides. /ʃ/ is often substituted for /ʧ/ in typical misarticulations, making *chew* become [ʃu]. The /ʧ/ may also be misarticulated by some speakers of English as a second language.

/ʤ/

Cognate:	/ʧ/
Description:	Voiced (lingua-) palatal affricate
Key Words:	jump, badger, edge
Common Spellings:	j, dg(e)

/ʤ/ Production

The /ʤ/ is produced in the same way as /ʧ/ except for the use of a voiced air-stream.

/ʤ/ Words

Prevocalic		Intervocalic		Postvocalic	
jam	giant	lodges	gradual	age	village
jaw	gem	badger	merger	edge	bridge
joy	gentle	codger	agent	gauge	cottage
jelly	gene	agitate	ridges	ledge	college
Jim	general	ginger	magic	urge	strange
joke	jest	wager	merging	merge	surge

/ʤ/ Contrasts/Minimal Pairs Words

/ʤ/–/ʧ/		/ʤ/–/j/		/ʤ/–/dz/	
jar	char	jam	yam	budge	buds
jet	chet	jeer	year	rage	raids
gin	chin	juice	use	siege	seeds
joke	choke	Jell-O	yellow	age	aids
jump	chump	Jen	yen	wedge	weds
Jerry	cherry	jet	yet	barge	bards
ridges	riches	gel	yell	ridge	rids
age	h	major	mayor	hedge	heads

Additional Notes

Like its cognate /ʧ/, /ʤ/ may also be difficult to produce for some young children and is mastered later. Typically, a /ʒ/ is substituted for /ʤ/ when this phoneme is misarticulated so that *jump* would be heard as [ʒʌmp]. The /ʤ/ occurs more frequently than /ʧ/ but is, nevertheless, a very low occurrence consonant. Correct articulation may pose problems for some speakers of English as a second language.

Transcription

You will find listening and transcription exercises in Appendix A, Exercises 4.11–4.13. Remember to follow the guidelines for correct transcription of the affricates and to transcribe all the phonemes that you have learned to this point.

NASALS

The three nasal resonant consonants of American English are /m/, /n/, and /ŋ/. They are produced by alteration of the cavities of the vocal tract (as are approximants/ oral resonant consonants, which follow in the next section). The nasals differ from consonants with oral airflow in one particularly important way: the velopharyngeal port is open, permitting open resonation of the voiced airstream in the nasal cavity. At the same time, the oral cavity is completely closed off at some point, forcing the airflow through the nasal cavity. For /m/ production, the resonating cavity consists of the oral cavity occluded at the lips as well as the open nasal cavity. The resonating space for /n/ is smaller, with oral closure at the alveolar ridge. The resonating space for /ŋ/ uses even less oral cavity space because closure is made with the back of the tongue and the velum. Discrimination among the nasals usually does not cause difficulty except for /n/ and /ŋ/ in certain contexts. Also, /n/ is sometimes substituted for /ŋ/ in rapid speech and in some dialects, for example *runnin'* for *running*.

/m/

Description	(Voiced) bilabial nasal
Key Words:	my, coming, team
Common Spellings:	m, mm

/m/ Production

The lips are closed, and the velopharyngeal port is open. The voiced airstream is directed out through the nasal cavity and the nostrils. The tongue lies flat in the mouth or is prepared for the following vowel. The teeth are slightly open.

/m/ Words

Initial		Medial		Final		Sequences	
me	men	summer	coming	am	storm	small	stormed
may	much	hammer	amen	whom	time	smile	snail
meat	might	animal	among	lamb	diaphragm	amber	Christmas
miss	mat	family	steaming	hymn	team	empty	someone
more	moon	America	humid	palm	roam	lamp	blimp

/m/ Contrasts/Minimal Pairs

/m/–/b/		/m/–/n/		/m/–/ŋ/	
mite	bite	me	knee	ham	hang
mean	bean	mine	nine	hum	hung
mare	bear	might	night	whim	wing
mate	bait	more	nor	ram	rang
rum	rub	hem	hen	swim	swing
lambs	labs	terms	turns	Sam	sang
come	cub	ram	ran	Kim	king
rum	rub	ohm	own	rum	rung

Additional Notes

The /m/ is one of the first sounds mastered by children and is seldom misarticulated. Like /h/, it is found in the first 50 vocabulary words of early speech development. It is also one of the most frequently occurring sounds in English.

/n/

Description	(Voiced) (lingua-) alveolar nasal
Key Words:	no, many, green
Common Spellings:	n, nn

/n/ Production

Production of /n/ is just like that of /m/ except that oral closure is made with the tip of the tongue against the alveolar ridge and the sides of the tongue against the upper molars. The velopharyngeal port is open and the voiced airstream passes through the nasal cavity.

/n/ Words

Prevocalic		Intervocalic		Postvocalic		Sequences	
not	gnat	funny	banana	can	ripen	snail	snow
knife	north	many	peanut	align	cotton	snare	snack
new	gnarled	any	enemy	sign	kitten	under	builder
know	nap	tiny	annotate	inn	on	Andy	Indiana
name	nice	Annie	Dennis	been	seen	pines	round
Nile	nor	sunny	running	one	line	hunt	pint

/n/ Contrasts

/n/–/d/		/n/–/m/		/n/–/ŋ/	
need	deed	Nate	mate	ban	bang
no	doe	night	might	fan	fang
knock	dock	nine	mine	win	wing
owner	odor	turns	terms	pin	ping
bin	bid	dine	dime	thin	thing
can	cad	own	ohm	lawn	long
kin	kid	main	maim	run	rung
bean	bead	sane	same	sun	sung

Additional Notes

Like /m/, the /n/ is one of the first sounds mastered by children and is seldom misarticulated. After /t/, /n/ is the most frequently occurring consonant in English.

/ŋ/

Description	(Voiced) (lingua-) velar nasal
Key Words:	song, ringer
Common Spellings:	ng, n

/ŋ/ Production

The /ŋ/ is produced like the /n/ except that oral cavity closure is made by the back of the tongue against the front part of the velum or the back part of the hard palate. Tongue pressure at the velum is less than it is for /k/ or /g/.

/ŋ/ Words

Note that /ŋ/ does not occur in the prevocalic position in English.

Intervocalic		Postvocalic		Sequences	
singer	hanger	tongue	along	linger	longer
ringer	singing	sang	lung	anger	thanking
pinging	winging	awning	working	rings	banked
stinger	zinger	among	string	think	longed
longing	ringing	long	sang	younger	kangaroo
		ring	meaning	drank	dangle

/ŋ/ Contrasts/Minimal Pairs

/ŋ/–/g/		/ŋ/–/n/		/ŋ/–/m/	
wing	wig	stung	stun	hung	hum
tongue	tug	long	lawn	ding	dim
long	log	fang	fan	clang	clam
bang	bag	sing	sin	sung	sum
rung	rug	hung	Hun	hanger	hammer
lung	lug	pang	pan		
ring	rig	stung	stun		

Additional Notes

The /ŋ/ is also mastered early by children (though later than /m/ and /n/). It is seldom misarticulated. In informal speech, the /n/ often replaces the /ŋ/ in words such as *running* ([ɹ ʌ n ɪ n]) and *jumping* ([dʒ ʌ m p ɪ n]). Remember that /m/ and /n/ resemble their lower case alphabetic counterparts. The /ŋ/ resembles the /n/ but with a "tail" extended below the symbol.

Transcription of Nasals

Turn to Appendix A to complete Exercises 4.14–4.17. You will find exercises for recognition and discrimination of the nasals as well as transcription. The transcription exercises include extra practice for words with similar spellings. Remember to follow the correct forms and transcribe all the phonemes you have learned.

APPROXIMANTS/ORAL RESONANT CONSONANTS

This manner or articulation category encompasses four phonemes: /j/ (as in *yes*), /w/ (*wing*), /l/ (*lend*), and /ɹ/ (*rug*). They are characterized by alterations of the resonating cavities for their distinctive identities. The four consonants are often subdivided into two smaller classes: **glides** (/w/ and /j/, also sometimes referred to as **semivowels**) and **liquids** (/l/ and /ɹ/).

/w/

Description	(Voiced) (lingua-) velar bilabial glide
Key Words:	we, away
Common Spellings:	w, wh

/w/ Production

With the velopharyngeal port closed, the lips are rounded (labial placement) for an opening slightly smaller than for the vowel /u/. At the same time, the tongue is elevated (velar placement) in the back of the mouth as for /u/. The voiced airstream is directed into the oral cavity and the articulators move or "glide" from this initial posture into the position of the vowel that must follow the /w/. The /w/ is of short duration and is always released into a vowel.

Some speakers differentiate between the /w/ in *witch* and the /ʍ/ in *which*. It was once an important distinction for speakers who were very strict about their pronunciation of English. However, most mainstream American English speakers use /w/ for both forms. Consequently /w/ will be used in this section and the remainder of the book.

/w/ Words

Prevocalic		Intervocalic		Sequences	
we	wash	away	unwind	twin	twist
way	weed	always	seaweed	queen	quick
were	wet	anyone	byway	Gwen	swell
won	one	forward	nowhere	sweater	sweet
wood	would	reward	otherwise	twilight	quest
web	whistle	rewind	highway	quiet	quota

/w/ Contrasts/Minimal Pairs

/w/–/l/		/w/–/ɹ/		/w/–/v/	
wed	led	wed	red	we	vee
weed	lead	when	wren	wary	vary
wake	lake	wind	rind	wet	vet
wise	lies	wake	rake	went	vent
why	lie	west	rest	wail	vale
win	Lynn	white	right	wow	vow
white	light	wheel	reel	west	vest
wick	lick	wick	Rick	wick	Vic

Additional Notes

The /w/ is mastered very early by children, usually appearing as a phoneme in the first 50 words acquired by children as they develop speech. It is often substituted for /l/ and/or /ɹ/ in children's early speech development. Thus, words like *light* and *balloon* might be produced as [w aɪ t] and [b əw u n].

/j/

Description	(Voiced) (lingua-) palatal glide
Key Words:	you, bayou
Common Spellings:	y

/j/ Production

The velopharyngeal port is closed and the tip of the tongue is positioned behind the lower front teeth with the tongue body flat. The front of the tongue is raised high toward the palate. The voiced airstream is directed through the oral cavity for a brief period as the tongue and lips assume the position for the following vowel. The space between tongue and palate is similar to that for /i/. The duration of /j/ is short, and it is always released into a vowel.

/j/ Words

Note that /j/ does not occur in the postvocalic position of words.

Prevocalic		Intervocalic		Sequences	
yard	young	loyal	beyond	few	music
year	yes	bayou	mayor	cute	onion
yet	yellow	royal	hallelujah	feud	dominion
yolk	useful	foyer	higher	muse	million
use	unit	rayon	voyage	pupil	canyon
yell	yarn	layer	lawyer	venue	barnyard

/j/ Contrasts

/j/–/w/		/j/–/ /		/j/–/ʤ/	
yet	wet	yam	am	yam	jam
yoke	woke	year	ear	yell	jell
yield	wield	yearn	earn	yet	jet
yell	well	beauty	booty	yak	jack
yes	Wes	cute	coot	year	jeer
ye	we	fuel	fool	yes	Jess
yen	when	mewed	mooed	ye	G
yip	whip	feud	food	Yule	jewel

Additional Notes

Some phoneticians consider /j/ as a diphthong when it is released into /u/, for example /ju/ in *cute, few*. We will treat it as part of a consonant sequence in this book. The /j/ is acquired fairly early and is seldom misarticulated. It is not a frequently occurring sound.

/l/

Description	(Voiced) (lingua-) alveolar liquid
Key Words:	lamp, balloon, bell
Common Spellings:	l, ll, le

/l/ Production

The velopharyngeal port is closed and the airstream is voiced throughout production. There are two articulatory positions for /l/, with use depending on the position (prevocalic, postvocalic) of the consonant in a word. For prevocalic /l/, the tongue tip closes with slight pressure against the alveolar ridge, with opening on both sides. This allows the voiced airstream to escape laterally around the tongue and out the oral cavity. (Hence, **lateral phoneme** is another term that is used to describe /l/.) When /l/ occurs in the postvocalic position, the back of the tongue is also raised toward the velum, in addition to the tongue-tip elevation. For prevocalic /l/, the tongue tip leaves the alveolar ridge to form the next phoneme. The tongue tip stays at the alveolar ridge for postvocalic /l/.

/l/ Words

Prevocalic		Intervocalic		Postvocalic		Sequences	
lay	loose	yellow	hollow	oil	bell	climb	clock
leaf	lunch	tulip	dollar	all	fall	flower	glass
low	lamb	eleven	fellow	mill	school	glee	plant
like	leg	lily	jelly	hole	tell	slide	sled
lion	lift	along	teller	motel	fail	aglow	onslaught
listen	lost	melon	mellow	seal	pool	gold	field

/l/ Contrasts/Minimal Pairs

/l/–/w/		/l/–/ɹ/		/l/–/n/	
let	wet	lane	rain	lead	need
Lou	woo	lair	rare	low	no
line	wine	load	road	load	node
lack	whack	leak	reek	lice	nice
Lee's	wheeze	cried	Clyde	line	nine
lair	where	splay	spray	tell	ten
lest	west	play	prey	slow	snow
lead	weed	ply	pry	slide	snide

Additional Notes

The /l/ is mastered late by children. It is often replaced by a /w/ (or sometimes a /j/) in early speech development. Thus, *lamb* could be heard as [w æ m] or [j æ m]. It is one of the sounds that may continue to cause difficulty for young children, though not as often as /s/. Speakers of Asian English may confuse /l/ and /ɹ/.

/ɹ/

Description	(Voiced) (lingua-) palatal liquid
Key Words:	run, caring, car
Common Spellings:	r, rr

/ɹ/ Production

The /ɹ/ can be produced in several different ways, even within the same speaker. All productions require velopharyngeal closure and a voiced airstream. Regardless of the specific position, the key to /ɹ/ production is that the tongue is held high in the oral cavity but does not touch the roof of the mouth. This allows a central flow of air from the oral cavity (as opposed to the lateral airflow of /l/). Three positions have typically been described:

Tongue-Tip Up Position. The sides of the tongue are against the upper molars. The tongue tip is raised toward the palate just behind the alveolar ridge but does not make contact with it. The voiced airstream escapes between the tongue and the palato-alveolar area, out of the oral cavity. The lips may be slightly protruded in a position similar to that for /ʊ/, but they usually take the position of the following vowel. For example, for the /ɹ/ in *rain*, the lips are spread for [eɪ], but in *room,* the lips are rounded in anticipation of the [u]. (You can see this for yourself if you say the two words while looking in a mirror.)

Retroflex Position. This is a variation of the tongue-tip-up position. It is produced in the same way except that the tongue tip is curled up and back.

Tongue-Tip Down Position/"Bunched." The sides of the tongue are against the upper molars. The front of the tongue is raised toward the palate with the tip neutral or pointing downward behind the maxillary incisors. The tongue is retracted or "bunched," hence the alternative name.

/ɹ/ Words

Note that postvocalic /ɹ/ is transcribed as a consonant, rather than as part of a centering diphthong in this section and throughout the remainder of the book.

Prevocalic		Intervocalic		Postvocalic		Sequences	
ran	write	very	marry	car	or	bring	bright
red	wrist	arrow	terrible	air	dear	drain	draw
rub	rhyme	berry	orange	four	chair	pray	pride
rake	right	story	airy	near	are	travel	trust
rose	roam	carrot	sorry	fire	dare	straw	street
rock	wren	carry	eerie	hair	bar	already	toothbrush

/ɹ/ Contrasts/Minimal Pair Words

/ɹ/–/w/		/ɹ/–/l/		/ɹ/–/ɝ/ or /ɚ/	
rip	whip	rest	lest	train	terrain
rich	witch	red	led	bray	beret
run	one	Rick	lick	dress	duress
raid	wade	room	loom	crest	caressed
rock	wok	ride	lied	broke	baroque
trig	twig	brink	blink	throw	thorough
trice	twice	crone	clone	creed	curried
tryst	twist	cram	clam	crowed	corrode

Additional Notes

The /ɹ/ is acquired later in speech development and is often among residual error sounds in young children. Substitution of /w/ for /ɹ/ ([w u m] for *room*) is common in early childhood. The /ɹ/ is also subject to dialectic variation depending on the type of English (e.g., British, Hispanic) and region of the United States. For example, intervocalic /ɹ/ is trilled in British English, making words like *very* sound like [vɛdi]. In New England and Southern English, the postvocalic /ɹ/ may be omitted or re-placed by a vowel, for example, resulting in park being produced as [pɑk] or *here* being produced as [hijə]. Although /ɹ/ is the official IPA symbol for this consonant, the symbol used to be /r/, which is now the symbol for a trilled sound characteristic of Spanish. Because /r/ is easier to transcribe, many American-English transcribers continue to use the symbol. You should ask what preference your instructor may have. If you use the /r/ symbol, remember that it is not a phoneme typical of American English. Further information on multicultural speech variations will be found in Chapter 6.

The consonant /ɹ/ differs from the **rhotic** vowels /ɝ/ and /ɚ/ in three ways: (1) it is shorter in duration, (2) it never constitutes a syllable, and (3) it entails movement away from the /ɹ/ position (as opposed to the rhotic vowels movement toward the /ɹ/ position).

Transcription of Liquids and Glides

Turn to Exercises 4.18–4.23. These exercises are designed to help you recognize and transcribe the liquids and glides. They also contain exercises to help you distinguish and transcribe the /ɝ/ and /ɚ/ vowels from the consonantal /ɹ/. Be sure to follow the conventions for correct formation of all the phonemes in your transcription.

CONCEPT QUESTIONS

1. Identify the consonants in the following words with regard to position and makeup (singleton or sequence)

			Position	Singleton/Sequence
a.	ring			
	r	/ɹ/	_____	_____
	ng	/ŋ/	_____	_____
b.	stove			
	st	/st/	_____	_____
	v	/v/	_____	_____
c.	chicken			
	ch	/ʧ/	_____	_____
	k	/k/	_____	_____
	n	/n/	_____	_____
d.	basket			
	b	/b/	_____	_____
	sk	/sk/	_____	_____
	t	/t/	_____	_____

    e. **telephone**

t	/t/	_____	_____
l	/l/	_____	_____
ph	/f/	_____	_____
n	/n/	_____	_____

2. Write the IPA symbol that matches each of the following brief descriptions:
    a. Bilabial nasal: _____
    b. Voiceless alveolar stop: _____
    c. Voiceless palatal fricative: _____
    d. Voiceless velar stop: _____
    e. Voiceless (inter)dental fricative: _____
    f. Palatal glide: _____
    g. Voiceless labiodental fricative: _____
    h. Voiceless palatal affricate: _____
    i. Bilabial-velar glide: _____
    j. Voiced (inter)dental fricative: _____
    k. Voiced velar stop: _____
    l. Velar nasal: _____
    m. Voiced palatal fricative: _____
    n. Voiced labiodental fricative: _____
    o. Voiced bilabial stop: _____
    p. Alveolar liquid: _____
    q. Voiceless bilabial stop: _____
    r. Voiceless glottal fricative: _____
    s. Alveolar nasal: _____
    t. Voiced alveolar stop: _____
    u. Voiced palatal affricate: _____
    v. Palatal liquid: _____

3. List the cognate for each of the following:
    a. /p/: _____   b. /z/: _____   c. /ʤ/: _____   d. /f/: _____
    e. /t/: _____   f. /ʒ/: _____   g. /θ/: _____   h. /k/: _____

4. List all the consonants included in each group described below:
    a. Voiced alveolar consonants: _____
    b. Palatal consonants: _____
    c. Voiced stop consonants: _____
    d. Voiceless fricative consonants: _____
    e. Nasal consonants: _____
    f. Voiced velar consonants: _____
    g. Labial consonants: _____
    h. Voiced affricate: _____

5. For each group of phonemes listed, indicate the characteristic(s) they share in common, for example /b w v/— labial, voiced.
    a. /s l n d/: _____
    b. /ʤ ʒ/: _____
    c. /r l/: _____

d. /r ʒ ʧ j/: _____

e. /k ŋ/: _____

f. /z t d/: _____

g. /g d n ʒ/: _____

h. /p b w/: _____

CONNECTED SPEECH: SEGMENTAL AND SUPRASEGMENTAL EFFECTS

INFLUENCES OF CONTEXT: COARTICULATION
DIACRITICS AND NARROW TRANSCRIPTION
SPEECH RHYTHM AND SUPRASEGMENTAL FEATURES
CONCEPT QUESTIONS

INFLUENCES OF CONTEXT: COARTICULATION

Up to this point, you have learned to analyze speech in terms of its **segmental** (phoneme) components, and then only in a somewhat artificial way. Each phoneme has been described as a segment with a specific description of formation for each. The intent was to provide a fundamental understanding of the units that make up connected speech. You had many terms and symbols to learn, and they were best learned as individual entities, one group at a time. But speech does not occur in distinctly separated segments. In normal (real, connected) speech, phonemes don't follow each other separately the way beads on a string do. That is, you don't produce a word or phrase by simply producing an individual phoneme and then moving on to the next phoneme, and so on. Instead, there is a constant, overlapping effect of the movements of the articulators so that each phoneme's production overlaps and is therefore influenced by the ones surrounding it. There is a term to refer to this influence of adjoining sounds on each other: **coarticulation**. Coarticulation means that the vocal tract can take more than one position at the same time, so that connected speech occurs as a continuous flow rather than as a series of individually produced phonemes. Coarticulation also means that the movements of the articulators are efficient and make connected speech easier to produce. Before we discuss the different types of coarticulatory effects, let's start with a few examples that you can try for yourself.

First, look in a mirror and say these two words in succession: /ʃ i/ and /ʃ u/. Notice the position of your lips as you produce each word. You should notice that your lips are spread for /ʃ/ in production of *she* but rounded for the /ʃ/ in *shoe*. The identity of the consonant /ʃ/ is not changed, but its manner of formation differs slightly, depending on the vowel that follows it. This is one example of coarticulation. In this example, the lip rounding (an articulatory feature of the vowel /u/) is coarticulated with the consonant /ʃ/.

Next, try saying this phrase quickly three times: *so easy*. Pay careful attention to the sound that appears between /o/ and /i/. Did you notice a /w/ "sneaking in" so that *easy* sounded a little like *wheezy*? In this case, coarticulation can produce an additional or intrusive sound as the articulators transition from the /oʊ/ position to the /i/ position (see Addition/Epenthesis, later in this chapter). The appearance of /w/ shouldn't be too surprising because the transition involved is from a rounded vowel position (/o/) to a spread vowel (/i/). The movement involved is very much like the description for /w/ formation found in Chapter 4. You may also notice /w/ intrusion due to coarticulation in phrases such as *to each* [t u w i ʧ] and *to a* [t u w ə]. The coarticulation effects discussed in this chapter are among the most commonly occurring in American English. Some will require the use of diacritic markings to clarify the coarticulatory effect. In addition to the examples in this chapter, you will find exercises in Appendix A to help you understand these effects.

The diacritic markings associated with assimilation (resulting from coarticulation) are covered in the first section of this chapter, accompanied by additional exercises in Appendix A. In addition to coarticulation, **suprasegmentals** (accent, stress, phrasing, emphasis, intonation, and tempo) of speech affect the phoneme segments produced and listeners' perceptions of a speaker's meaning. Information on this topic is discussed in the second section with exercises in Appendix A to help you understand the concepts involved.

DIACRITICS AND NARROW TRANSCRIPTION

As you learn to transcribe phonemes in context and in connected speech, you will find that their sound properties can shift. This section demonstrates such changes and how to record them. In some cases, you will transcribe a different phoneme than the one you might have expected. In other cases, you will learn to use **diacritic markings** to signal the alteration (but not complete change) of one or more phoneme characteristics. Diacritic markings allow you to specify the nature of an allophonic variation in your transcription. We will cover some, but not all, of the diacritic markings used in the International Phonetic Alphabet (IPA). (**Table 5.1** shows the IPA chart for all diacritic markings.) The markings that are emphasized are particularly useful in applying phonetics to everyday work in speech-language pathology. They are also necessary for phonetic/narrow transcription as opposed to phonemic/broad transcription. In this chapter, the examples are drawn from normal adult speech. Later, in Chapter 7, we return to this topic with examples from the speech of children with normally developing speech as well as speech sound disorders.

ASSIMILATION PROCESSES

The effect of coarticulation may be rather minimal (as in the differences in /ʃ/ lip shaping for *she* (spread) versus *shoe* (rounded)). Or it may cause changes in the identity of a phoneme, for example, in place, manner, or voicing. In these cases, the effect is referred to as **assimilation**.

Phoneticians sometimes disagree over the concepts of coarticulation and assimilation. Some use the terms interchangeably, whereas others view coarticulation as the gestures that underlie pronunciation changes (Ohde & Sharf, 1992; Shriberg & Kent,

TABLE 5.1 IPA DIACRITIC MARKINGS FOR NARROW TRANSCRIPTION
DIACRITICS MAY BE PLACED ABOVE A SYMBOL WITH A DESCENDER, E.G., ŋ̊

̥ Voiceless n̥ d̥	̤ Breathy voiced b̤ a̤	̪ Dental t̪ d̪
̬ Voiced s̬ t̬	̰ Creaky voiced b̰ a̰	̺ Apical t̺ d̺
ʰ Aspirated tʰ dʰ	̼ Linguolabial t̼ d̼	̻ Laminal t̻ d̻
̹ More rounded ɔ̹	ʷ Labialized tʷdʷ	̃ Nasalized ẽ
̜ Less rounded ɔ̜	ʲ Palatalized tʲ dʲ	ⁿ Nasal release dⁿ
̟ Advanced u̟	ˠ Velarized tˠdˠ	ˡ Lateral release dˡ
̠ Retracted e̠	ˤ Pharyngealized tˤdˤ	̚ No audible release d̚
̈ Centralized ë	~ Velarized or pharyngealized ɫ	
̽ Mid-centralized ě	̝ Raised e̝ (ɹ̝ = voiced alveolar fricative)	
̩ Syllabic n̩	̞ Lowered e̞ (β̞ = voiced bilabial approximant)	
̯ Non-syllabic e̯	̘ Advanced tongue root e̘	
˞ Rhoticity ɚ ɑ˞	̙ Retracted tongue root e̙	

From the International Phonetic Association (http://www.langsci.ucl.ac.uk/ipa/). Copyright 2005 by International Phonetic Association. Reprinted with permission.

1982, 2013; Small, 2012). These pronunciation changes, then, are seen as examples of assimilation (Ohde & Sharf, 1992). Ohde and Sharf (1992) point out that the disagreement is related to limited understanding of the nature of speech motor control. For our purposes, we will view assimilation as a product of coarticulation.

Assimilation may be **progressive** or **regressive**, **contiguous** or **noncontiguous**. In progressive assimilation, an earlier occurring phoneme affects a phoneme that follows it in a word or phrase. The opposite is true of regressive assimilation. In this case, a later occurring phoneme alters the characteristic(s) of a phoneme preceding it. Assimilation is called contiguous if the phonemes involved are immediately adjacent to each other. If one or more phonemes separate the phonemes involved in assimilation, it is considered noncontiguous.

One way that assimilation can be found is in contexts where a phoneme takes on one or more of the characteristics of an adjacent phoneme but still retains its essential identity. For example, in Chapter 4 you learned that the liquids /l/ and /ɹ/ are both produced with a voiced airstream. This is true, in the "pure" sense of their identities. However, if /ɹ/ or /l/ is part of a prevocalic consonant sequence with a voiceless consonant, for example *pray* or *clay,* it becomes **devoiced.** The essential identity of the palatal liquid or alveolar liquid is maintained despite the voicing alteration. The devoicing is a form of assimilation that occurs because of the overlapping articulatory movements involved when /ɹ/ and /l/ are combined with voiceless consonants like /p/, /k/, /f/, /θ/, /s/, or /ʃ/. (You can try this by putting your hand across your larynx so that you can feel vocal fold vibration. Say *lay* and then *play,* and note the difference in the timing of vibration for the /l/.) In these examples, assimilation is considered **progressive** because the earlier occurring phoneme (/p/, in this case) causes a change in the phoneme that follows it. It is also considered **contiguous** because the /p/ and liquid /l/ are directly adjacent to each other.

An example of **regressive assimilation** can be found in the relationship between the alveolar nasal /n/ when it immediately precedes /k/ or /g/, as in words like *handkerchief*. Coarticulation results in the simplification of the [n d k] consonant sequence to [ŋ k]. (Note that the stop, /d/, is lost, another example of coarticulation.) Then, the expected alveolar placement for /n/ becomes velar, producing an /ŋ/ due to the influence of the velar /k/ that follows it. The velar placement of the later sound (/k/) "backs up" onto the place of an earlier sound (/n/).

We can also find examples of noncontiguous assimilation in the speech of children. Indeed, such effects are especially noticeable in the earliest stages of language development. As a toddler, the author's child sometimes produced the word *penny* as [pɛmi]. In this case, alveolar [n] shifted to a bilabial nasal [m] because of progressive, noncontiguous assimilation (the effect of the bilabial [p]). It could also be referred to as **bilabial assimilation** because the change was caused by the first bilabial phoneme in the word. Such assimilatory alterations often occur in the speech of very young children.

PLACE OF ARTICULATION

There are a number of alterations in place of articulation that may occur as a result of assimilation. Some result in a complete change of place of articulation; others, in a slight shift of place. Typical examples follow.

One common example is that of **dentalization**. You have learned that there are two interdental phonemes: /θ/ and /ð/. If /θ/ or /ð/ is adjacent to an alveolar phoneme (/t/, /d/, /s/, /z/, /n/, /l/) the alveolar phoneme may shift to a *dental* place of articulation. Try this for yourself by saying these two phrases and noting your tongue placement for /s/: *less time, less thought*. Notice that your tongue tip remains on your alveolar ridge for the first phrase because the alveolar /s/ is followed by another alveolar consonant, /t/. When /s/ is followed by /θ/, however, the position for /s/ shifts so that the tongue is more against the teeth. The diacritic marking for dentalization is [̪], and *less thought* would be narrowly transcribed as [l ɛ s̪ θ ɔ t]. You can find additional examples of narrow transcription of assimilation effects in **Table 5.2**.

TABLE 5.2 EXAMPLES OF ASSIMILATION: PLACE OF ARTICULATION

Example	Transcription	Progressive/ Regressive	Contiguous/ Noncontiguous	Place Term
*bath **s**oap*	[b æ θ s̪o p]	Progressive	Contiguous	Dentalization
*both **s**tars*	[b o θ s̪t ɑɪ z]	Progressive	Contiguous	Dentalization
*hor**s**eshoe*	[h ɔ ɪ ʃː u]	Regressive	Contiguous	Palatal assimilation
*pla**c**e change*	[p l eɪ ʃ ʧ e n ʤ]	Regressive	Contiguous	Palatal assimilation
*co**n**quest*	[k ɑ ŋ k w ɛ s t]	Regressive	Contiguous	Velar assimilation
*ba**n**quet*	[b æ ŋ k w ə t]	Regressive	Contiguous	Velar assimilation

Note: the phoneme that changes is underlined and in bold type in the orthographic representation of each example.

You have already read about another example of place change: the shift of /n/ to velar /ŋ/ when it directly precedes a velar /k/ or /g/, (as in *handkerchief* [h æ ŋ k ɚ ʧ ɪ f]). Additional examples are found in words that are spelled with *n* but in which assimilation from the velar /k/ causes a shift to /ŋ/. In narrow transcription, *bank*, *ink*, and *sank* would be transcribed as [b æ ŋ k], [ɪ ŋ k], and [s æ ŋ k], respectively.

There are many other examples of assimilation in English involving other places of articulation as well. One everyday example can be found in the pronunciation of *Grandma* and *Grandpa* as [g ɹ æ m ə] and [g ɹ æ m p ə]. Notice that it's much easier to say the transcribed words than to try to pronounce every phoneme in *Grandma* and *Grandpa*. The demands of rapid speech require economy of movement. In this case, the /d/ is omitted (see Omissions/Elision/Haplology, below), and the alveolar /n/ becomes a bilabial /m/, just like the place of the phonemes that follow it (/m/ and /p/). This regressive assimilation effect could also be referred to as **labial assimilation**.

Another change in place of articulation can affect alveolar phonemes /s/ and /z/ when they are adjacent to a palatal phoneme in phrases such as *Bridge Street* or *flash stick*. If only a slight change in place occurs, the narrow transcription symbol [ʲ] may be used, for example [b ɹ ɪ ʤ sʲ t ɹ i t] and [f l æ ʃ sʲ t ɪ k]. With a more complete assimilatory shift, the phrases would be transcribed as [b ɹ ɪ ʤ ʃ t ɹ i t] and [f l æ ʃ t ɪ k], respectively. (Again, see **Table 5.2** for additional examples of assimilation involving place of articulation.)

PRACTICE: EXERCISES 5.1A AND B: PLACE CHANGES

For practice in recognizing and transcribing the occurrence of dentalization, go to Exercise 5.1A in Appendix A. When you're finished, check your answers against the answer key in Appendix C. Exercise 5.1B in Appendix A has additional examples of phrases in which an alveolar /s/ or /z/ may shift to a palatal place of articulation. Listen to your instructor's presentation of these words or produce them yourself. Complete the answers using narrow transcription. When you are finished, refer to the answer key in Appendix C.

VOICING EFFECTS

We noted earlier that voicing can also be affected by assimilation. Not only can a voiced phoneme become partially voiceless, but a voiceless phoneme can become partially voiced, depending on phonetic context. We begin with the first type, devoicing of a voiced consonant.

You learned in Chapter 4 that /ɹ/, /l/, /w/, and /j/ are voiced consonants. As noted in the beginning of this section, however, assimilation can cause a change in voicing. When a liquid or glide is blended with a preceding voiceless consonant (forming a consonant sequence), these consonants are produced almost without voicing. You might try saying the following word pairs and noticing that /ɹ/ and /l/ are definitely voiced in the first word of each pair and have almost no voicing in the second word. Again, to do this, place your hand on your neck at the level of the larynx. You should feel vibration immediately for the words that begin with the singleton sound; you should feel a slight delay in voicing for those words with the consonant sequence.

ray [ɹ eɪ] – *pray* [p ɹ̥ eɪ]   *row* [ɹ oʊ] – *crow* [k ɹ̥ o ʊ]
lay [l eɪ] – *play* [p l̥ eɪ̥]   *coot* [k u t] – *cute* [k j̊ u t]
lie [l aɪ] – *ply* [p l̥ aɪ]   *rye* [ɹ aɪ] – *fry* [f ɹ̥ aɪ]
rue [ɹ u] – *true* [t ɹ̥ u]   *Lee* [l i] – *flee* [f l̥ i]
foo [f u] – *few* [f j̊ u]   *low* [l oʊ] – *slow* [s l̥ oʊ]

Because none of these phonemes has a voiceless cognate, a diacritic marking must be used to indicate the partial loss of voicing. The symbol used to account for this assimilatory effect is [̥] for phonetic symbols that extend above the line (/ɹ/ /l/ /w/) and [̊] for symbols that extend below the line /j/. (Also see **Table 5.1**, the IPA diacritics chart.) The marking looks like a very small, open circle, placed directly under or over the phoneme affected. Thus, appropriate narrow transcription of *tree* and *sleet* would be [t ɹ̥ i] and [s l̥ i t], respectively. Narrow transcription of *cube* and *few*, however, would look like this: [k j̊ u b] and [f j̊ u].

Another voicing effect appears as **intervocalic voicing**. In this case, a voiceless singleton phoneme in the intervocalic position is surrounded by voiced phonemes, for example the /t/ in *butter*. As a result, the allophone of /t/ in this word may be heard with a range of voicing. It could be produced as an audibly aspirated stop [tʰ], as in [b ʌ tʰ ɚ]. Or, the /t/ might become totally voiced, sounding like [b ʌ d ɚ]. It is quite likely, however, that a partially voiced [t] will result because of the voiced sounds around it [b ʌ t̬ ɚ]. The diacritic marking to indicate partial voicing looks like a lower case orthographic *v* [̬], and it is placed under the affected phoneme. Another alternative symbol to use in these cases is an alveolar allophone of /t/ and /d/ known as the **alveolar tap**. The tongue makes a very quick movement against the alveolar ridge, resulting in a very brief stop, shorter than a /t/ or /d/. The symbol is /ɾ/. Examples using both symbols follow.

heater   [h i t̬ ɚ]   [h i ɾ ɚ]
water   [w ɑ t̬ ɚ]   [w ɑ ɾ ɚ]
matter   [m æ t̬ ɚ]   [m æ ɾ ɚ]
liter   [l i t̬ ɚ]   [l i ɾ ɚ]
utter   [ʌ t̬ ɚ]   [ʌ ɾ ɚ]

Check with your instructor to see which symbol you should use in your class. Some instructors prefer the use of the voicing symbol; others prefer the use of /ɾ/.

One more consonant frequently affected by intervocalic voicing is /h/ in words like *birdhouse* and *behind* (transcribed as [b ɝ d ḥ aʊ s] and [b i ḥ aɪ n d], respectively). Because /h/ has no voiced cognate, use the [̬] symbol to indicate the partial voicing that occurs as a consequence of assimilation.

PRACTICE: EXERCISE 5.2

Exercise 5.2 has practice items for narrow transcription of devoicing and voicing of phonemes. You can listen to your instructor produce the words or say them yourself.

Remember to use the [॒], [°], and [॒] symbols (or [ɾ]) to note devoicing and voicing, respectively. When you have finished your transcription, check your answers against the answer key in Appendix C.

RESONANCE / NASALITY

There is also an assimilatory effect that can affect vowels in conversational speech. This effect involves the nasal consonants /m n ŋ/. Often in connected speech, a vowel sound adjacent to a nasal consonant also takes on nasal resonance. Try saying these two words and listening for a difference in vowel resonance: *boot* ([b u t]), *moon* [m ũ n]. Even though the vowel is the same (/u/) in each word, it is more "nasal-sounding" in *moon*. The diacritic marking used to indicate this **nasal assimilation** is [˜]. The symbol is placed over the vowel affected. Thus, *moon* would be transcribed as [m ũ n].

Several rules tend to govern this assimilatory effect. In these cases nasalization of a vowel will occur if:

1. The vowel is preceded *and* followed by a nasal consonant.
   Examples: *man* [m æ̃ n], *mink* [m ĩ ŋ k], *Nan* [n æ̃ n], *none* [n ʌ̃ n]

2. The vowel immediately follows the nasal consonant and forms an open syllable ending the word.
   Examples: *honey* [h ʌ n ĩ], *hammer* [h æ m ɚ̃], *bandana* [b æ n d æ̃ n ə̃].

See **Table 5.3** for additional examples of assimilation nasality.

PRACTICE: EXERCISES 5.3 AND 5.4

The first of these exercises in Appendix A gives you practice in recognizing and transcribing vowels affected by nasality. When you have finished, check your transcriptions with the answer key in Appendix C. Then go to Exercise 5.4. This exercise requires you to use almost all the narrow transcription symbols that you have learned in this section, including dentalization, palatal assimilation, and assimilation nasality.

TABLE 5.3 CONTEXTS FOR ASSIMILATION NASALITY

Example	Transcription	Example	Transcription
bean	[b i n]	buddy	[b ʌ d i]
mean	[m ĩ n]	bunny	[b ʌ n ĩ]
dune	[d u n]	hang	[h æ ŋ]
moon	[m ũ n]	hanging	[h æ ŋ ĩ ŋ]
sign	[s aɪ n]	muddy	[m ʌ d i]
mine	[m ãɪ n]	money	[m ʌ̃ n ĩ]
merry	[m ɛ ɹ i]	Mickey	[m ɪ k i]
many	[m ɛ̃ n ĩ]	Minnie	[m ĩ n ĩ]

When you have finished the exercises, compare your transcriptions to those in the answer key.

ASPIRATION OF STOPS

You learned in Chapter 4 that the audible release (aspiration) phase of stops is optional. In mainstream American English, *prevocalic* and *intervocalic voiceless* stops are audibly released. Voiceless singleton postvocalic stops and voiceless singleton stops, which occur at the ends of utterances, however, are not always audibly released. Or, they may be released so gently that audible aspiration is unnoticeable. The voiced stops are unreleased.

Audible stop aspiration is transcribed using the diacritic marking [ʰ] following the consonant. The symbol [̚] following a stop indicates that it was not released. A third symbol, [̄], is used to indicate the difference in aspiration found in stops contained in /s/ sequences. Notice the appropriate narrow transcription for the following words:

pie	[pʰ aɪ]	*pipe*	[pʰ aɪ p ̚]	or	[pʰ aɪ pʰ]
toe	[tʰ oʊ]	*tote*	[tʰ oʊt ̚]	or	[tʰ oʊ tʰ]
Kay	[kʰ eɪ]	*Kate*	[kʰ eɪ t ̚]	or	[kʰ eɪ tʰ]
pie	[pʰ aɪ]	*spy*	[s p ̄aɪ]		
tow	[tʰ oʊ]	*stow*	[s t ̄oʊ]		
key	[kʰ i]	*ski*	[s k ̄i]		

The presence of audible aspiration varies for consonant sequences containing stops. In general, these rules can be followed in transcription:

1. /s/ + stop prevocalic blends: stop will not be audibly released: [̄].
   Examples: *spin* [sp ̄ɪ n], *steam* [st ̄i m], *skim* [sk ̄ɪ m]

2. Nasal + stop postvocalic blends: stop will be audibly released: [ʰ]
   Examples: *lamp* [l æ m pʰ], *sent* [s ɛ n tʰ], *sink* [s ɪ ŋ kʰ]

3. Fricative + stop postvocalic blends: stop will be audibly released: [ʰ].
   Examples: *lisp* [l ɪ s pʰ], *least* [l i s tʰ], *mosque* [m ɑ s kʰ]

4. Postvocalic sequences composed of two stops: first stop will not be audibly released but the second one will: [̚ʰ]
   Examples: *kept* [kʰ ɛ p ̚tʰ], *slacked* [s ḷ æ k ̚tʰ], *soaked* [soʊk ̚tʰ]

5. Intervocalic sequences composed of stops:
   a. If the stops differ in place of articulation, the first stop will not be audibly released, but the second one will: [̚ʰ]
      Example: *potpie* [pʰ ɑ t ̚pʰ a ɪ]
   b. If the stops share place of articulation, the first stop will not be released and will be held longer than usual before the second stop is audibly released: [̚: ʰ].
      Example: *black cat* [blæk ̚:ʰaetʰ]

Further examples of narrow transcription of voiceless stops can be found in **Table 5.4**.

TABLE 5.4 ASPIRATION OF STOPS

when	[w ɛ n]	went	[w ɛ n tʰ]	slip	[s ḷ ɪ p˺]	slipped	[s ḷ ɪ p˺tʰ]
pane	[p ʰeɪ n]	paint	[p ʰeɪ n tʰ]	cook	[kʰ ʊ kʰ]	cooked	[kʰ ʊ k˺tʰ]
ping	[pʰɪ ŋ]	pink	[pʰɪ ŋ kʰ]	rock	[ɹ ɑ kʰ]	rocked	[ɹ ɑ k˺tʰ]
hem	[h ɛ m]	hemp	[h ɛ m pʰ]	peek	[pʰ i k ʰ]	peeked	[pʰ i k˺t ʰ]
wren	[ɹ ɛ n]	rent	[ɹ ɛ n tʰ]	look	[l ʊ kʰ]	looked	[l ʊ k˺tʰ]

To be completely accurate, narrow transcription of voiceless stops should always indicate whether or not a stop is aspirated. In clinical application, however, these symbols are most often used when aspiration is used inappropriately. This most often happens in transcription of disordered speech and of speakers of English as a second language (refer to Chapters 6 and 7 for further details.) Ask your instructor about the amount of detail required for narrow transcription in your class. (The author has always required students to learn to apply all relevant narrow transcription symbols, just as her instructor required when she was a beginning phonetics student. In everyday practice, however, she uses the symbols to indicate changes in sound production that are not necessarily the result of coarticulation.)

OTHER PHONOLOGICAL PROCESSES

The remaining topics in this section of the chapter are concerned with coarticulatory effects associated with duration. These topics also are tied to the next section on suprasegmentals and prosody. The first subsection discusses changes in phoneme duration; the second, sound omissions or additions that can occur in connected speech.

CHANGES IN DURATION

You have probably already noticed that phonemes naturally vary in duration; for example, vowels are longer in duration than stops. In connected speech, the length of vowel sounds is also influenced by the manner of articulation of the consonant that follows them. Vowels are typically shorter before a stop consonant or affricate than before a fricative or resonant consonant. Try saying these word pairs and note the difference in vowel duration for each pair member:

loot [l u t] – loose [l u s]   Ted [t ɛ d] – tell [t ɛ l]
let [l ɛ t] – less [l ɛ s]   beg [b ɛ g] – bell [b ɛ l]
up [ʌ p] – us [ʌ s]   match [m æ ʧ] – mash [m æ ʃ]
it [ɪ t] – if [ɪ f]   latch [l æ ʧ] – lash [l æ ʃ]

Vowel duration may also be affected by the voicing of the consonant that follows it in connected speech. A vowel has a *shorter* duration before a *voiceless* stop or affricate than before its voiced counterpart, made in the same position. Compare the difference in vowel duration in the following pairs of words:

etch [ɛʧ] – edge [ɛʤ]   sup [s ʌ p] – sub [s ʌ b]
at [æt] – ad [æd]   back [b æ k] – bag [b æ g]

lap [l æ p] – *lab* [l æ b]   *niece* [n i s] – *knees* [n i z]
neat [n i t] – *need* [n i d]   *ice* [aɪs] – [aɪz] – ice

In the following examples, notice how vowel duration differs in each set of words as a result of manner and voicing of the following consonant (note that the place of articulation is the same for each word set):

at [æt]   *ad* [æd]   *an* [æn]
cup [kʌp]   *cub* [kʌb]   *come* [kʌm]
luck [lʌk]   *lug* [lʌg]   *lung* [lʌŋ]
seat [s i t]   *seed* [s i d]   *seen* [s i n]

Effects on Consonants

In the previous examples, it was not necessary to use any narrow transcription symbol to indicate the difference in vowel duration that resulted from coarticulation. However, there are several symbols that are used to indicate durational changes, particularly those affecting consonants. They may be used with vowels as well if vowel duration extends beyond the normal variation found in connected speech.

The first example requiring a narrow transcription symbol occurs when the same consonant is produced at the end of one word and the start of another. Contrast the duration of /m/ in these expressions: *summon* (/m/ articulated as one nasal consonant) and *some more* (/m/ prolonged). In expressions of the second type (same consonant ending a word and beginning the following word), the two consonants will be produced as one sound, but the duration is usually extended. This difference is indicated in narrow transcription with the symbol [:] (which looks like a colon and follows the phoneme with increased length). Try saying the following phrases. Notice how the sound that ends the first word lasts longer in the second set of phrases than in the first set.

summon [s ʌ m ə n]   *some men* [s ʌ m: ɛ n]
calling [k ɑ l ɪ ŋ]   *call light* [k ɑ l:aɪ t]
topping [t ɑ p ɪ ŋ]   *top pair* [t ɑ p: ɛ r]
lighting [l aɪ t ɪ ŋ] *light tap* [l aɪ t: æ p]
liking [l aɪ k ɪ ŋ]   *like cats* [l aɪ k: æ t s]

Another characteristic of connected speech affects resonant consonants (specifically /m/, /n/, /l/). They may be increased in duration to take the role of a syllable nucleus (vowel) under certain conditions. These **syllabic consonants** are marked by the diacritic [ˌ] placed under the affected consonant. These effects most often occur in two particular coarticulatory contexts. In one, the resonant consonant and the consonant preceding it share the same place of articulation, for example words like *mitten* and *candle* (alveolar place of articulation). In these cases, an intervening vowel is unnecessary because the tongue tip can maintain its alveolar position for both the phonemes. Thus, lengthening the /n/ or /l/ forms a syllable nucleus. (See the next paragraph for examples.) The other context occurs when the articulators are free to move to the syllabic consonant while the preceding consonant is being made. Examples include *apple* [æ p l̩] and *driven* [d ɹ ɪ v n̩]. In these words, the alveolar position for [l] or [n] can be taken during production of the labial [p] or labiodental [v].

Try saying the following words, first with /ə/ and then with a syllabic consonant for the syllable nucleus. Notice the difference in transcription.

ridden	[r ɪ d ə n]	[r ɪ d n̩]
huddle	[h ʌ d ʊ l]	[h ʌ d l̩]
blossom	[b l ɑ s ə m]	[b l ɑ s m̩]
mitten	[m ɪ t ə n]	[m ɪ t n̩]
happen	[h æ p ə n]	[h æ p n̩]

Did you notice how much more "natural" the words with syllabic consonants sounded? That is typical of coarticulatory effects; they make connected speech more efficient and easier to produce.

A number of syllabic consonants also occur in rapid connected speech as a result of sound omissions and lengthening of [n] or [l]. Some examples are given below:

stop them	[s t ɑ p ð ɛ m]	[s t ɑ p m̩]
you and me	[j u æ n d m i]	[j u n̩ m i]
it will do	[ɪ t w ɪ l d u]	[ɪ d l̩ d u]
burger and fries	[b ɝ g ɚ æ n d f ɹ a ɪz]	[b ɝ g ɚ n̩ f ɹ a ɪ z]

Look for further information and more examples in the section Omissions/Elision/Haplology, below. These concepts will also be applied in the second half of the chapter on speech rhythm and suprasegmentals.

PRACTICE: EXERCISE 5.6A,B

Now turn to Exercise 5.6A,B in Appendix A. Exercise A consists of phrases in which the same sound ends one word and begins another, requiring prolongation of the last sound in the first word, for example [s ʌ m: ɪ l k] for *some milk*. You may listen to your instructor produce these phrases or produce them yourself to transcribe them. Exercise B focuses on syllabic consonants. You need to listen to your instructor's presentation of these words. After you have finished each section, check your answers with those in the answer key in Appendix C.

OMISSIONS/ELISION/HAPLOLOGY

A number of speech sounds and even syllables may be omitted in connected speech as a result of coarticulation. The /h/ and /ð/ are two consonants especially prone to this effect. They are frequently dropped in rapid connected speech, as in *Where is he?* ([w ɛ ɹ ɪ z i]) and *Stop them!* ([s t ɑ p m]). Final consonants of words may occasionally be omitted during rapid speech, such as *Let me go!* ([l ɛ m i g oʊ]). When just one consonant or a few consecutive consonants are omitted in this way, the term applied is **elision**. Sometimes elision may also lead to assimilation as in our previous examples of *handkerchief* [h æ ŋ k ɚ ʧ ɪ f] (/d/ elided, velar assimilation of /n/, and *grandpa* [g ɹ æ m p ə] (/d/ again elided but labial assimilation of /n/.

Words such as *sixths* and *guests* also provide us with examples of elision occurring in response to the demands of rapid connected speech. With consonant sequences such as -*sts* (*nests, wasps*), two sounds that are essentially the same (/s/) are separated by an intervening sound. The demands of rapid speech often result in the loss of the intervening consonants along with elongation of the first sound. For example, *sixths* ([s ɪ k s θ s]) may be produced as [s ɪ k s:] (remember that the symbol [:] indicates increased duration). Similarly, *desks* ([d ɛ s k s]) is more easily produced as [d ɛ s:]. Production of *asks* ([æ s k s]) as [æ s:] is another example of this type of omission, as is the production of *mirror* [m ɪ ɹ ɚ] as [m ɪ ɹ:].

Sometimes in connected speech, whole syllables may be omitted. **Haplology** is the term used to describe what can happen when two very similar syllables occur in close succession. *Mississippi* (four syllables) is often pronounced as [m ɪ s ɪ p i] (three syllables) by natives of the state. Similarly, *CocaCola* (four syllables) may become [k o k oʊ l ə]. In Cuyahoga County in northeast Ohio, speakers often reduce the four syllables of Cuyahoga to three [k aɪ j ɔ g ə]. Generally, listeners will understand these changes without difficulty. See **Table 5.5** for additional examples of elision and haplology.

TABLE 5.5 EXAMPLES OF ELISION AND HAPLOLOGY

Word/Phrase	Transcription	Elision/Haplology
masks	[m æ s:]	Elision: /ks/
sifts	[s ɪ f s:]	Elision: /t/
nests	[n ɛ s:]	Elision: /ts/
That's her.	[æ t s ɚ]	Elision: /ð/ /h/
Is he here?	[ɪ z i i ɹ]	Elision: /h/ (twice)
vegetable	[v ɛ dʒ tə b l]	Haplology: 2nd syllable
mineral water	[m ɪ n ɹ ə l w ɑ ɾ ɚ]	Haplology: 2nd syllable

ADDITION/EPENTHESIS

At the beginning of this chapter, you were shown examples of a consonant addition (intrusive /w/) in the expressions *so easy* ([s o w i z i]) and *to each* ([t u w i ʧ]). In connected speech, the /w/ and /j/ are sometimes intruded in order to separate vowels that end one word and begin another. The type of intruded consonant depends on the height and position of the first vowel. In the examples below, notice that /w/ follows high back vowels like /u/ and /j/ follows high front vowels like /i/:

New England	[n u w ɪ ŋ g l ə n d]	*see Ann*	[s i j æ n]
so old	[s o w oʊ l d]	*my apple*	[m aɪ j æ p l̩]
bow out	[b aʊ w aʊ t]	*stay in*	[s t e j ɪ n]
go in	[g oʊ w ɪ n]	*be anybody*	[b i j ɛ n i b ə d i]

A **glottal stop** may intrude instead of a /w/ or a /j/ in these same types of coarticulatory environment. The glottal stop is produced at the glottis by rapidly closing the vocal folds tightly and then releasing them to continue voicing. It is especially needed to separate *the* from a following vowel-initiated word. For example, the phrase *the apple* needs an intrusive /ʔ/ or /j/ to be most easily understood: [ð i ʔ æ p l] or [ð i j æ p l]. In phrases such as *hi eats* ([h i ʔ i t s] or [h i j i t s]), an intrusive [ʔ] or [j] is important to distinguish the phrase from the word *heats* [h i: t s] produced with an elongated vowel. Notice how a glottal stop or a glide may intrude in the following phrases:

we even	[w i ʔ i v n̩]	[w i j i v n̩]
the only	[ð i ʔ oʊ n l i]	[ð i j oʊ n l i]
two apples	[t u ʔ æ p l̩ z]	[t u w æ p l̩ z]
buy all	[b aɪ ʔ ɔ l]	[b aɪ j ɔ l]
we are	[w i ʔ ɑ ɹ]	[w i j ɑ ɹ]

The glottal stop /ʔ/ or /j/ can also occur in /ɪ ŋ/ combinations in words like *seeing*: [s i ʔ ɪ ŋ] or [s i j ɪ ŋ].

Another manner of articulation, an intrusive stop, may intrude if a nasal resonant consonant immediately precedes a voiceless fricative such as /s/ or /θ/. The stop will be voiceless, with closure in the same place of articulation as the nasal consonant. Thus, in the word *warmth*, a /p/ may intrude: [w ɔ ɹ m p θ] In the word *chance*, an alveolar /t/ may intrude: [ʧ æ n t s]. Finally, the word *strength* gives us an example of possible /k/ intrusion due to coarticulation: [s t ɹ ɛ ŋ k θ]. Not all phoneticians agree on the regularity of occurrence of these intrusive stops in these contexts (Small, 2012). Check with your instructor for transcription preferences with regard to this type of coarticulation.

PRACTICE: EXERCISE 5.7A AND B

You can now turn to these exercises in Appendix A. They are designed to help you recognize and transcribe occurrences of elision, haplology, and intrusive glides and /ʔ/. You can listen to your instructor's presentation or say them aloud yourself. For each transcription, be sure to indicate sound loss or addition as you've learned in the previous section. When you have finished these exercises, check your answers against the answer key in Appendix C.

EXERCISE 5.8: USE OF ALL NARROW TRANSCRIPTION SYMBOLS

This exercise is designed to help you to integrate all the information that you have learned about diacritics and narrow transcription. As you say the words in the exercise, be sure to include all appropriate narrow transcription symbols: place, voicing and resonance changes, duration changes, and aspiration of stops. When you have completed the exercise, compare your answers to the answer key in Appendix C.

SUMMARY: INFLUENCE OF CONTEXT

By now you are very aware of how phonemes can vary in production in connected speech. Phonemes may be omitted, added, or completely/partially change their identity depending on the demands of connected speech. Stops may or may not be audibly released depending on phonetic context. We noted earlier that these adjustments make speech production more efficient. They also have another effect: they make a speaker sound more "natural" or "native." Some speakers of English as a second language tend to produce speech as if they were reading words, slowly and deliberately, giving full pronunciation to each vowel. This decreases coarticulatory effects and makes the speaker sound less fluent. In the next section of the chapter, we discuss another important part of the "naturalness" of speaking a language: supra-segmentals.

SPEECH RHYTHM AND SUPRASEGMENTAL FEATURES

If you listen to speakers of languages other than English, for example French, Hindi, or Swedish, you will undoubtedly first note that you can't understand the words! But if you keep listening to these speakers, you may notice that some of their phonemes (also known as **segments** of speech) don't sound like anything you've ever heard in English. You'll also notice that, regardless of the phonemes and words, the language doesn't necessarily sound like English. French has more of a "flow" or a different "melody" than English. For that matter, British English doesn't sound exactly like mainstream American English. An important part of the way that different languages sound is the result of the **suprasegmental aspects** of speech. Other terms that have been applied to this phenomenon include speech **melody** or **prosody**. Supra-segmental aspects of speech are most simply defined as features of speech over and above phoneme segments, especially aspects of speech rhythm. They include accent, emphasis, phrasing, and tempo.

THE SYLLABLE AS A UNIT IN SPEECH RHYTHM

The basic unit of speech rhythm is the **syllable**. Although this sounds simple, the concept of what constitutes a syllable has been a source of intense study and scientific argument over the years. Most recently, Shriberg and Kent (2013) have described sonority as "the *sine qua non* of syllabicity" (p. 100). **Sonority** refers to the relative loudness of speech sounds. Some phonemes, especially vowels, have greater sonority than other phonemes because they are produced with more energy. A phoneme's sonority is determined in relation to the relative loudness of other phonemes that share similar length, pitch, and stress. For each spoken syllable, Shriberg and Kent note that there is a speech segment of maximum energy or greater sonority, most often a vowel. Consonants (which may or may not surround a vowel) form a **trough**, with less energy.

A syllable may consist of only a vowel or it may consist of a vowel and adjacent consonant(s). Consonants can begin and end a syllable, but they do not function as the essential part, or sonorant crest (except for syllabic consonants, mentioned earlier in this chapter). Syllables that end in a vowel are termed **open** (e.g., *tea*, *my*), whereas those that end in a consonant are **closed** (e.g., *mat*, *sit*). The most common syllable shape in English is the CV (consonant + vowel). Examples would be the *re-* in *refill* and the *pa-* in *paper*. Another commonly occurring syllable shape is the CVC (consonant + vowel + consonant), such as the *-ton* in *Washington*, and the *-sic* in *music*. The VC (vowel + consonant) syllable shape (e.g., *on-* in the word *onset*) occurs less often. The most complex syllable shape found in English is CCCVCCCC. An example of this syllable shape is found in the word *strengths* ([s t ɹ ɛ ŋ k θ s]. However, a syllable cannot contain more than one vowel or sonorant peak. If it does, it will be perceived as more than one syllable. For example, the word *seeing* contains a CV ([s i]) and a VC ([ɪ ŋ]). *Seeing* would sound very similar to *sing* if it weren't for the unisyllable-bisyllable dis-tinction. For additional examples of monosyllable shapes, see **Table 5.6**.

TABLE 5.6 EXAMPLES OF AMERICAN ENGLISH SYLLABLE SHAPES AND ONSET AND RHYME

Word	Transcription	Shape	Onset	Rhyme	Nucleus	Coda
eye	/aɪ/	V		/aɪ/	/aɪ/	
pie	/paɪ/	CV	/p/	/aɪ/	/aɪ/	
pies	/paɪz/	CVC	/p/	/aɪz/	/aɪ/	/z/
spies	/spaɪz/	CCVC	/sp/	/aɪz/	/aɪ/	/z/
spry	/spɹaɪ/	CCCV	/spɹ/	/aɪ/	/aɪ/	
sprite	/spɹaɪt/	CCCVC	/spɹ/	/aɪt/	/aɪ/	/t/
sprites	/spɹaɪts/	CCCVCC	/spɹ/	/aɪts/	/aɪ/	/ts/
sprints	/spɹɪnts/	CCCVCCC	/spɹ/	/ɪnts/	/ɪ/	/nts/
strengths	/stɹɛŋkθs/	CCCVCCCC	/stɹ/	/ɛŋkθs/	/ɛ/	/ŋkθs/

Another way of looking at the concept of a syllable is in terms of internal structure. In this context, a syllable is viewed as having an underlying structure, composed of **onset** and **rhyme**. An onset consists of all the phonemes that precede the vowel or **nucleus** in a syllable. The onset is an *optional* element. Thus, it could be nonexistent (vowel-initiated syllables such as *eat* or *ale*), a singleton consonant (*seat* or *tale*), or a consonant sequence (*sleet* or *stale*). The **rhyme** in a syllable has two parts: the nucleus or vowel (required) and the **coda**. The coda is also optional so that a word may have no coda or a coda consisting of a singleton consonant or consonant sequence. Examples would include *see* /s i/, *seat* /s i t/, and *seats* /s i t s/, or *beau* /b oʊ/, *boat* /b oʊ t/, and *boast* /b oʊ s t/. Shriberg and Kent (2013) combine these two concepts of sonority and internal structure to define a syllable as "a sonorant crest in the auditory pattern of speech" (p. 100). Again, refer to **Table 5.6** for additional examples of onset and rhyme in monosyllabic words.

PRACTICE: EXERCISE 5.9 CV STRUCTURE, ONSET, AND RHYME

After looking at the examples in **Table 5.6**, complete Exercise 5.9 in Appendix A. In it you should classify each word according to CV structure, onset and rhyme, and shape (open/closed). When you have finished, check your answers against the answer key in Appendix C. The first example is completed for you.

Syllable composition or shape influences coarticulation and relates to the timing of speech. Average American-English syllable duration is two-tenths of a second (Calvert, 1986; Calvert, Garn-Nunn, & Lynn, 2004; Small, 2005). Of course, this is just an average; there are some variations of syllable duration because of individual speaker differences and stress patterns. If you pronounce two similar syllables with equal stress, they will have roughly the same duration. For example, try saying the words *catch* and *scratch* with the same amount of stress. With equal stress, they will be almost the same duration. Here's another example: The words *buy* and *bite*, when spoken with equal stress, will be very similar in duration. The /aɪ/, which has longer duration in *buy*, is shortened by the intrinsic coarticulation required in a syllable in the CVC word *bite*. Consequently, the duration of each of the two-syllable shapes is similar. Rather than hearing phonemes presented individually and irregularly, you hear them coarticulated in syllable units. These units help you recognize each phoneme because of the transitional characteristics of consonant–vowel and vowel–consonant **junctures**. These junctures supply you with important auditory perceptual information.

The remainder of this chapter focuses on American-English **accent/word stress**, **emphasis/sentence stress**, **phrasing**, **intonation**, and **rate/tempo**. These **nonlinguistic** aspects of speech result from the interaction of variations in loudness, pitch, and duration of syllables as they occur in connected phrases and pauses. The result is a speech signal with additional information that influences meaning, assists in listening and understanding, and makes speech more interesting.

ACCENT/WORD STRESS

Accent is one form of speech stress. **Stress** points out, sets apart, focuses on, or otherwise gives *vocal prominence* to a unit of speech. Accent, in particular refers to the stress given a syllable within a word when compared with other syllables. (Stress can also vary across words in a phrase or sentence, as you'll discover later in this chapter.) Some authors use the term **word stress** rather than accent (Bauman-Waengler, 2009; Small, 2012).

In a stress-timed language, one syllable is stressed above the others in words of two or more syllables. Stressed syllables are perceived as audibly different from those with less stress. English is primarily a stressed-timed language as opposed to a language like Spanish, which is more syllable-timed (Shriberg & Kent, 2013). Syllable-timed languages have a more regular beat and do not observe variable stressing. Even within English dialects, the difference between heavily stressed and unstressed syllables can vary. American English uses less difference between heavily stressed and unstressed syllables than British English. As a result, syllables that are pronounced in American English may be omitted in British English. For example, the word *secretary* is produced with four syllables [s ɛ k ɹ ə t ɛ ɹ i] in American English. British English speakers may use only three syllables [s ɛ k ɹ ə t r i].

You will learn to identify three basic levels of accent or word stress in American English: primary, secondary, and unaccented syllables. The sonorant peak, or vowel, is the syllable element that changes with accent, not the consonants. An accented syllable is made with greater physiological force, which produces a syllable perceived as having (1) greater loudness (intensity), (2) greater duration, and (3) a rise in pitch (higher frequency). Research, however, has not been able to determine a direct correspondence between level of loudness and stress (Black, 1949; Fairbanks, House, & Stevens, 1950; Lehiste and Peterson, 1959; Liberman, Cooper, Harris, & MacNeilage, 1963). Unaccented syllables have reduced force in production, resulting in the perception of production with reduced loudness and shorter duration as well as a lowered pitch. Many speakers use a combination of both stressing and de-stressing syllables to produce accenting in their connected speech. Thus, the contrast or ratio between accented and unaccented syllables can be made by expanding (accenting) a stressed syllable or reducing force of production (deaccented syllable) or a combination of both. Different speakers can vary in their use of accent levels, depending on the utterance. Also, accenting can sometimes vary according to dialectic variation (see Chapter 6). Despite these individual variations, you can still learn some general rules for assigning accent levels and practice with the exercises in this chapter to help you develop this skill. Understanding of accent is crucial to effective communication. It also is important in programming for individuals with speech disorders, particularly children with intelligibility problems (see Chapter 7).

PRACTICE: EXERCISE 5.10

Before you begin determining accented and unaccented syllables, it may help to complete Exercise 5.10 in Appendix A. It is designed to help you recognize the number of syllables in a word, an important step in determining the level of accent. It may help to say each syllable separately rather than saying the word quickly. For each set of words, underline the words that contain the number of syllables indicated at the top of the column. The first example is completed for you. When you have finished, compare your answers with those in the answer key in Appendix C.

Given our emphasis on the IPA in this book, we will use IPA diacritical marking symbols to mark accent differences (**Table 5.7**). You mark a syllable with primary accent by placing a vertical mark ['] above and to the left of it; for example, *hanger* is transcribed as ['h æ ŋ ɚ]. For secondary accent, you place a vertical mark [ˌ] below and to the left of the affected syllable. Unaccented syllables are unmarked. Thus, narrow transcription of the word *peppercorn* would be ['pʰ ɛ p ɚ ˌkʰ ɔ ɹ n]. The counterparts of these marks in a dictionary would be a heavy accent mark over the vowel with the primary accent and a lighter accent mark over the syllable with secondary accent. Depending on your reasons for taking a phonetics course, you or your instructor may find one set of markings preferable or more useful than the other. This book uses the standard IPA symbols.

Rules for assigning stress in English can seem erratic because deciding which syllable to accent is largely a matter of following conventional usage. There are some general rules that can be observed in assigning syllable stress. First, in bisyllabic (two-syllable) words, there is a strong tendency for the first syllable to receive the primary accent (e.g., *making* ['m eɪ k ɪ ŋ], *mainly* ['m ẽɪ n l i]). This rule holds especially true when the accented syllable precedes suffixes such as *-ing*, *-er*, *-est*, *-cious*, and *-tion*. In contrast, the accented syllable usually follows unaccented prefixes such as *a-*, *be-*, *re-*, *de-*, *ad-*, *ex-*. **Table 5.8** lists examples of stress assignment for different bisyllabic words.

TABLE 5.7 IPA SYMBOLS FOR SUPRASEGMENTALS

ˈ Primary stress
ˌ Secondary stress
ˌfoʊnəˈtɪʃən
ː Long eː
ˑ Half-long eˑ
˘ Extra-short ĕ
| Minor (foot) group
‖ Major (intonation) group
. Syllable break ɹi.ækt
‿ Linking (absence of a break)

TABLE 5.8 EXAMPLES OF STRESS ASSIGNMENT FOR DIFFERENT BISYLLABIC WORDS

cupcake	[ˈk ʌ pˌkek]	happy	[ˈh æ p i]	above	[əˈb ʌ v]
under	[ˈʌ n d ɚ]	debate	[d iˈb eɪ t]	reply	[ɹ iˈp l aɪ]
apart	[əˈp ɑ ɹ t]	market	[ˈm ɑ ɹ k ə t]	sunny	[ˈs ʌ n i]
taco	[ˈt a k oʊ]	detain	[ˌd iˈt eɪ n]	admit	[ˌæ dˈm ɪ t]
faded	[ˈf eɪ d ə d]	station	[ˈs t e ɪʃ ə n]	extent	[ˌɛ kˈs t ɛ n t]

PRACTICE: EXERCISE 5.11

Exercise 5.11 is designed to help you determine primary accent in the least complicated context: two–syllable/bisyllabic words. If you have difficulty determining the syllable with primary accent, try saying the word with stress on a different syllable each time. For example, try saying the word *many* with varying syllable accents: [ˈm ɛ n i], [m ɛˈn i]. Which one "sounds" correct? The first pronunciation, with primary stress on the first syllable: [ˈm ɛ n i]. (Feeling discouraged? Remember, you've come a long way in learning the IPA since you started with the vowels; marking for accent/word stress is just another step along the way!) When you finish this exercise, check your answers against the answer key in Appendix C.

Words of more than two syllables may have several accent levels distributed among the syllables. In general, the vowels in syllables with primary and secondary accent are likely to follow their usual vowel spelling pronunciation. Unstressed syllables tend to have /ə/ for their nucleus; the full vowel identity is "neutralized" by lack of stress. Not all multisyllabic words have all levels of stress, however. Primary accent should always be marked; a word may not have a syllable with secondary accent. And the vowel in a syllable can change depending on whether or not it receives secondary accent. For example, consider the word *sandwich*. If you pronounce it as [ˈs æ n dˌw ɪ ʧ], both vowels maintain their identity, with primary accent on the first syllable and secondary accent on the second syllable. However, if you pronounce the word as [ˈs æ n d w ə ʧ], with /ə/ as the vowel in the second syllable, you have only a primary accented syllable and an unaccented syllable.

In addition, the vowels in unaccented syllables can change. The diphthongs /eɪ/ and /oʊ/ become pure vowels /e/ and /o/ when unstressed, except when they occur in final, open syllables. Thus, transcription of -o- in *location* would be [ˌl oˈk eɪ ʃ ə n], but *window* would be transcribed as [ˈw ɪ nˌd oʊ]. For the vowels /i/, /æ/, /u/, and /ɑ/, loss of primary stress leads to their pronunciation as /ɪ/, /ɛ/, /ʊ/, and /ʌ/, respectively. Further de-accenting reduces these vowels to /ə/. Thus, you might hear *relief* as [ˌɹ iˈl i f], [ˌɹ ɪˈl i f], or [ɹ əˈl i f], depending on the degree of de-accenting of the first syllable. Notice that for every variation, the primary accent remains on the second syllable. Another example would be found in these three words: *photo, photograph, photography*. In them, the primary and secondary accents can shift, depending on the number of syllables and your individual pronunciation: [ˈf oʊˌt oʊ], [ˈf oʊ t əˌg ɹ æ f], [f əˈt a g ɹ ə ˌf i]. In *photograph*, the primary accent remains on the first syllable with a secondary accent on the third syllable. But in *photography*, primary accent shifts to the second syllable and the first vowel becomes /ə/.

TABLE 5.9 EXAMPLES OF WORD STRESS ASSIGNMENT FOR MULTISYLLABIC WORDS

friction	[ˈf ɹ ɪ k ʃ ə n]	mosquito	[m ə ˈs k i ˌt oʊ]	marigold	[ˈm ɛ ɹ ə ˌɡ o l d]
appeared	[ə ˈpi ɹ d]	ornament	[ˈɔ ɹ n ə ˌm ɛ n t]	beginner	[ˌb i ˈɡ ɪ n ɚ]
fellow	[ˈf ɛ ˌl oʊ]	telephone	[ˈt ɛ l ə ˌf o n]	nasality	[ˌn e ˈz æ l ə t i]
standard	[ˈs t æ n d ɚd]	gigantic	[ˌdʒ aɪ ˈɡ æ n t ɪ k]	overboard	[ˈoʊ v ɚˌb ɔ ɹ d]
matchbook	[ˈm æ tʃˌb ʊ k]	computer	[k ə m ˈp j u t ɚ]	antithesis	[ˌæ n ˈt ɪ θ ə s ə s]

Special note should be made of compound words formed from two other words. In these words, a secondary accent is also present in compound words. The second syllable is almost never reduced to /ə/. Examples include *airplane* [ˈɛ ɹ ˌp l e n], *hotdog* [ˈh ɑ t ˌd ɑ ɡ], *cowboy* [ˈk aʊ ˌb ɔɪ], and *baseball* [ˈb eɪ s ˌb ɑ l]. **Table 5.9** lists additional examples of multisyllabic words to help you hear the differences in word stress.

PRACTICE: EXERCISES 5.12

Exercise 5.12 in Appendix A includes two- and three-syllable words. Some have primary accent only; others have both primary and secondary accents. After you complete the exercise, check your answers against the answer key in Appendix C.

Accent can also be **phonemic**; that is, a change in syllable accent, which changes syllable pronunciation, can change the meaning of the word. Examples of phonemic accent occur in the following words when primary accent shifts from the first to the last syllable: *survey, suspect, torment, transport, subject, reject, produce, digest, escort, insult, exile, content,* and *recess.* For example, *survey* may be a noun ([ˈs ɝ v e ɪ] (a thing surveyed/looked over) or a verb ([s ɚ ˈv e ɪ] (to complete a survey). Someone might be a *suspect* ([ˈs ʌ s p ɛ k ̚tʰ], a noun) in a crime or you could *suspect* ([s ə ˈs p ɛ k ̚tʰ], a verb) that something is wrong. **Table 5.10** gives additional examples of phonemic stress.

Word meaning can also change depending on the presence or absence of secondary shift in pronunciation. This is especially noticeable in words that take the suffix *-ate.* **Table 5.11** shows the vowel change (/ə/ to /e/) that occurs when the addition of *-ate* adds a syllable with secondary accent.

Of course, syllable accent can also change *and not* alter meaning. Such pronunciation differences often reflect dialect variations. In American English, for example, you may say *adult* as [ə ˈd ʌ l t] or [ˈæ d ə l t] without altering meaning. The word *theater* may be said as [θ i j ə ɾ ɚ] (mainstream English) or [ˌθ i ˈj eɪ ɾ ɚ] (Southern English), but the meaning does not change. Compare your pronunciation of these words with those of a friend or acquaintance: *automobile, cigarette, concrete, contrary,*

TABLE 5.10 WORD PAIRS FOR PHONEMIC STRESS

perfect	Adjective: [ˈp ɝ ˌf ɪ k t]	→	perfect	Verb: [p ɚ ˈf ɛ k t]
progress	Noun: [ˈp ɹ ɑ ˌɡ ɹ ɛ s]	→	progress	Verb: [ˌp r o ˈɡ ɹ ɛ s]
conflict	Noun: [ˈk ɑ n ˌf l ɪ k t]	→	conflict	Verb: [k ə n ˈf l ɪ k t]
abstract	Adjective: [ˈæ b ˌs t ɹ æ k t]	→	abstract	Verb: [ˌæ b ˈs t ɹ æ k t]
complex	Noun: [ˈk ɑ m ˌp l ɛ k s]	→	complex	Adjective: [k ə m ˈp l ɛ k s]

TABLE 5.11 PRONUNCIATION CHANGES WITH SHIFT OF SECONDARY ACCENT

No Secondary Accent		Secondary Accent Present	
deliberate	Adjective: [d ə'l ɪ b ɚ ə t]	deliberate	Verb: [d ə'l ɪ b ɚ ˌe t]
affiliate	Noun: [ə'f ɪˌl i j ə t]	affiliate	Verb: [ə'f ɪ l i ˌj e t]
delegate	Noun: ['d ɛ l ə g ə t]	delegate	Verb: ['d ɛ l ə ˌg e t]
graduate	Noun: ['g ɹ æˌdʒ u ə t]	graduate	Verb: ['g ɹ æ dʒ u ˌe t]

defense, dictator, gasoline, illustrate, and *locate.* For these words, the accent may be different, but it is not a **phonemic** change.

For unaccented syllables, de-stressing may even lead to the loss of /ə/ as you learned in the earlier section of this chapter on syllabic consonants. This is most likely to occur when the following resonant consonant is **homorganic** (made in the same position with the same articulator) with the previous consonant. For example, because /d/ and /l/ are both lingua-alveolars in the word *middle,* pronunciation may be either ['m ɪ d ə l] or ['m ɪ d l]. In this case (and others like it), the stress is so reduced that the syllabic [l] can take on the function of a syllable nucleus. Other familiar examples of this phenomenon are found in *kitten* ['k'ɪ ɾ n] and *button* ['b ʌ ɾ n]. (See Changes in Duration, earlier in chapter.)

In the most extreme form of stress reduction, an unstressed syllable is completely omitted. This occurs quite often in British English, as noted earlier in this chapter. There are a number of words that may lose syllables in mainstream American English. Look at the examples that follow.

Word	**Formal Speech**	**Conversational Speech**
annual	['æ n j u ə l]	['æ n ə j ʊ l]
evening	['i v ə n ɪ ŋ]	['i v n ɪ ŋ]
family	['f æ m ə l i]	['f æ m l i]
miniature	['m ɪ n i j ə ʧ ɚ]	['m ɪ n j ə ɪʧ ɚ]

(See the related sections Omissions/Elision/Haplology and Addition/Epenthesis earlier in this chapter.)

PHRASAL AND SENTENCE STRESS

This type of stress affects units larger than the syllable. In particular, it refers to the stressing of a word or words within a phrase or sentence. As with accent, sentence stress is produced primarily by greater physiologic force in production. This results in increased loudness and duration of syllables within the stressed word(s), along with an accompanying pitch change. Conversely, some other words may be de-emphasized because of reduced force. You may also achieve emphasis by using pauses surrounding words or by elongating the duration of a particular syllable. As with levels of word stress, levels of phrasal stress are variable. Sentence or phrasal stress may be marked in different ways, most often by the use of <u>underlining</u> and <u>double underlining</u>. Use of **bold type** may also mark stressed elements.

Unlike accent/word stress, application of sentence/phrasal stress does not follow either consistently recurring patterns or conventional usage. How you apply stress in your speech is personal and relates to your communicative intent. If your communicative intent changes, you will change your stress as a result. Sentence stress thus adds information to an utterance over and above the phoneme segments, their grouping into syllables, and their syllable accent pattern. If you want to draw attention to a particular word label, then you emphasize the label accordingly. Consider the sentence: "That's a big dog." With stress on *dog* ("that's a big <u>dog</u>.") you are signaling the type of animal (a dog, not a cat). Or, you could say it this way: "That's a <u>big</u> dog." Now the emphasis is on size (it's big, not little). If you are trying to reiterate or stress a point, you might use emphasis this way: "I <u>said</u>, I <u>don't</u> want to go." (Interpretation: "Maybe you didn't hear me the first time; I'm not interested in going!") Perhaps you are contrasting parallel thoughts: "I can be here at <u>six</u>, but she can't come until <u>seven</u>." Notice how the meaning of the following sentence can change, depending on phrasal stress:

"<u>I</u> need some sleep!" (Emphasis: <u>who</u> needs sleep; you may not, but I do.)

"I <u>need</u> some sleep!" (I'm exhausted; I need rest.)

"I need <u>some</u> sleep!" (Emphasis on minimum amount needed; without rest, I can't function.)

"I need some <u>sleep</u>!" (I've had enough to eat/drink; now I need to rest.)

PRACTICE: EXERCISE 5.13A–C

These exercises will help you learn to interpret sentence stress in transcription as well as adding stress to transcribed word sets. You should use single underlining or accent marks to indicate stressed words. Check with your instructor to see if one or the other type of marking is preferred. When you finish the exercise, check your answers against the answer key in Appendix C.

Sometimes this type of stress is used to distinguish a compound word from an adjective + noun combination. For example, a baby may sit in a <u>high</u>*chair* [ˈh aɪ ˌʧɛ ɹ], but you may choose to sit in a *high chair* [ˌh aɪ ˈʧ ɛ ɹ] at the breakfast counter in a restaurant. You might specifically see a red-winged <u>black</u>*bird* (compound word) [ˈb l æ k b ɚ d] in springtime or you might see just some unidentifiable *black bird* (adjective + noun) [ˌb l æ k ˈb ɚ d] (as opposed to some other type of animal, e.g., a dog or cat). Word pairs such as <u>green</u>*house* [ˈg ɹ i n ˌh aʊ s] (where plants are grown) and *green house* [ˌg ɹ i n ˈh aʊ s] (the house painted green) also follow this pattern. *Hotdog* [ˈh ɑ t ˌd ɑ g] (something to eat) and *hot dog* [ˌh ɑ t ˈd ɑ g] (a panting poodle) are another example.

De-emphasis of a word is also possible. When it occurs, it is similar to reduction of unaccented syllables. Frequently used, short, connective words such as *was, of, the,* and *a* are almost never emphasized. Instead, they are usually produced as /ə/ in connected speech. Thus, "Do you have to go?" would most likely be transcribed as [d u j ə h æ f t ə g oʊ]. This de-emphasis explains why expressions such as *want to, have to,* and *got to* are most often pronounced as *wanna, hafta,* and *gotta* in the connected speech of both adults and children.

A **speech phrase** consists of a continuous utterance, bounded by silent intervals. Intervals between phrases are called **pauses**. Your speech phrasing is related to your breathing but does not necessarily reflect your breathing pattern. When you inhale for speech in conversation, you do it in a pause between phrases. You don't have to inhale for each phrase, however. More than one phrase can be said on a single breath; for example, "She saw the guests arrive and then she went downstairs." In this example, you may pause between *arrive* and *and*, but you should be able to complete the sentence (and more!) on a single breath.

In writing, phrases can be marked be punctuation marks such as commas, periods, semicolons, colons, question marks, and exclamation marks. These written punctuation conventions do not necessarily correspond to your speech phrasing, though. For example, the written expression "red, white, and blue" has commas to separate elements. More than likely, however, you would say a continuous phrase in speech [r ɛ d w a ɪ t n̩ b l u] rather than pausing between each color name (also notice the realization of *and* as a syllabic [n̩]). On the other hand, you might insert pauses when punctuation would not signal their presence; for example, "Today (pause) is the last day (pause) of class!"

Several methods have been suggested for marking phrases. You can use either method with orthographic symbols or with IPA symbols. Pauses can be signaled by inserting one or two lines between words, depending on length of pause. Again, with the previous sentence, we could mark phrasing this way:

"Today (pause) is the last day (pause) of class!"

[t u d eɪ] ‖ [ɪ z ð ə'l æ s t d eɪ] | [ə v k l æ s]

Notice that the phonetic symbols within a phrase are transcribed consecutively, without interruption for word boundaries. This indicates junctures that are coarticulated. There is more than one way to indicate phrasing in connected speech. Your choice of system will probably depend on your purpose(s) for transcribing as well as your instructor's preference. Marking for phrasing is much more frequently used by radio broadcasters for speaking scripts than for error transcription by speech-language pathologists, for instance. Also, phrasing will be linked to intonation (see next section).

You or any other speaker will determine which and how many words to link together in a phrase, as well as the duration of pauses. These decisions affect the listener's ability to understand the message. Reasons for using phrasing patterns include the following:

1. To group the words of a thought into a unit
2. To create emphasis
3. For parenthetical comments
4. To accommodate to difficult listening situations

The use of phrasing to present units of meaning is particularly important for listener understanding. "We went to the store/because we were hungry" makes sense. But, "We went to the/store because we/were hungry" interferes with, rather than facilitates, understanding. Similarly, pauses can be used for emphasis: "I want to go now ‖ not later." (Translation: Let's get moving!) In addition, the word *now* will probably be uttered with longer duration and a higher pitch. Parenthetical remarks (conversational "asides") will also be marked by pauses. For example: "The weather

‖ I hope ‖ is going to get better." In this case, "I hope" will also probably have reduced loudness and pitch compared to the rest of the utterance.

A sensitive speaker also takes listeners and listening conditions into account. If you were speaking in a noisy room to people with a hearing loss, you would probably use shorter phrases and more pauses to aid their understanding. In class, your instructor (ideally) uses shorter phrases and longer pauses when presenting new, unfamiliar, or especially difficult material. Listener age, ability to listen, and speaking environment can all influence the use of phrasing.

You also use pauses to formulate your next phrase or phrases when you are speaking extemporaneously. If you are speaking rapidly in conversation, you may need to pause to gather your thoughts. Sometimes such pauses are marked with fillers such as "um," "uh," "well," "I guess. . ." These pauses give you time to think and formulate exactly what you wish to say as well as add emphasis and meaning.

Overall, sentence stress and phrasing are another aspect of speech that you must control as a speaker. Your message is not just composed of words made up of phonemes. Effective communication also requires use of accent, emphasis, phrasing patterns, and intonation (covered in the next section).

PRACTICE: EXERCISE 5.14

This exercise will help you to recognize pauses to logically separate speech phrases. Each example consists of a pair of utterances, one with appropriate pauses and one without. Determine which of the utterances shows the appropriate phrasing that makes it easier to understand.

By now it should be obvious to you that transcription of connected speech requires much more detail than transcription of single words. If you read a transcribed utterance you have to use what you know about coarticulation and stress. The next exercise is designed to give you practice in **transliteration**, putting transcribed speech into orthographic symbols.

PRACTICE: EXERCISE 5.15

In this exercise you will find transcriptions of continuous utterances. Remember that sounds and words can get altered or even omitted in connected speech. Read each utterance aloud to yourself; then write the sentence orthographically. When you have finished, check your answers against the answer key in Appendix C.

INTONATION

You have previously learned that accent or word stress reflects changes in syllables within a word, whereas sentence stress or emphasis reflects changes in the words in a phrase. Intonation, however, involves changes over an entire phrase. What changes in intonation is the rising and falling of pitch, determined by the frequency of the vocal fold vibration. In English, these pitch inflections result in audible **intonation contours,** which can add meaning over and above the phonemes, accent pattern, and emphasis pattern used (**Table 5.12**). Thus, the contours typically enhance, but do not change, meaning in English. However, in tonal languages, such as Chinese or

TABLE 5.12 TYPICAL INTONATION CONTOURS IN ENGLISH

Contour	Applicable Phrases/Sentences	Examples
Rising	Questions:	
	Yes/no	Are you coming?
		Did you see him
	Wh-	Where is he?
		Who's coming?
	Tag	It's his, isn't it?
		You like Oreos, don't you?
	Item lists	I like chocolate, vanilla, and orange.*
		I had a burger, fries, and a shake.
Falling	Statements	It's time to leave.
		He's inside.
	Exclamations	I'm not coming.
		Put it down!

*Although intonation rises through the utterance, it falls for the last syllable of the last word.

Japanese, syllable pitch changes can indicate differences in meaning. That is, the same CVC syllable [gaɪ] can have different meanings, depending on the pitch level at which it is said or if there is a pitch change as it is said. We will focus here on the intonation characteristics typical of English, however.

An utterance can be composed of one or more **intonational phrases** (Small, 2012). An intonational phrase can be as small as word or as long as a sentence. An utterance can contain one or more intonational phrases. Within that framework, the main levels of intonation in English are rising and falling. However, there can be more than one of these levels within an utterance. Because your fundamental voice pitch varies as you speak (centering on an average), intonation is marked by pitch changes that are relatively different from each other, not from an absolute, unchanging pitch. Direction and rate of pitch change can be depicted by using straight and slanting lines to mark the levels. The examples below illustrate use of this marking system:

"Hurry up! He's coming! My goodness!"

Remember that these markings, while sufficient for indicating intonation, correlate only roughly with measured variations in fundamental voice frequency. Nevertheless, they can be particularly useful when such a system is needed.

Many intonation patterns result, in part, from pitch changes caused by application of accent and emphasis. The following sentence illustrates this: "I lost my cellphone." The word *cellphone* is a key word to be emphasized above the rest of the sentence by greater intensity and duration, and by a rise in fundamental voice frequency. These parts of the intonation contour are dictated by accent and emphasis. A drop in pitch on the final syllable, *phone*, however, is the result of intonation that tells the listener something new. Here, it says, the utterance is now completed. Compare the intonation contours in these sentences:

I lost my/cellphone.
I lost my/cellphone, my/keys,\and my/backpack.

In the second sentence, the rising intonation on *cellphone*, with the help of appropriate phrasing, tells the listener to keep listening, as there's more to come. Consider the sentence "We bought knives, forks, dishes, and spoons." Use of rising pitch on *knives*, *forks*, and *dishes* signals your listener that there is more to come in the series. Conversely, the lowering pitch for *spoons* indicates the completion of the series and the utterance. In this example, the end of the series is also marked by the word *and*, occurring just before the last word. Consequently, both the word *and* as well as the intonation contour provide complementary and redundant information to aid the listener. Try to say this sentence again, without *and* but still using appropriate intonation. Now, try it again, including *and* but using unvaried intonation on *knives*, *forks*, *dishes*, and *spoons*. Last, use both *and* as well as varied intonation to say this sentence. Which version of the sentence is easiest to understand: (1) the one without *and*, (2) the one containing *and* but accompanied by consistent intonation across all items, or (3) the one with both *and* as well as the varied intonation contour? Notice how the sentence is most easily understood when it includes *and* with the varied intonation contour.

You have now learned two uses of intonation: to indicate a series and to indicate termination of an utterance. Another important use of intonation is in signaling a question. Consider the statement, "They will." If it is said with a slight drop in intonation, you hear it as a statement. But if it is said with rising intonation, it becomes a question: "They will?" Because we don't have question marks in speaking, as we do in writing, we mark the difference by intonation contour.

In "They will?" the intonation contour influences the meaning very strongly. Another example of the intonation contour altering meaning can be found in the expression "oh" [oʊ]. The syllable does not have a meaning of its own but can convey meaning through intonation. The following common intonation messages demonstrate this point:

Carrier	Message
oh	"I'm still listening to you."
oh\	"I understand."
o͡h\	"Now I finally understand it."
oh⌡	"Really, are you sure?"
u͡h-oh	"Now you're in trouble."

You may use intonation carriers in conversation, especially to signal your conversational partner that you are listening but that you don't want to interrupt them. Carriers such as *uh-huh* [ə h ʌ], *mmm* [m:], and *yeah* [j æ] are commonly used. Use of *mmm-hmm* [m: hm:] even allows you to keep your mouth closed while still indicating that you're paying attention! Notice how intonation contours carry meaning in the following:

Carrier	Information
uh-huh	"I'm still listening."
uh-huh	"I understand."
uh-huh	"I didn't know that" or "That's really interesting."
mmmmmm	"I'm still listening."
mmmmmm	"Is that so?"
mmmmmm	"I didn't know that" or "That's really interesting."

Intonation is another suprasegmental that adds to meaning over and above the speech segments making up words. The combination of word stress, phrasal stress, and intonation all combine to differentiate meaning and aid the listener. Speakers of English as a second language (ESL) often find it difficult to master these suprasegmental characteristics, which makes it harder for native English speakers to understand them. This difficulty can especially interfere with understanding if the ESL speaker also speaks at a very fast rate or tempo.

RATE/TEMPO

Tempo or rate refers to speaking speed. We usually measure the **rate** at which speech is produced in the number of words or syllables per unit of time. The average duration of a syllable is 0.18 seconds. This corresponds to a rate of 5 to 5.5 syllables/second. In oral reading, most adults produce 150 to 180 words/minute. In conversational speech, you may produce 200 or more words/minute. Individuals vary, of course, in their speaking rate. The maximum rate of speech production appears to be influenced by articulatory control. We can improve our articulatory control (as evidenced by skillful speakers and debaters), but there is a limit to how much. Even though the duration of different phonemes varies, you average a rate of 10 sounds/second in conversation (Calvert, 1986). At 15 words/second, however, errors are frequent, and speech is distorted. On the other hand, speech understanding occurs at a much faster rate. So do silent reading and thinking. In fact, we can understand up to 30 sounds/second when paying careful attention. As with word stress and intonation, a careful speaker will adjust tempo according to the listener's understanding of a topic and apparent ability to understand. Individuals with hearing loss or cognitive impairment may benefit from a slower rate, careful pauses, and repetition of important information. Shouting, however, only distorts the speech signal. Even if listeners cannot understand all the words, suprasegmentals and redundancy can make it easier for them to understand.

SUMMARY: SPEECH RHYTHM AND SUPRASEGMENTAL FEATURES

Have you ever tried to communicate with someone via email and discovered that he or she totally misunderstood your message? Then you have some idea of the role that suprasegmental aspects of speech play in conjunction with actual speech segments. Email does not allow you to hear the speaker's rate, stress, or intonation, nor does it allow you to observe facial expression. All these cues are crucial in making your listener understand your communicative intent and message. Coarticulation and assimilatory effects make speech more fluent and "native English" sounding. They allow you to speak more easily and with less effort. Over time we have all adjusted to the effects of coarticulation in connected speech. In addition, we constantly use suprasegmental cues to help us interpret speakers. As noted before, one of the reasons that ESL speakers may not sound like native English speakers is their misunderstanding of American-English coarticulation and prosody. They may pronounce all vowels as full vowels rather than as /ə/, as native English speakers usually do. The prosody of their native language may affect the sound of their English as well. Individuals with hearing loss may also have altered prosody. Patients with neurological damage may have problems not just with speech sounds but also with prosody. You will learn more about coarticulation and phonological processes in the next chapter.

CONCEPT QUESTIONS

PART I

Are the following statements true or false?

_____ 1. Intervocalic voicing is an example of assimilation.

_____ 2. Velar assimilation is a change in manner of articulation when /n/ is adjacent to /k/.

_____ 3. Connected speech is a series of coarticulated movements, not a phoneme-by-phoneme process.

_____ 4. Transcription of *plane* as [p ḻ e n] is an example of progressive contiguous assimilation.

_____ 5. Stops are always produced with audible aspiration or release of air.

_____ 6. *Eight owls* would be transcribed as [e t: aʊ l z].

_____ 7. The word *record* provides an example of phonemic accent, e.g., ['ɹ ɛ k ɚ d] vs. [ɹ i ˈk ɔ ɹ d].

_____ 8. Rising intonation is characteristic of statements and commands.

_____ 9. Two-syllable words always have both primary and secondary accent.

_____ 10. Speaking rate can be measured in words per minute.

PART II: DIACRITICS

1. *Voicing:* for the following transcriptions, mark those items for which transcription is correct.

a.	three→[θ ɹ̥ i]	_____		e.	little→[l ɪ ɾ ə l]	_____
b.	crew→[k ɹ̥ u]	_____		f.	slim→[s l̥ ɪ m]	_____
c.	play→[p l̥ eɪ]	_____		g.	rehire→[ɹ i ḥ aɪ ɹ̥]	_____
d.	sitting→[s ɪ d ɪ ŋ]	_____		h.	Lehigh→[l i ḥ aɪ]	_____

2. *Lengthening:* mark those examples that are transcribed correctly.

a.	soon now→[s u n: aʊ]	_____		d.	big glass→[b ɪ g l: æ s]	_____
b.	about time→[ə b aʊ: t aɪ m]	_____		e.	ripe pears→[ɹ aɪ p:ɛ ɹ z]	_____
c.	bad days→[b æ d: eɪ z]	_____		f.	black cab→[b l æ k: æ b]	_____

3. *Syllabic consonants:* the following examples should all be transcribed using syllabic consonants. Mark those that are transcribed correctly. The first one is marked for you.

   a.   Eden-→[i d n̩]   X

   b.   bread 'n' butter→[bɹ ɛ d n̩ b ʌ ɾ ɚ] _____

   c.   driven→[d ɹ ɪ v ɛ n̩] _____

   d.   modem→[m oʊ d m̩] _____

   e.   bundle→[b ʌ n d ʊ l] _____

4. In the following sets of transcription words, only one of the three has correct narrow transcription. Choose the correct one and explain why it is correct.

Word	Transcriptions			
a. *plank*	[p ˡ æ n kʰ]	[p ˳ æ ŋ kʰ]	[b l æ ŋ k˺]	_____
b. *slipped*	[s ˡ ɪ p d]	[s ˡ ɪ pʰ tʰ]	[s ˡ ɪ p˺tʰ]	_____
c. *banana*	[b ə n æ n ɔ̃]	[b ɔ̃ n æ n ɔ̃]	[b ə n æ n ə]	_____
d. *spinning*	[s pʰ ɪ n ɪ̃ ŋ]	[s p‾ ɪ n ɪ̃ ŋ]	[s p˺ ɪ n ɪ̃ ŋ]	_____
e. *miss things*	[m ɪ s θ ɪ ŋ z]	[m ɪ ş θ ɪ ŋ s]	[m ɪ ş θ ɪ ŋ z]	_____

PART III: SPEECH RHYTHM AND SUPRASEGMENTAL FEATURES

1. Transcribe the following words in IPA symbols as you would say them, and mark the primary accent in each word.

  suspect (verb) _____   *suspect* (noun) _____

  insult (verb) _____   *insult* (noun) _____

  combine (noun) _____   *combine* (verb) _____

  reward _____   *cobra* _____

2. Match the stressed word in the following repeated sentences with the question/intent it signals to the listener.

	Statement		Question/Intent
_____	1. <u>I'm</u> too busy to handle that now.	a.	I'm even busier than usual.
_____	2. I'm <u>too</u> busy to handle that now.	b.	I might have time later.
_____	3. I'm too busy to handle that <u>now</u>.	c.	All I could do is look at it, not deal with it.
_____	4. I'm too <u>busy</u> to handle that now.	d.	I could handle a smaller, different task.
_____	5. I'm too busy to handle <u>that</u> now.	e.	Someone else might be able to do it.

3. Transcribe the following speech units in connected IPA symbols as you (or another speaker) would say them, observing coarticulation effects, and marking phrasing and pause duration, using [|] and [‖] symbols.

   a.   I don't believe it. I got an A.

   b.   Oh, my. It's time to go.

   c.   Did you hear about that? I didn't.

   d.   They came in first and second, respectively.

   e.   Please bring me a pen, some paper, and a dictionary.

4. Indicate whether the following sentences would be characterized by rising, falling, or level intonation.

    a.   Are you coming?

    b.   I'm sorry.

    c.   I'm in here.

    d.   Who wants to know?

    e.   What's the difference?

MULTICULTURAL VARIATIONS: DIALECTS

INTRODUCTION TO DIALECTS

DEFINITIONS

VIEWS OF DIALECTS

EVOLUTION OF AMERICAN-ENGLISH DIALECTS

REGIONAL DIALECTS

CULTURAL AND ETHNIC DIALECTS

CONCLUSION

CONCEPT QUESTIONS

Do you remember the roommates example from Chapter 1? If not, you might want to go back and briefly read it again to prepare yourself for the information in this chapter. That example illustrated some of the differences in regional dialects, specifically Southern American, Midland American, and Eastern New England dialects. Most of the pronunciation differences in that example affected vowels, but there was also a difference in pronunciation of postvocalic /ɹ/ across the two dialects. Despite these differences, it's quite likely that you and your roommate would quickly adjust to these differences in pronunciation and have no difficulty understanding each other. Or, you might (unconsciously) start to change your pronunciation to become more like that of your roommate from Eastern New England. Quite often, when people move to a new dialect area, they find that adopting some of the dialectic characteristics makes them fit in better and be more easily understood. Another example may help reinforce this point.

I lived and taught college-level phonetics and phonology courses in southwestern Virginia for 18 years. The dialect most characteristic of this area was Appalachian English, now considered a variant of Southern English (Labov et al, 2006; Wolfram, 1991). It made for some interesting discussions in my phonetics classes, especially as we covered American-English vowels. In particular, many of my students used the same vowel, /ɪ/, in words like *pin* and *pen* in their speech. They often pronounced *hi* as [h ɑ:]. Many also had difficulty hearing a contrast between /ɑ/ and /ɔ/. (This confusion is not unique to speakers of Southern English.) Many dialects do not make a distinction between these two vowels. I vividly remember undergraduate classmates from central and southern Ohio who struggled to hear the difference in our introductory phonetics course. So when we covered these phonemes, they had to work harder at hearing the contrasts between them. Although they learned to distinguish the vowels and produce them according to the textbook in class, they did not necessarily change the way they talked outside of class. Even so, many of my students did change their pronunciation depending on whether they were on campus or in their home community. As noted previously, speakers may change their pronunciation to better fit in and be understood within a speech community. My students were a prime example.

INTRODUCTION TO DIALECTS

Throughout this book the pronunciation characteristic of what has often been referred to as **Standard American English** or **General American English** have been used. Another term sometimes used is **mainstream English (ME)**, particularly by professionals who study and work with a variety of regional or cultural dialect speakers. In general, Standard America English or mainstream is supposed to be relatively free of any regional characteristics (Wolfram, 1991). However, the authors of *The Atlas of North American English* (Labov et al, 2006) suggest that "the Atlas data do not justify the labeling of any one dialect as 'General American.'" (p. 263). The findings of their extensive research project are discussed later in this chapter.

How do we decide what is standard or mainstream? Typically, the American-English pronunciation and grammar used in textbooks and school instruction has been the source. This academic English has been labeled as **formal standard English** by Wolfram and Schilling-Estes (2006). National television broadcasters also usually provide an example of what would be called mainstream American English. These pronunciations and grammar usage are understood by the widest possible number of Americans. In most instances, we speak using what Wolfram and Schilling-Estes refer to as **informal standard English**. This variation can also exist on a continuum, depending on communicative situation, familiarity and background of the listeners, and other factors. Most often, this means that the English spoken in the Midwest and central regions of the United States tends to be the model for ME. If you are from the South (Southern English) or eastern New England (Eastern New England English), you know that your pronunciation varies in some ways from ME. For example, in both Southern English and Eastern New England English, speakers may omit or neutralize postvocalic /ɹ/. Thus, *park the car* [p ɑ ɹ k ð ə k ɑ ɹ] could become or [p ɑ: ð ə k ɑ:]. Although loss of postvocalic /ɹ/ may characterize workers in the rural South, newer research has shown that speakers in urban areas of the south do use postvocalic /ɹ/ (Labov et al, 2006). Many speakers in Eastern New England continue to vowelize this phoneme.

This chapter introduces you to dialects and their transcription. In some cases, you will learn new phoneme symbols; in others, you will learn to use diacritic markings to indicate dialectic variations from ME.

DEFINITIONS

Let's begin by discussing key terms for this chapter. The terms **dialect** and **accent** are often used in describing speech variations. Although the definitions can vary, this book will follow those of several professional associations (Montgomery, 1999). **Dialect** refers to a set of differences that make the speech of one American English speaker differ from another (Montgomery, 1999; Wolfram & Fasold, 1974). These differences can include *phonological*, *morphological*, and *grammatical* differences. Even though American-English dialects do differ, the vast majority of their characteristics are the same. (That's why you can usually understand someone who speaks a different dialect, although you may have to adjust to their speaking pattern.) **Accent** most often refers to the *phonetic* and *suprasegmental* traits that characterize a person's speech. Thus, accent is concerned with fewer features of speech than dialect. Typically, what the mainstream American speaker notices in eastern New England English is related to accent or pronunciation changes. As we noted earlier, ME uses full pronunciation of /ɹ/ in all word positions; eastern New England English does not. In addition, speakers from this region may use what is referred to as a broad a (sounds in words like *half* and *calf*). In mainstream American English, speakers would use /æ/ for these words and others like them. An example of a dialectic difference affecting syntax occurs in the Hispanic English or Spanish-influenced phrase, *the coat of my father* (rather than *my father's coat* in ME). In this chapter you will find examples and information on both accent and dialect. Because this is a phonetics textbook, the emphasis is on pronunciation effects rather than on morphology and syntax.

Several types of dialects have been studied extensively: **regional** and **cultural** or **ethnic** dialects. So far this chapter has discussed regional dialects—those speech patterns that are characteristic of a particular geographic region. These developed for a variety of reasons, including patterns of immigration and settlement, the English dialect spoken by original settlers, and geographic isolation. Cultural or ethnic dialects are speech patterns characteristic of a particular cultural or ethnic group. In this chapter, you will learn about African-American English vernacular, Spanish-influenced English (SIE), and several varieties of Asian English. These are the most prevalent cultural dialects used in the United States. Each is associated with a cultural group with a common background and a sense of community. More detail will be found in the section on cultural dialects. Similarities in pronunciation, rather than syntax, will be emphasized, however.

VIEWS OF DIALECTS

With regard to attitudes about dialect, two opposing views are commonly found: **sociolinguistic** and **deficit**. The sociolinguistic view, advocated by linguists and other professionals who study languages, characterizes dialect as a difference in the way a person speaks, not a disorder. Professional organizations that advocate the sociolinguistic view of dialect include the American Dialect Society (2001), the Linguistic Society of America (1996), and the National Council of Teachers of English (2001) (Farr, 1991). All these organizations stress the legitimacy of mainstream American English-alternative dialects and the importance of allowing their use. In addition, the American Speech-Language-Hearing Association (1983, 2003) has stated that no dialectal variety of English is a disorder or a pathological form of speech or language. Thus, if a person's language usage is communicatively appropriate to other speakers in the community, but different from another's (non–community member) language usage, it is considered a language *difference* not a language deficit or disorder.

Unfortunately, for many non-ME speakers, the general public may view alternative dialects from a deficit viewpoint. From this perspective, dialect is viewed as a deviation from ME that needs to be changed or even eliminated so that the non-ME speaker "talks like everyone else." Some dialects enjoy higher regard by much of the American public. Similarly, some accents may be viewed as more acceptable than others. There are documented cases of social bias and negative reactions based solely on a person's use of non-ME dialect or accent (Buck, Maynard, Garn-Nunn, & Seyfried, 1996; Massey & Lundy, 2001; Purnell, Idsardi, & Baugh, 1999; Rosenthal, 1974; Terrell & Terrell, 1983). In reality, *everyone* speaks with an accent (Cheng, 1999), and each accent is viewed as acceptable within a person's speech community.

I am originally from central Ohio and I spent my late childhood and adolescence living in the Chicago suburbs. My dialect thus contrasts in some ways from speakers in southern Illinois (where I later lived as an adult for 6 years). As a northern Illinoisan, I pronounce *Illinois* as [ɪ l ə n ɔɪ]. My rural elementary school students in the southern part of the state pronounced the state name as [ɪ l ə n ɔɪ z]. I also notice speakers who talk about [s t ɑ ɹ m z] (*storms*) coming in from the [n ɑ ɹ θ w ɛ s t] (*northwest*). This particular use of [ɑɹ] rather [ɔɹ] is associated with St. Louis and southeast Missouri speakers, which I again discovered while I lived and worked in southern Illinois. Thirty years later, this dialect characteristic, though fading, is still used by a number of speakers in that geographic area (Labov et al, 2006).

Sometimes, alternative dialect speakers find it necessary to **code switch**. That is, they change their dialect characteristics according to their listening audience. My students in Virginia often used a different dialect at college (more ME-sounding) but continued to use Appalachian English/Southern English in their home environment. As they explained it, community (college or home) acceptance required that they speak that community's dialect. Other students continued to use Southern English in all settings. They felt that the dialect expressed who they were and that people should have to accept them that way!

As we noted earlier, most professional organizations view dialects as different, but equally valid, ways to communicate. Speech-language pathologists who work with dialect speakers do not do so because the person's speech is disordered. Rather, they help their clients to use ME in certain situations while valuing the original dialect in appropriate settings. The idea is to expand a person's dialect capacities rather than stamp out any evidence of the non-ME dialect.

EVOLUTION OF AMERICAN-ENGLISH DIALECTS

In addition to the previously mentioned dialectic influences such as geographic area and ethnic background, other factors may influence dialect usage. These include level of education and socioeconomic status. In addition, the very nature of spoken language contributes to language changes and dialectic variation. Quite simply, spoken language is constantly evolving (Boberg, 2001; Boberg & Strassel, 2000; Curzan & Emmons, 2004; Graddol et al, 1996; Labov, 1991, 1994, 2001, 2010; Labov et al, 2006). Pronunciation differences that were emphasized generations ago (e.g., usage of /w/ vs /ʍ/) may become unimportant. My father (a product of "speech and diction" classes in the 1920s and 1930s) always found it difficult to reconcile the "collapse" of those two phonemes into one, even in ME. For me, the next generation, it was much simpler to use just one phoneme. By now, the use of /w/ for both phonemes is so prevalent that many phonetics books devote very little attention to the /ʍ/ phoneme. Recent research has indicated that very few speakers make this distinction, regardless of regional dialect (Labov et al, 2006).

Dialects may even evolve from the pronunciation characteristics originally described years earlier. This is apparent in *The Atlas of North American English* (Labov et al, 2006). Prior to this project, the landmark work was Kurath and McDavid's *The Pronunciation of English in the Atlantic States* (1961), which had been one of the primary references on regional dialects. Labov et al's newer, more extensive work (2006) enables us to confirm not only regional dialect characteristics but also more recent historical changes in vowel pronunciation in different geographic areas.

Some of the differences noted in this atlas are related to the authors' method of gathering data and their area of research emphasis. Previous studies focused on vocabulary and grammar contrasts as well pronunciation (Carver, 1987; Kurath, 1949; Kurath, Hanley, Bloch, & Lowman, 1943). But Labov et al (2006) focused almost exclusively on American English pronunciation characteristics. Earlier researchers used face-to-face interviews with speakers from both urban and rural areas. Labov and his associates used highly trained researchers to conduct telephone interviews (the TELSUR project), which were also audio-recorded for acoustic analysis. Thus, the report relies on more than human interviewers; spectrographic analysis was used to confirm trends. In addition, Labov et al focused on major metropolitan areas across the country. Because they were especially interested in the evolution and change of American-English pronunciation, they reasoned that urban areas would be at the forefront of such change. The result is a picture of ongoing merging of dialects with some definite regional characteristics still obvious. **Table 6.1** delineates the major (and some smaller) regional dialects of English.

REGIONAL DIALECTS

The most recent research on regional dialects (Labov et al, 2006) has identified four *primary* dialectic regions—North, South, Midland, and Western—with smaller subdivisions in each. This research has found several types of changes in vowel production over time, including **chain shifts** and **mergers**. **Chain shifts** occur when place of articulation of one vowel moves; the other vowels follow to "fill in" the vowel quadrilateral so that separate positions are maintained. **Mergers** refer to sounds that were previously distinguished or produced as different phonemes but are now represented by one phoneme. The previously mentioned "collapse" of /w/ and /ʍ/ into one phoneme is an example of a consonant merger. Mergers can be complete or conditional, the latter occurring only in specific phonetic environments.

Three major shifts in place of vowel production were noted: the **Northern Cities Chain Shift**, the **Southern Cities Chain Shift**, and the **Back-Up Glide Shift** (Labov et al, 2006). Three regional dialects were identified on the basis of these vowel shifts and mergers alone: the inland North, the South, and the West. The following discussion includes these dialects as well as several others, which have some distinctive characteristics.

As shown in **Table 6.1**, which delineates the major regional groups and their constituents, a number of regions are included within the area described *geographically* as the North. However, the dialect for all residents of the northern United States is not completely uniform. Although these areas generally have more pronunciation similarities than differences, the most notable differences are outlined in this section. Before beginning to discuss these areas, however, it is important to discuss the Northern Cities Chain Shift, which has affected vowel production in the both the North and the inland North regions.

TABLE 6.1 U.S. REGIONAL DIALECTS AND THEIR AREAS OF USAGE

Primary Dialect Area/Subdivisions	Areas of Usage (State Abbreviations)
Northern	
Eastern New England	ME, NH, RI; eastern portions of CT, MA, VT
Western New England	Central and western VT, western half of MA, central and western CT
Inland North	New York State, major cities in the Great Lakes region (excluding Erie, PA)
New York City	
Middle Atlantic	Major urban and surrounding areas of Philadelphia and Reading, PA, Atlantic City, NJ, Wilmington, DE, and Baltimore, MD
North Central	Northern MI, MN, MT, ND
North	Central and southern MN and IA, eastern SD, northeast NE, central and western WI
Midland	Central and southern OH, IN, IL; north and central MO; southern IA; southeast NE; central and eastern KS
Southern	NC, SC, GA, FL, AL, MS, northern OK; LA; TX; VA
Inland South	Northern AL, eastern TN, western NC and SC
Texas South	(North) central TX
Western	AZ, CA, CO, ID, NM, NV, OR, UT, WA, WY, central and western MT, west KS, west NE, west OK, west SD

Source: Modified from Labov, W., Ash, S., and Boberg, C. (2006). *The Atlas of North American English.* Berlin: Mouton de Gruyter.

Six vowels show a shift from their traditional places of production in the vowel quadrilateral: the front vowels /ɪ/ /ɛ/ /æ/, the central vowel /ʌ/, and the back vowels /ɔ/ and /ɑ/. As with the other shifts identified in current research, the movement of one vowel causes the vowel next to it to shift, which causes the adjacent vowel to shift, and so on. In the northern cities chain shift, the first change affects the vowel /æ/, which moves up to sound more like [iə]; for example, *cat* and *sack* would sound like [kiət] and [siək], respectively. The movement of /æ/ allows /ɑ/ placement to move forward, so that words like *hot* and *nod* now sound more like [hæt] and [næd], respectively. This means that there is room for /ɔ/ to move downward, making words like *hawk* and *dawn* sound like [hɑk] and [dɑn]. Additionally, the low back merger of /ɑ/ and /ɔ/ is found in a number of dialect regions; depending on your dialect, you may not produce word pairs like *hock* and *hawk* or *Don* and *dawn* with different vowels but with /ɑ/ for all four words.

The other vowels affected by this shift are /ʌ/, /ɛ/, and /ɪ/. Placement for /ʌ/ moves back and up so that *duck* and *luck* will sound more like [dɔk] and [lɔk]. Movement for /ɛ/ shifts centrally, closer to /ʌ/, so that words like *bed* and *net* will sound more like [bʌd] and [nʌt]. Placement for /ɪ/ lowers slightly and moves centrally so that it, too, sounds more like /ʌ/. See **Tables 6.2, 6.3,** and **6.4** for examples of vowel contrast according to the Northern Cities, and Southern Cities, and Upland Glide Shifts.

TABLE 6.2 NORTHERN CITIES CHAIN SHIFT AND EXAMPLES OF VOWEL EFFECTS

Vowel Affected	Nature of Shift	Narrow Transcription	Vowel Similarity	
/æ/	Raising	[æ]		
/ɑ/	Fronting	[ɑ̈]	cot→cat	[kɑt] →[kɑ̈t] or [kæt],
			Don→Dan	[dɑn]→[dɑ̈n] or [dæn]
			odd→add	[ɑd]→[ɑ̈d] or [æd]
/ɔ/	Lowering	[ɔ̞]	hawk→hock	[hɔk]→[hɔ̞k] or [hɑk],
			naught→not	[nɔt]→[nɔ̞t] or [nɑt]
			cawed→cod	[kɔd]→[kɔ̞d] or [kɑd]
[ʌ ɛ ɪ]	Backing	[ʌ̠]	cud→cawed	[kʌd]→[kʌ̠d] or [kɔd]
			done→dawn	[dʌ̠n]→[dʌ̠n] or
[dɔ̞n]		[ɛ̠]	bed→bud	[bɛd]→[bɛ̠d] or [bʌd]
			ten→ton	[tɛn]→[tɛ̠n] or [tʌn]
		[ɪ̠]	lit→let	[lɪt]→[lɪ̠t] or [lɛt]
			fin→fen	[fɪn]→[fɪ̠n] or [fɛn]

Source: Modified from Labov, W., Ash, S., and Boberg, C. (2006). *The Atlas of North American English.* Berlin: Mouton de Gruyter.

TABLE 6.3 SOUTHERN CITIES SHIFT AND EXAMPLES OF VOWEL EFFECTS

Vowel Affected	Nature of Shift	Narrow Transcription	Vowel Similarity	
/aɪ/	Monophthong	/a/	light→lot	[laɪt]→[lat] or [lɑt]
			hide→hod	[haɪd]→[had] or [hɑd]
			my→ma	[maɪ]→[ma] or [mɑ]
/æ/	Raised	[æ̝]	sat→set	[sæt]→[sæ̝t] or [sɛt]
			mad→med	[mæd]→[mæ̝d] or [mɛd]
			lad→led	[læd] [læ̝d] or [lɛd]
/ɛ/	Raised	[ɛ̝]	let→late	[l ɛ t]→[lɛ̝t] or [let]
			set→sate	[s ɛ t]→[sɛ̝t] or [set]
			bell→bail	[bɛl]→[bɛ̝l] or [bel]
/ɪ/	Raised	[ɪ̝]	lid→lead	[l ɪ d]→[lɪ̝d] or [lid]
			mitt→meet	[mɪt]→[mɪ̝t] or [mit]
			sit→seat	[sɪt]→[sɪ̝t] or [sit]
/i/	Lowered	[i̞]	wheat→wit	[wit]→[wi̞t] or [wɪt]
			lead→lid	[lid]→[li̞d] or [lɪd]
			deep→dip	[dip]→[di̞p] or [dɪp]

Source: Modified from Labov, W., Ash, S., and Boberg, C. (2006). *The Atlas of North American English.* Berlin: Mouton de Gruyter.

TABLE 6.4 COMPARISON OF VOWEL CHANGES ACROSS CHAIN SHIFT REGIONS

Vowel Phoneme	Northern Cities Chain Shift	Southern Cities Shift
/æ/	[æ]	[æ]
/ɛ/	[ɛ] or [ʌ]	[ɛ] or [e]
/ɪ/	[ɪ] or [ʌ]	[ɪ] or [i]
/i/	NA	[i̞] or [ɪ]
/ʌ/	[ʌ] or [ɔ]	
/ɑ/	[ɑ] or [æ]	
/ɔ/	[ɔ̈] or [ɑ]	[aʊ]
/aɪ/	NA	[a:] or [ɑ]
/aʊ/		[æ̂ʊ]

NORTHERN DIALECT REGIONS

INLAND NORTH DIALECT REGION

This region is particularly notable for the role of the Northern Cities Chain Shift in defining vowel production except for the merger of /ɑ/ and /ɔ/. Speakers in this region still contrast the vowels in words like *Don* ([d ɑ n]) and *Dawn* ([d ɔ n]). This region appears to be resistant to this merger, which is found in a number of other dialects (Labov et al, 2006).

NORTH DIALECT REGION

Like speakers in the inland North dialect region, speakers in this area also demonstrate the Northern Cities Chain Shift in their vowel production. Unlike the inland North speakers, however, North dialect speakers *do* show a merger of /ɑ/ and /ɔ/, so that *hock* and *hawk* and *Don* and *Dawn* would all be produced with virtually the same vowel, sounding very much like /ɑ/.

NORTH-CENTRAL DIALECT REGION

As shown in **Table 6.1**, this region includes parts of Minnesota, Montana, and South Dakota. Vowel productions characteristic of this region include a backward shift in placement for the vowels /u/ and /o/. Researchers have also noted that speakers in these areas tend to change the vowel /æ/ to an elongated /e/ in words containing postvocalic /g/ or /ŋ/ (Labov et al, 2006). Thus, words like *nag* and *sang* may sound more like [ne:g] and [se:ŋ], respectively.

NEW ENGLAND DIALECT REGION

As a dialect region, New England includes two subdivisions, Eastern New England and Western New England (Labov et al, 2006). Northern speakers from areas outside New England may notice some very specific differences from their dialects, especially for some of the vowels and for usage of postvocalic /ɹ/, /ɝ/, and /ɚ/.

Previous studies of dialectic variation found New England dialect to be characterized by vowelization of postvocalic /ɹ/, so that *car* or *heart* might be realized as [ka:] and [ha:t], respectively. Correspondingly, the vowels /ɝ/ and /ɚ/ showed a loss of rounding, with *bird* and *earth* produced as [bɜd] and [ɜθ], respectively. The unstressed /ɚ/ was often realized as /ə/, so that *winter* and *summer* would be heard as [wɪntə] and [sʌmə], respectively. More recent research (Labov et al, 2006) has indicated that these changes are still characteristic of eastern, but not western, New England speakers. Also, in eastern New England, speakers may produce /ɑ/ and /ɔ/ as one vowel. In contrast to other regions, however, the single vowel sounds like /a/ rather than /ɑ/, so that *dawn* and *Don* are both produced as [dan].

NEW YORK CITY

New York City maintains dialect characteristics that are distinct from a number of other northern dialect regions (Labov et al, 2006). In particular, New Yorkers do not use postvocalic /ɹ/. Instead they vowelize the /ɹ/ to an /ə/ (compare to Eastern New England English). Despite being in the North geographically, New York City English has not been affected by the northern cities chain shift. Some vowel variations found in this dialect area vary according to the phonetic environment of the vowel.

MIDDLE ATLANTIC

Labov et al (2006) identify the Middle Atlantic dialect region as demonstrating a combination of South and Midland dialect characteristics. It is another regional dialect that appears resistant to the back vowel merger of /ɑ/ and /ɔ/. Additional similarities to other regional dialects will be mentioned in the following sections.

MIDLAND DIALECT REGION

This dialect region, according to Labov et al (2006), may very well be the "default system" (p. 35) of North American English. Another way to look at it might be to see it as the closest dialect to "mainstream English." Only a few vowel characteristics are unique to this area: fronting of /u/ and [oʊ] and the merger of /ɑ/ and /ɔ/ to be produced as the vowel /ɑ/, just like in the West and parts of the South.

THE SOUTH

Two chain shifts have been found to characterize the speech of this dialect region (Labov et al, 2006). First, the Southern Cities chain Shift has affected place of production of all the front vowels (/æ ɛ e ɪ i/), the diphthong /aɪ/, and the monophthong vowel /a/. The first step in this shift occurs when /aɪ/ becomes a monophthong vowel /ạ/ (similar to /ɑ/). Correspondingly, /e/ is lowered and takes a more central position. This means that placement for both /a/ and /e/ are much closer together than in the traditional vowel quadrilateral. /i/ placement is also lowered, whereas placements for /æ/, /ɛ/, and /ɪ/ are higher. The result is a distinctive vowel pattern depicted with examples in **Table 6.3**.

The second chain shift characteristic of southern dialect is the Back Up-Glide Shift (Labov et al, 2006). Two vowels are affected: the diphthong /aʊ/ and the back monophthong vowel /ɔ/. The /ɔ/ is both raised and unrounded so that it sounds much like /aʊ/. Correspondingly, /aʊ/ also changes, sounding like [æʊ]. Consequently, the word *ought* ([ɔ t]) could sound like *out* ([æ ʊ t]). Words like *down* and *mouse* might be heard as [dæʊn] and [mæʊs], respectively.

In addition to the vowel changes caused by the southern shift and the back up-glide shift, other pronunciation differences have been noted between speakers in the South and North. Although some of these differences appear to be disappearing in urban areas (Labov et al, 2006), this is not necessarily the case with more rural speakers. In particular, these include monophthongization of /aɪ/ and /ɔɪ/, although the latter appears to be disappearing in urban speakers in the South (Labov et al, 2006).

Monophthongization of /aɪ/ is probably heard by most non-southern speakers as a key characteristic of southern dialect. The /aɪ/ becomes /a:/ (an elongated /a/, sounding like /ɑ/). Words like *buy* and *nine* will sound like [b a:] and [m a: n]. I still clearly remember a new neighbor's gift of [ɹ a t n a s g ɹ i n b i n z], that is, *right nice green beans* when my family first moved to Virginia. If monophthongization of /ɔɪ/ occurs, it is produced like /ɔ/ so that words like *oil* and *boil* may sound like [ɔ l] and [b ɔ l].

An additional dialect variation in the South is a conditional merger affecting /ɪ/ and /ɛ/ (Labov et al, 2006). When /ɛ/ is followed by a nasal /m/ or /n/, it is produced as [ɪ]. Thus, you would write with a [p ɪ n] *(pen)* and also fasten something with a [p ɪ n] *(pin)*. Sometimes southern speakers will clarify the difference between these as an *ink pen* [ɪ ŋ k p ɪ n] versus *a safety pin* [s eɪ f t i p ɪ n]. Similarly, the *hem* might sound like *him*, with both words produced with /ɪ/.

Some southern speakers may also substitute /ɪ/ for /ə/ in the second syllable of a two-syllable word. For example, *salad* and *lettuce* would be pronounced as [s æ l ə d] and [l ɛ t ə s] by those in dialect regions outside the South. In SE, these words would be pronounced as [s æ l ɪ d] and [l ɛ t ɪ s], respectively.

THE WEST

It is obvious from **Table 6.1** that this dialect area is very large, especially compared to some of its closest neighbors, the Midland, North, and North Central dialect areas. Labov et al (2006) note that it is less homogeneous as a dialect region than the other regional dialects they studied. This should not be surprising, because so many of the original settlers in the West came from varied parts of the eastern half of the United States. Parts of this region that border closely on other dialect regions show some shared characteristics with those regions. One of the most noticeable features of this dialect area is consistent appearance of the low back merger, that is, loss of the distinction between /ɔ/ and /ɑ/. Speakers in the West also show complete merger of /ʍ/ and /w/, producing them as the single phoneme /w/.

CULTURAL AND ETHNIC DIALECTS

Another source of dialectic variation in the United States is the different cultures and ethnic backgrounds of Americans. These dialects are strongly associated with a person's sense of identity and "peoplehood." The pronunciation characteristics of a speaker of African-American English or Spanish-influenced English, for example, differ from mainstream American English in certain characteristics. Nevertheless, each dialect is a systematic, rule-governed system that shares both similarities and differences with mainstream American English. This section discusses the three main cultural dialects found in the United States today: African-American English (vernacular), Spanish-influenced English (also known as Hispanic English), and several varieties of Asian/Pacific Islands English. Note that individuals from one of these cultures may not necessarily use all the dialect characteristics listed. Use can vary according to family customs, conversational partners, and situational factors. Code-shifting, mentioned earlier in the chapter, may also affect speakers of African American English, Spanish-influenced English, and Asian English. In addition, the regional dialect can affect any cultural dialect used (Wolfram, 1994). Consequently, an African American English speaker living in the South will not sound exactly like an African American English speaker who lives in Minnesota. Nevertheless, there are certain characteristics of each of these dialects that have been identified as occurring more frequently among their users, and they are included in the following subsections.

AFRICAN-AMERICAN ENGLISH (VERNACULAR)

Variously referred to as African-American English, black English, and ebonics, this dialect is the most prominent linguistic system associated with African Americans (Battle, 2002). African-American English shares characteristics with the languages of West Africa (VanKeulen, Weddington, & DeBose, 1998) and southern American English (Wolfram, 1994). Although African American English, too, is evolving, Labov et al (2006) have noted that it remains much more consistent in its usage than the regional dialects covered previously in this chapter. African-American English includes verbal and nonverbal factors, but emphasis in this chapter is on pronunciation characteristics.

A variety of factors can influence the nature of African American English usage among speakers, especially listener identity and situational contexts. The ethnic background of African American English listeners and the degree of formality of the speaking situation, for example, can affect dialect use. Like speakers of some regional dialects, African American English speakers may find it necessary to "code switch" or be "bidialectical" (VanKeulen et al, 1998). African-American English differs somewhat from mainstream American English in certain aspects of phonology, morphology, and syntax. Phonological differences affecting consonants have been documented according to three primary rules (Battle, 2002): (1) silencing or substitution of selected intervocalic or postvocalic consonants in words, (2) silencing of unstressed prevocalic phonemes and syllables, and (3) silencing of the last consonant in a postvocalic consonant sequence.

Phonemes most affected by the first rule include stops, voiced and voiceless fricatives, nasals, and liquids /l/ and /ɹ/ (Battle, 2002). **Table 6.5** presents these rules in detail with examples to illustrate them. The second rule, affecting unstressed prevocalic phonemes, can be found in expressions such as *he was coming* (African American English: *he uz comin*) or *that one* (African American English: *that 'un*). Syllables affected by the second rule are most easily seen in production of *potatoes* as

TABLE 6.5 FREQUENTLY CITED PRONUNCIATION CHARACTERISTICS OF AFRICAN-AMERICAN ENGLISH: SINGLETON CONSONANTS

Consonant	Prevocalic	Intervocalic	Postvocalic	Example
Stops				
Voiceless			May be omitted	hat→[h æ] top→[tɑ]
Voiced			May be voiceless with elongated vowel preceding	had→[h æː t] red→[[ɹ ɛː t]
Fricatives:				
/θ/		/f/	/f/	birthday→ [b ɜ f d eɪ] tooth→[t u f]
/ð/	/d/	/d/	/d/ or /v/	them→[d ɛ m] either→[i d ə] breathe→ [b ɹ i d] or [b ɹ i v]
Nasals: /m/ /n/			Possible omission with preceding vowel nasalized	pin→[p ĩ] fin→[f ĩ]
/ŋ/			Unstressed *–ing*→ /n/	seeing→[s i ɪ n] being→[b i ɪ n]
Liquids				
/l/			Vowelized	bell→[b ɛ ə] will→[w ɪ ə]
/ɹ/			Omitted or /ə/	car→[k ɑ] or [k ɑ ə]

Sources: Battle, 2002; Bauman-Waengler, 2012; Kamhi, Pollack, & Harris, 1996; Stockman, 1996; Williams & Wolfram, 1977; Wolfram, 1994.

tatoes and '*pears* for *appears*. **Table 6.6** gives examples of the third rule affecting consonant sequences. Thus, *fold* might be heard as [f oʊ l] and *mask* might be produced as [m æ s]. In addition to consonant differences, African American English vowels may be different from mainstream American English, as shown in **Table 6.7**. In particular, notice the effects on postvocalic /ɹ ɝ ɚ/ (changes once very characteristic of all Southern English speakers) as well as effects on /ɛ/ before nasal consonants.

TABLE 6.6 FREQUENTLY CITED PRONUNCIATION CHARACTERISTICS OF AFRICAN-AMERICAN
ENGLISH: CONSONANT SEQUENCES

Position/Sound	Usage	Example	
Prevocalic			
/θ ɹ/	/θ/	throw	[θ oʊ]
/ʃ ɹ/	/s ɹ/	shrimp	[s ɹ ɪ m p]
/s t ɹ/	/s k ɹ/	street	[s k ɹ i t]
Postvocalic			
/l/ + nasal	/l/ omitted	helm	[h ɛ m]
		film	[f ɪ m]
/l/ + stop	/l/ omitted	help	[h ɛ p]
		hold	[h oʊ d]/[h oʊ t]
/l/ + fricative	/l/ omitted	self	[s ɛ f]
Nasal + stop	Stop omitted	dent	[d ɛ n]
		hand	[h æ n]
Fricative + /p/, /t/	Stop omitted	laughed	[læf]
		last	[l æ s]
/k/ + /s/	Segments reversed	ask	[æ k s]
Three-element sequences	Variable phoneme omission	length	[l ɛ ŋ k θ]→[l ɛ n f]
		sinks	[s ɪ ŋ k s]→[s ɪ n s]
		text	[t ɛ k s t]→[t ɛ k s]

Sources: Battle, 2002; Bauman-Waengler, 2012; Kamhi, Pollack, & Harris, 1996; Stockman, 1996; Williams & Wolfram, 1977; Wolfram, 1994.

TABLE 6.7 FREQUENTLY CITED PRONUNCIATION CHARACTERISTICS OF AFRICAN-AMERICAN
ENGLISH: VOWELS

Vowel	Usage	Examples
/ɛ/	Shift to /ɪ/ before nasals	pen→[p ɪ n]
		Ben→[b ɪ n]
/ɝ/	/ɜ/	bird→[b ɜ d]
		turn→[t ɜ n]
/ɚ/	/ə/	brother→[b ɹ ʌ d ə]
		under→[ʌ n d ə]
/ɔɪ/	/ɔ/	oil→[ɔ l]
		foil→[f ɔ l]

Sources: Battle, 2002; Bauman-Waengler, 2012; Kamhi, Pollack, & Harris, 1996; Stockman, 1996; Williams & Wolfram, 1977; Wolfram, 1994.

SPANISH-INFLUENCED ENGLISH

Americans of Latino or Hispanic origin are among the fastest growing ethnic groups in the United States. Consequently, the number of individuals who speak English as a second language continues to grow. However, just because someone is of Latino origin or uses Spanish-influenced English does not mean that all speakers of this dialect will sound alike. Factors affecting Spanish-influenced English use include the speaker's country of origin and the type and dialect of Spanish spoken. Not all Spanish-influenced English speakers come from the same country, of course. Immigrants and first-generation citizens come from Cuba, Puerto Rico, Mexico, Central America, and South America, as well as from Spain and other countries. There are also different varieties of Spanish, just as there are different dialects in English. Depending on the person's original Spanish language, Spanish-influenced English can vary. Usage also differs according to the language (English or Spanish) spoken in the home and by extended family and friends. Some speakers are fully bilingual, but others are not (Goldstein & Iglesias, 2009). The degree of English proficiency can vary according to all these factors as well as the amount of time spent in the United States and the nature and extent of the speaker's schooling. As with African American English speakers, Spanish-influenced English speakers' characteristics vary according to the geographic region of the United States (Wolfram, 1994). Even with all these factors, a core of phonological characteristics has been identified as most typical of Spanish-influenced English speakers. These are displayed in **Tables 6.8** and **6.9**.

Some Spanish-influenced English characteristics are easier to understand if you know something about Spanish. First, Spanish uses fewer vowels than English. Con-

TABLE 6.8 FREQUENTLY CITED CHARACTERISTICS OF SPANISH-INFLUENCED ENGLISH: VOWELS

Vowel	Usage	Examples
/i/	/ɪ/	eat→[ɪ t]
		seat→[s ɪ t]
/ɪ/	/i/	sit→[s i t]
		hit→[h i t]
/ɛ/	/eɪ/ or /æ/	said→[s eɪ d or [s æ d]
		bed→[b eɪ d] or [b æ d]
/æ/	/ɛ/	hat→[h ɛ t]
		sad→[s ɛ d]
/u/	/ʊ/	news→[n ʊ z]
		soon→[s ʊ n]
/ɔ/	/oʊ/	caught→[k oʊ t]
		hawk→[h oʊ k]
/ʌ/	/ɑ/	duck→[d ɑ k]
		puppy→[p ɑ p i]
/ɝ/	/ɛ r/	her→[h ɛ r]
		turn→[t ɛr n]

Sources: Goldstein & Iglesias, 2009; Perez, 1994.

TABLE 6.9 FREQUENTLY CITED CHARACTERISTICS OF SPANISH-INFLUENCED ENGLISH: CONSONANTS

Consonant	Initial	Medial	Final
Singletons: stops			
/p/ /t/			Omitted/distorted
/b/ /k/ /g/			Omitted/distorted/cognate
/d/		Dentalized	
Singletons: fricatives			
/f/			Omitted
/v/	/b/	/b/	Distorted
/θ/	/t/ /s/	Omitted	/t/ /s/
/ð/	/d/	/d/ /z/ /v/	/d/
/z/	/s/	/s/	/s/
/ʃ/	/ʧ/	/s/ /ʧ/	/ʧ/
Singletons: affricates			
/ʧ/	/ʃ/	/ʃ/	/ʃ/
/ʤ/	/d/	/j/	/ʃ/
Singletons: nasals			
/m/			Omitted
/ŋ/		/d/	/n/
Singletons: liquids and glides			
/w/	/h u/		
/j/	/ʤ/		
/r/	Distorted	Distorted	Distorted
Consonant sequences			
/s/	/ɛ/ + sequence		

sequently, substitutions of similar sounds can result. Note in **Table 6.8** that both /i/ and /ɪ/ may be interchanged. Spanish phonology includes /i/ but not /ɪ/, which explains how the two phonemes may be used variably in English.

Some mainstream American English-Spanish-influenced English consonant differences result from Spanish consonant phonemes being substituted for similar English phonemes. Other substitutions result because an English phoneme is absent in Spanish. In particular, substitutions will be found for /v/, /z/, /θ/, /ð/, and /ʒ/. Also, the alveolar stops /t/ and /d/ and the alveolar nasal /n/ may be dentalized in SIE, as they are in Spanish. Other commonly observed SIE characteristics include deletion of most final consonants (only /s n r l d/ occur in the final word position in Spanish) (Perez, 1994). See **Table 6.9** for additional consonant characteristics.

ASIAN-PACIFIC ISLANDER/ASIAN ENGLISH

Americans who trace their origins to Asian countries and the Pacific Islands constitute another fast-growing ethnic group in the United States. Like any other minority dialect group, Asian English speakers may experience communication interference and discrimination, based on their dialect. However, the term *Asian English* is misleading because it sounds as if it is referring to one uniform dialect for all Asian Americans. Although some common characteristics have been found, a variety of factors can affect the person's actual dialect.

First, Americans of Asian English extraction come from a large number of countries and represent an even larger number of languages. Speakers of Asian English come from China, Japan, Southeast Asia (including Vietnam, Cambodia, Laos, Thailand, Malaysia, and others), India, Pakistan, or one of a number of different Pacific Islands. Even Asian English speakers from the same country will not necessarily share all dialect characteristics. Asian English speakers from China may speak Mandarin or Cantonese in addition to any number of local dialects. Americans of Indian origin may speak Hindi, Punjabi, or Bengali and other local dialects as well as English. Their English pronunciation may be British English, which also contrasts with mainstream American English. Asian languages differ from one another and from English in the number of consonants and vowels, as well as in permissible phonemic arrangements (phonotactics). Chinese and Laotian, among others, are tonal languages in which intonation signals a difference in meaning. The same CVC (consonant—vowel—consonant) can vary in meaning depending on which tonal pattern is used to produce it, for example "upper even" or "lower even" (Cheng, 1994). Thus, Asian English characteristics depend heavily on the speaker's native language and any other languages that might have affected the native languages.

Other influences on Asian English are similar to those affecting speakers of other ethnic dialects. Is the speaker newly arrived in the United States or a longtime resident? First or second generation in this country? What dialect of English did he or she learn? At what age did the speaker learn English? What language is used at home and in the extended family? What language is spoken at school? All these factors and more can affect Asian English speaker characteristics. Because there is no single, uniform Asian English dialect, the following subsections include information on some of the Asian English characteristics by country of origin. **Table 6.10** depicts the consonants shared between mainstream American English and several Asian languages: Mandarin and Cantonese Chinese, Korean, and Vietnamese. In addition, some common

TABLE 6.10 ASIAN LANGUAGES CONSONANT COUNTERPARTS OF MAINSTREAM ENGLISH CONSONANTS

Language	Stops	Fricatives	Affricates	Nasals	Glides	Liquids
Mainstream English	p b t d k g	f v θ ð s z ʃ ʒ h	ʧ ʤ	m n ŋ	w j	l ɹ
Mandarin	p pʰ t tʰ k kʰ [a]	f	s	m n ŋ		l
Cantonese	p pʰ t tʰ k kʰ [b]	f	s [c]	m n ŋ	w j	
Korean	p b t d k g[d]	s	h	m n	j	l
Vietnamese	p b t d k g[e]	f v s z ʃ ʒ h[f]		m n ŋ[g]	w j	l

Note: Only mainstream English equivalents are shown. These languages all have additional phonemes that are not found in English.

Sources: Cheng, 1991; Fang & Ping-an, 1992; Hwa-Froelich, Hodson, & Edwards, 2002).

characteristics have been found among the languages listed in **Table 6.10** (Cheng, 1991; Hwa-Froelich, Hodson, & Edwards, 2002):

1. Consonant clusters do not occur in these languages.

2. Words are usually monosyllabic (Mandarin and Cantonese are strictly mono-syllabic).

3. /l/ is the only liquid represented across all these languages and may be con-fused with /ɹ/.

4. No interdental phonemes (/θ ð/ occur in these languages).

Mandarin Chinese

Mandarin is a tonal language, one of two primary dialects spoken by Chinese English learners in the United States (Cheng, 1991). The only phonemes used in the post-vocalic position in Mandarin are /n/ and /ŋ/ (Fang & Ping-an, 1992); consequently, the Mandarin Chinese speaker who is learning English may omit other postvocalic phonemes. Common phoneme substitutions in English may include /s/ replacing /θ/ in all prevocalic and intervocalic positions and /s/ or /f/ replacing /θ/ in the postvocalic position. Substitutions for /ð/ include /d/ and /z/ in prevocalic and intervocalic positions. The fricative /v/ may be replaced by /w/ in the intervocalic position. Lack of consonant clusters in Mandarin results in loss of phonemes in these phoneme sequences in English.

Cantonese Chinese

Also a tonal language, Cantonese is the other primary language used by Chinese learners of English. The use of postvocalic consonants is limited to the voiceless stops and the nasals (So & Dodd, 1997). Consequently, many postvocalic consonants may be deleted in English. Common sound substitutions in the Cantonese English speaker include the following (Cheng, 1991):

1. /θ/ replaced by /s/ (prevocalic) position /f/ (postvocalic)

2. /ð/ replaced by /d/ (prevocalic and intervocalic)

3. /z/ replaced by /s/ (any position)

4. /ʃ/ replaced by /s/ (any position)

5. /v/ replaced by /w/ (prevocalic and intervocalic)

6. /ɹ/ replaced by /s/ (any position)

In addition, prevocalic /n/ and /l/ may be interchanged (So & Dodd, 1997). As previously noted, there are no consonant sequences in Cantonese, so one or more elements of consonant sequences may be omitted in English.

Korean Phonology

As noted in **Table 6.10**, the following phonemes in English are not found in Korean: /f v θ ð ʃ ʒ ʧ ʤ ɹ w/ (Cheng, 1991, 1994). Consequently, other phonemes are substi-tuted for them by the Korean English speaker. Korean has more postvocalic pho-nemes that Mandarin and Cantonese; only fricatives and affricates may be omitted in the postvocalic position in English (Cheng, 1991). English consonant sequences may be reduced because Korean lacks prevocalic and postvocalic consonant sequences.

VIETNAMESE PHONOLOGY

Another tonal language, Vietnamese has three major dialects (Hwa-Froelich et al, 2002) that also affect the speaker's pronunciation of English. This discussion is limited to those characteristics found in all three dialects. Postvocalic consonants in Vietnamese are limited to the voiceless stops (/p t k/) and the nasal consonants (/m n ŋ/) (Cheng, 1991). Thus, final consonant deletion may occur frequently in the speech of Vietnamese English speakers. Omissions can occur in consonant sequences because Vietnamese does not have consonant clusters. Because Vietnamese lacks interdental fricatives (/θ/ and /ð/) and palatal affricates (/ʧ/ and /ʤ/), the Vietnamese English speaker substitutes other, similar phonemes for them.

Not only are there consonant differences in Asian-influenced English, there are vowel differences as well. Not all Asian languages have the same number of vowels, and Asian vowels do not necessarily correspond to their English counterparts. However, Cheng (1994) has noted that vowel confusions may be expected, often involving /ɪ/ (alternating with /i/) and /æ/ replaced by /e/. Other vowels that may be produced differently include /ʊ/ and /ɔ/. The vowel /ə/ may intrude (epenthesis) in consonant sequences, for example *black* produced as [b ə l æ k], because not all Asian languages have consonant sequences.

Because of the great variety of dialect variations among Asian English speakers, no exercises are included for this subsection. It is important, however, that professionals recognize that not all Asian English speakers sound alike. Country of origin, dialect, and other factors must be considered in distinguishing dialectic variation from a speech sound disorder.

PRACTICE: EXERCISES 6.1 TO 6.3

In addition to the concept questions at the end of this chapter, Appendix A has exercises to help you challenge your knowledge of multicultural dialects and the other material discussed in this chapter. The answers are provided in Appendix C.

CONCLUSION

As noted at the beginning of this chapter, a number of regional, cultural, and ethnic dialects have been identified in the United States. Each represents a valid, rule-based system that governs language usage in an individual's language community. Dialects are not static; they continue to evolve in pronunciation as well as other language characteristics. In addition, the number of speakers learning English as another language continues to grow in this country. Consequently it is imperative that health and educational professionals recognize and respect such dialectic differences. Valid dialectic differences are not speech disorders and should not be labeled as such. Professionals who work with speakers of any non-mainstream American English dialect must have knowledge of all the linguistic features of the dialect as well as children's developmental milestones within their dialect. Children who are English language learners should be evaluated in both their first and second languages in order to determine if a disorder is present. Therapy should be limited to disordered features, not valid dialectic features. Consequently, a child whose speech shows only dialectic variations is not a candidate for treatment. Sometimes adults who speak alternative dialects may seek professional help to sound "more American" or to be better understood by American listeners. The speech-language pathologists who offer such services are engaged in accent reduction, not therapy. It is an optional service, not a required one.

CONCEPT QUESTIONS

PART I

Are the following statements true or false?

_____ 1. Dialects are valid language systems appropriate for the language community in which they are used.

_____ 2. Regional and cultural dialects are rule-based systems rather than substandard varieties of a more "prestigious" dialect.

_____ 3. All dialects in the United States have equal prestige in the view of the average American.

_____ 4. A dialect is not a disorder that requires changing.

_____ 5. Regional dialects vary in their production of /ɔ/ and /ɑ/ as two distinct phonemes.

_____ 6. The Midland dialect is probably the closest to what would be described as mainstream American English.

_____ 7. Vowel shifts have affected Southern and Northern English dialects in exactly the same ways.

_____ 8. A dialect is not a disorder that requires changing.

_____ 9. The phonemes /θ/ and /ð/ are often subject to dialectic variation in African-American speakers.

_____ 10. Final consonants may be omitted by both Asian English and SIE speakers.

PART II: REGIONAL DIALECTS

For the following, indicate the most likely regional dialect of the speaker (e.g., INE, ME, SE, ENEE). More than one answer is possible.

Examples		Probable Regional Dialect(s)
a.	mine→[m a: n]	_____
	hide→[h a: d]	_____
b.	bird→[b ɜ d]	_____
	ladder→[l æ d ə]	_____
c.	handed→[h æ n d ɪ d]	_____
	palace→[p æ l ɪ s]	_____
d.	sent→[s ɪ n t]	_____
	men→[m ɪ n]	_____
e.	pond→[p ɑ n d]	_____
	pawned→[p ɔ n d]	_____

PART III: AFRICAN-AMERICAN ENGLISH

Using the tables in the text, transcribe the following words as they might be produced by the AAE speaker. (Sounds in bold type are those most subject to dialectic variation.)

a.	meant	[ ]	e.	first	[ ]
b.	other→	[ ]	f.	shelf	[ ]
c.	herself	[ ]	g.	birthday	[ ]
d.	desk	[ ]	h.	throw→	[ ]

PART IV: SPANISH-INFLUENCED ENGLISH

Using the tables in the text, transcribe the following words as they might be produced by the SIE speaker. (Again, sounds in bold type are those most subject to dialectic variation.)

a.	very	[ ]	e.	skirt	[ ]
	shovel	[ ]		scurry	[ ]
b.	breathe	[ ]	f.	call	[ ]
	teeth	[ ]		law	[ ]
c.	choose	[ ]	g.	shin	[ ]
	juice	[ ]		chin	[ ]
d.	which	[ ]	h.	thing	[ ]
	win	[ ]		sing	[ ]

APPLIED PHONETICS

SPEECH SOUND DISORDERS

ENGLISH-LANGUAGE LEARNERS AND SPEAKERS OF ENGLISH AS A SECOND LANGUAGE

VOICE AND DICTION TRAINING

CONCLUSION

CONCEPT QUESTIONS

So far this book has been devoted to developing basic and advanced skills in the transcription of American English, including dialectic variations. There are additional uses for phonetics beyond transcription of normal speech, however. Knowledge and application of phonetics are instrumental to the work of linguists, speech-language pathologists, English as a second language (ESL) instructors, and speech trainers/coaches, to mention some of the professionals who use applied phonetics in their work. This chapter discusses some of the applications of phonetics in different professions.

SPEECH SOUND DISORDERS

Traditionally, speech-language pathologists who work with clients with speech sound disorders must have a thorough knowledge of phonetics and phonology. Patients with **speech sound disorders** are unable to produce American-English phonemes after the chronological age at which they should have been mastered. There are two types of speech sound disorders: **articulation disorders** and **phonological disorders**. Patients with articulation disorders are unable to physically produce acoustically correct phonemes and usually have only a few phonemes in error, for example a problem with /s/ or /l/. Those with phonological disorders are unable to master the *sound system* of the language and have a rule-based problem. Speech sound disorders can range from a simple lisp (usually an articulation problem) to loss of whole sound classes (a phonological problem). Rule-based problems include **final consonant deletion** (*house*→[haʊ], *book*→[bʊ], *hill*→[hɪ]). Another pattern commonly found in rule-based speech sound disorders is **stopping,** that is, replacing fricatives with stops so that *fan* becomes [p æ n], *thumb* becomes [t ʌ m], and *sat* becomes [t æ t]. In order to treat such problems effectively, speech-language pathologists must be able to transcribe the client's speech, determine errors, and explain the placement and manner of phoneme formation to the patient in the course of treatment.

ASSESSMENT

The speech-language pathologist has several key determinations to make in testing a patient for a possible speech sound disorder. Even if a patient displays sound substitutions or omissions, a disorder is not necessarily present. Some types of substitutions are common in toddlers but not in older children. Children who are bilingual or adult ESL speakers may display sound productions that are different from standard American-English phonemes. Those productions would be considered a speech difference, not a disorder (American Speech-Language-Hearing Association, 1983, 2003). (See the next section for more information about this topic.)

To determine the existence of a speech sound disorder, the speech-language pathologist must collect a representative sample of the patient's speech. There are a number of ways to collect speech samples for analysis. Most often, the speech-language pathologist administers some type of speech sound inventory or formal test to older preschoolers, school-aged children, adolescents, and adults. Children are asked to name pictures or read words or sentences. Adolescents and adults are asked to read a series of sentences designed to assess production of all English phonemes in all word positions. All errors are transcribed phonetically. Some tests evaluate mastery of phonemes (**articulation tests**), whereas others are designed to examine the patient's understanding of phonological rules (**phonological tests**). A conversational sample must also be collected, transcribed, and analyzed.

TYPES OF TESTS

Articulation/phonetic tests or "one sound at a time" tests typically evaluate every English consonant in prevocalic, intervocalic, and postvocalic positions. These tests may or may not include words for evaluating vowel accuracy. Errors are transcribed phonetically and may be classified as substitutions, omissions, distortions, or (much less frequently) additions. If an **omission** occurs, the patient deletes or omits the tested phoneme, for example *house* is produced as [haʊ] (omission of /s/ in the postvocalic or final position). In a **substitution**, one standard speech sound replaces another standard speech sound, for example *house* may be produced as [h aʊ θ] (substitution of θ/s in the postvocalic position). A distortion occurs when a standard speech sound is replaced by a nonstandard speech sound. Often, transcription of distortions requires the use of narrow transcription symbols. A lateralized production of /s/ in *house* would be transcribed as [sˡ] for example. A lowered production of /l/ would be transcribed as [l̞]. **Table 7.1** lists additional International Phonetic Alphabet (IPA) symbols for characterizing speech sound disorders (Duckworth, Allen, Hardcastle, & Ball, 1990). (You were introduced to many of these symbols in Chapter 5.) Finally, an **addition** occurs when one or more phonemes are added to a word. Production of *house* as [h aʊ s t] would be an example of an addition in the postvocalic position. **Table 7.2** lists a number of examples of phonemic test error recording.

TABLE 7.1 INTERNATIONAL PHONETIC ALPHABET (IPA) SYMBOLS FOR CHARACTERIZING DISORDERED SPEECH

Voiceless	n̥ d̥	Breathy voiced	b̤ a̤	Dental	t̪ d̪
Voiced	s̬ t̬	Creaky voiced	b̰ a̰	Apical	t̺ d̺
Aspirated	tʰ dʰ	Linguolabial	t̼ d̼	Laminal	t̻ d̻
More rounded	ɔ̹	Labialized	tʷ dʷ	Nasalized	ẽ
Less rounded	ɔ̜	Palatalized	tʲ dʲ	Nasal release	dⁿ
Advanced	u̟	Velarized	tˠ dˠ	Lateral release	dˡ
Retracted	e̠	Pharyngealized	tˤ dˤ	No audible release	d̚
Centralized	ë	Velarized or pharyngealized	ɫ	
Mid-centralized	ě	Raised	e̝	(ɹ̝ = voiced alveolar fricative)
Syllabic	n̩	Lowered	e̞	(β̞ = voiced bilabial
Non-syllabic	e̯	Advanced Tongue Root	e̘	approximant)
Rhoticity	ɚ ɝ	Retracted Tongue Root	e̙	

Source: From the International Phonetic Association (http://www.langsci.ucl.ac.uk/ipa/). Copyright 2005 by International Phonetic Association. Reprinted with permission.

TABLE 7.2 EXAMPLES OF TRADITIONAL ERROR RECORDING

Test Phoneme/ Position		Stimulus Word	Production	Error Recording	Error Type
/s/	(I)	sun	[θ ʌ n]	θ/s (I)	Substitution
	(M)	bicycle	[b aɪ θ ɪ k ə l]	θ/s (M)	Substitution
	(F)	house	[h aʊ sˡ]	sˡ/s (F)	Distortion
/ʃ/	(I)	shoe	[su]	s/ʃ (I)	Substitution
	(M)	dishes	[d ɪ s ə z]	s/ʃ (M)	Substitution
	(F)	fish	[f ɪ ʧ]	ʧ/ʃ (F)	Substitution
/l/	(I)	lamp	[j æ m p]	j/l (I)	Substitution
	(M)	balloon	[b ə l̪ u n]	l̪/l (M)	Distortion
	(F)	bell	[b ɛ]	–/l (F)	Omission
/ɹ/	(I)	red	[w ɛ d]	w/ɹ (F)	Substitution
	(M)	carry	[k ɛ ɟ i]	ɟ/ɹ (M)	Distortion
	(F)	deer	[d i]	–/ɹ (F)	Omission

PRACTICE: EXERCISES 7.1 AND 7.2

These exercises, which are in Appendix A, are designed to help you learn to recognize speech sound errors, transcribe them in IPA symbols, and classify them according to position and error type. The words in the first exercise are from the *Test of Minimal Articulation Competence* (TMAC) (Secord, 1981). In the second exercise you will find responses to the *Goldman-Fristoe Test of Articulation* (GFTA-2) (Goldman & Fristoe, 2000). After you have completed the exercises, check your answers against the answer key in Appendix C.

Phonological tests (also known as rule-based tests or pattern tests) are designed to determine the English-language phonological rules that the child does not understand. Many phonological tests are also word tests, but they require that you transcribe *every* sound change, not just a single sound production in prevocalic, intervocalic, or postvocalic position. For example, the word *house* has three sounds to account for, as opposed to the postvocalic singleton /s/ in an articulation test. Given a response of [aʊ] for *house* on a phonological test, you would transcribe for loss of both /h/ and /s/. Later, when you completed test scoring, you would record for occurrences of both prevocalic and postvocalic consonant deletion, not just a single sound error. Once all patterns have been identified, the speech-language pathologist can determine percentages of occurrence for each process and develop a treatment plan to help the child learn to close words (final consonant deletion) or use the long sound (replacing fricatives with stops), or use the two-step word (consonant sequence omissions). See **Tables 7.3** and **7.4** for definitions, examples, and scoring of commonly occurring phonological patterns.

TABLE 7.3 DEFINITIONS AND EXAMPLES OF COMMON DEVELOPMENTAL PHONOLOGICAL PATTERNS

Pattern	Definition	Examples
Weak syllable deletion	Loss of unstressed syllable(s)	banana→[n æ n æ] elephant→[ɛ f ə n t]
Final consonant deletion	Omission of final/postvocalic consonant	beet→[b i] ice→[aɪ] house→[h aʊ]
Cluster reduction/ consonant sequence reduction	Loss of one or more consonants in a sequence	spoon→[p u n] blue→[b u] boats→[b oʊ t]
Stopping	Stop replaces fricative/affricate	Sue→[t u] feet→[p i t] shove→[t ʌ b] watch→[w ɑ t] jump→[d ʌ m p]
Velar fronting	Alveolar consonant replaces velar /k g ŋ/	key→[t i] egg→[ɛ d] ring→[ɹ ɪ n]
Liquid simplification Gliding	Affects /l/ and /ɹ/ /w/ or /j/ replaces /l/ and/or /ɹ/ in initial or medial position	leaf→[w i f] *or* [j i f] ring→[w ɪ ŋ] balloon→[bəwun] *or* [bəjun] carry→[k ɛ w i]
Vowelization	Vowel replaces /l/ or /ɹ/ in the final position	bell→[b ɛ o] bowl→[b oʊ ʊ] chair→[ʧ ɛ i]

TABLE 7.4 SCORING FOR OCCURRENCE OF PHONOLOGICAL PATTERNS

Target Word	Transcription	Syllable Reduction	Final Consonant Deletion	Stopping	Velar Fronting	Liquid Simplification	
						Gliding	Vowelization
sun	[t ʌ]		X				
bicycle	[t ɪ k oʊ]	X		X			X
house	[h aʊ]		X	X			
shoe	[t u]			X			
dishes	[d ɪ t ə]		X	X			
fish	[p ɪ]		X	X			
light	[w aɪ]		X			X	
balloon	[l u]	X	X				
bell	[b ɛ]		X				
red	[w ɛ]		X			X	
carry	[t ɛ w i]				X	X	
deer	[d i ɔ]						X

PRACTICE: EXERCISE 7.3

This exercise consists of sample responses to phonological test items. Check those patterns that appear to have occurred for each response. Refer to **Tables 7.3** and **7.4** in completing this exercise. Remember that more than one pattern can affect a phoneme or word. When you are finished, check your answers against the answer key in Appendix C.

Children with Limited Language Output

Some young preschoolers may have extremely limited language output and may be unable to respond to a standardized test. For example, they may communicate in one- and two-word utterances only, with many of their productions sounding the same. The author once had a 2-year, 9-month-old preschool patient who produced [h ʌ] for several different words (including *sun*, *house*, and *thumb*). *Boy*, *ball*, *baby*, and *big* were all produced as [b ʌ] or [b ɑ]. If a word contained a nasal phoneme, all other consonants became nasals (nasal assimilation); for example, *barn* was produced as [m ɑ n]. He never used more than two syllables in an utterance and obviously had an extremely limited phoneme repertoire. In cases like this it is necessary to transcribe the child's output and analyze it for comparison with developmental norms.

Sample Transcription

Any test responses and a conversational sample should be transcribed during the evaluation. For highly unintelligible children, it can help to use a book or familiar toys to collect the sample. In this way, you know what the child is talking about and you will be better able to record speech.

The evaluation should be video- or audio-recorded. Live transcription enables you to take advantage of all cues, auditory and visual. It is crucial to watch the patient as the words are produced and transcribe the response as accurately as possible. For children with phonological disorders and highly unintelligible speech, it can be extremely helpful to **gloss** each response, that is, to repeat the word they produced (Bauman-Waengler, 2012). For example, if the child says [aʊ t] for *house*, you would say, "Right, it's a *house*." Notice that you do not repeat the child's production but the intended test word. Later, as you review your taped sample, the glosses will help you interpret any responses that may be difficult to understand, ensuring that your transcription is accurate. Accurate transcription is a necessity for analysis of a speech sound disorder and for establishing treatment goals.

ANALYSIS

The analysis method used depends on a variety of factors, including the patient's age, language level, and type of speech sound disorder. The analysis time required for an older patient with an articulation disorder is generally much less than that needed for a preschooler with a phonological problem. Analysis of an articulation problem is generally less time-consuming than that of a phonological disorder. As previously mentioned, errors may be analyzed in terms of substitutions, omissions, distortions, and additions or as phonological patterns. In general, standardized test responses are part of a **relational analysis**, comparing the patient's productions with the expected adult model.

Children with limited language require a more detailed analysis than that found on a typical articulation test. For highly unintelligible children or children at very low language levels, **independent analysis** may be necessary to set appropriate goals. An independent analysis is based on the child's conversational speech without regard to the phonemes expected in the adult model. It can reveal a number of important characteristics of the child's speech, including speech sound inventory, syllable and word shapes, and any sequential limitations/rules demonstrated by the child (Bernthal, Bankson, & Flipsen, 2013; Stoel-Gammon & Dunn, 1985). For example, an independent analysis of the speech of the author's previously mentioned 2-year, 9-month old patient would include the following:

Consonant inventory:	/b/ (initial/prevocalic)
	/m/ (initial/prevocalic)
	/n/ (final/postvocalic)
Vowel inventory:	/ʌ/ /ɑ/
Syllable shapes:	CV, CVC
Constraints:	nasal assimilation in words containing nasal consonants

See **Table 7.5** for additional examples of independent analyses.

TABLE 7.5 INDEPENDENT ANALYSIS OF RESPONSES

Word	Transcription	Consonants (I) (M) (F)	Vowels	Syllable Structure
dog	[d ɑ]	d	ɑ	CV
cat	[d æ]	d	æ	CV
spoon	[b u]	b	u	CV
knife	[n ɑ p]	n p	ɑ	CVC
fork	[b ɑ]	b	ɑ	CV
doll	[d ɑ]	d	ɑ	CV
baby	[b ɑ b ɑ]	b b	ɑ	CVCV
eyes	[ɑ]		ɑ	V
nose	[n oʊ]	n	oʊ	CV
ears	[i]		i	V

Summary:

Vowel inventory:	/i u æ ɑ oʊ/	Syllable shapes:	
Consonant inventory:	/b d n/ (Initial)	V	2
	/b/ Medial	CV	6
	/p/ (Final)	CVC	1
		CVCV	1

Note: The stimulus words used in this table are characteristic of words often elicited from children who are unable to respond to a conventional test.

PRACTICE: EXERCISE 7.4

This exercise is designed to help you analyze patient responses in terms of phonemes produced, position, and syllable structure. Refer to **Table 7.5** as you complete this exercise. Then compare your answers to those in the answer key in Appendix C.

DEVELOPMENTAL NORMS

Numerous studies have been conducted to identify the ages of phoneme acquisition (Otomo & Stoel-Gammon, 1992; Porter & Hodson, 2001; Prather, Hedrick, & Kern, 1975; Sander, 1972; Smit et al, 1990; Stoel-Gammon, 1985, 1987; Templin, 1957) and dissolution of phonological patterns (Grunwell, 1982; Haelsig & Madison, 1986; Hodson & Paden, 1981; Ingram, 1976; Lowe et al, 1985). Other useful research studies have investigated acquisition of syllable shapes (Dodd, 1995; Flipsen, 2006; Stoel-Gammon, 1985; Watson & Scukanec, 1997a,b). These norms indicate ages of mastery for vowels and consonants and are designed to provide a reference for determination of normalcy of a patient's speech sound development. **Table 7.6** compares several key studies; you will notice that mastery of the speech sound system is generally complete by age 8. Thus, any consistent errors past that age indicate a speech sound disorder. (This does not include productions that reflect dialectic variation.) As you look at **Table 7.6,** be aware that studies can differ in how they define "mastery." All the studies cited were **cross-sectional** and based on single-word responses. In a cross-sectional study, different groups of children at specific age levels are tested, and results are taken as evidence of phoneme mastery for each age group.

Results of relational analysis can be examined in a variety of ways, including type of error; word position; place, manner, and voicing contrasts; and use of phonological patterns. The speech of a patient with a simple articulation problem does not require phonological pattern analysis, but the speech of a patient with a phonological problem does.

TABLE 7.6 AGES (IN YEARS) FOR MASTERY OF CONSONANT SOUNDS BY MANNER OF ARTICULATION: SELECTED RESEARCH STUDIES

Researcher(s)	Chronological Age				
	<3-0	4-0	5-0	6-0	7-0
Arlt et al (1976)[1]	m n ŋ w p b t d k g h f	v s z ʒ ʧ ʤ l	θ ð ʃ ɹ		
Prather et al (1975)[2]	m n ŋ w j p b t d k g h f s	v θ ð z ʒ ʧ ʤ			
Smit et al (1990)[3]	m n w p b t d k g h f	ŋ j v ʃ ʧ ʤ	ð	θ s z l	
Templin (1957)[4]	m n ŋ w p h f	j b d k g ɹ	s ʧ ʤ	t v θ l	z ʒ ð ʤ

Note: Studies varied in ages studied and criteria for "mastery."
[1]Cross-sectional study conducted with 240 children in the U.S. for half-year intervals from ages 3-0 to 5.
[2]Cross-sectional study conducted with 147 children in the U.S. between ages 2 and 4.
[3]Cross-sectional study conducted with 997 children in the U.S. ranging in age from 3-0 to 9-0.
[4]Cross-sectional study conducted with 480 children in the U.S. between ages 3 and 8.

There are several key questions to be answered in determining if a speech sound disorder exists:

1. Does the patient produce all the phonemes expected for her or his chronological age?
2. Does the patient still use any phonological rules (e.g., final consonant deletion) that are not age-appropriate?
3. How understandable (intelligible) in the patient?

Intelligibility refers to understandability. It does not necessarily mean that all sounds are produced correctly. Children's speech intelligibility grows throughout the preschool and early school-age period. A 36-month-old should be understandable to outside listeners at least 50% of the time. The speech of a kindergartener should be 100% understandable. The number of error sounds or use of age-inappropriate patterns, accompanied by poor intelligibility, are key indicators of a need for treatment.

TREATMENT

The type of treatment for a patient with a speech sound disorder depends on a variety of factors, including types of errors, patterns, intelligibility, and etiology. **Etiology** refers to the cause of the speech sound disorder. In general, simple articulation disorders can be treated using a phonetic treatment approach that is based on motor-based intervention (McDonald, 1964; Secord, 1989; Van Riper & Erickson, 1996; Winitz, 1975, 1984). Some, but not all, phonetic approaches also include auditory training/ear training. The patient learns to identify the phoneme, for example /s/ or /l/, in isolation and then in progressively larger units, and finally learns to distinguish correct sound production from incorrect production in words. All phonetic methods include production training. The patient is shown where and how to place the articulators to produce the correct phoneme. A series of steps to production mastery follows, usually starting with the isolated phoneme, then syllable production, word production, and so on. The final goal is carryover of the new sound into conversational speech.

Linguistic, or rule-based, approaches to treatment are used for patients with phonological disorders. A number of approaches have been devised (Gierut, 1990, 2001; Hodson & Paden, 1991; Howell & Dean, 1991; Weiner, 1981; Williams, 2000a,b, 2003). Rather than focusing on motoric production of a single phoneme, they emphasize the meaning signaled by a phoneme or group of phonemes. For example, a child who deletes final consonants may learn to listen and then produce words that differ in final consonant production, for example *bow-boat*, *E-eat*, or *pie-pipe*. A child who reduces consonant clusters may listen to and then produce word pairs like this: *pot-spot*, *pie-spy*, *pill-spill*. The advantage of these phonemic treatment methods is that they promote generalization of correct production to groups of sounds, rather than a single phoneme (typical of phonetic methods). Consequently, they are more effective and time efficient for children with phonological disorders.

Etiology of speech sound disorders can also affect how treatment is structured and delivered. A child with a hearing loss requires amplification as part of treatment.

For a patient with **childhood apraxia of speech (CAS)**, work on sequencing and transitioning of phonemes may receive primary emphasis. In addition to all the speech tests previously described, speech-language pathologists also perform a **hearing screening** and **oral mechanism exam** to determine possible etiological factors of the problem. A hearing screening is a brief test designed to determine if a patient's hearing is within normal limits for speech acquisition and production. In an oral mechanism exam, the speech-language pathologist determines if there are any structural or functional problems that appear to be contributing to the problem. The results are incorporated into the design of the patient's treatment plan.

PHONOLOGICAL AWARENESS

One additional consideration should be mentioned in discussing speech sound disorders. It concerns children with phonological disorders whose intelligibility is very poor. Research studies have indicated that such children can be at risk for reading problems because of poor **phonological awareness skills** (Foy & Mann, 2001; Mann & Foy, 2007; Nathan, Stackhouse, Goulandris, & Snowling, 2004; Rvachew, Ohberg, Grawburg, & Heyding, 2003; Schuele, 2004; Stackhouse & Snowling, 1992). This is especially true when a child also has additional language difficulties (Bird, Bishop, & Freeman, 1995; Catts, Fey, Tomblin, & Zhang, 2002; Larrivee & Catts, 1999; Snowling, Bishop, & Stothard, 2000). Phonological awareness refers to the ability to deal with language components apart from meaning. Rhyming is a phonological awareness skill that develops in preschool and is highly correlated with later reading success. Additional examples of phonological awareness skills include identifying beginning and ending sounds in words or blending sounds together for reading. A child who tells you that a bird can fly is demonstrating basic vocabulary (meaning) skills, but if she can also tell you that *bird* rhymes with *word* and begins with the /b/ sound, then she also has developed some basic phonological awareness skills (rhyming and sound segmentation). Similarly, a child who can tell you that a banana is something to eat (vocabulary) and that *banana* has three syllables (syllable segmentation skills) is showing you his mastery of certain phonological awareness skills.

When a child is enrolled in treatment for a phonological disorder, phonological awareness should also be assessed. Of course, the level of assessment depends on the child's age. Some experts have recommended that phonological awareness work should be implemented as the child's speech becomes more intelligible (Hodson, 1994; Stackhouse, 1992). The author has supervised treatment for a large number of children with phonological disorders over her career. Preschoolers with phonological disorders are regularly evaluated for rhyming and segmentation skills. When possible, rhyming is incorporated into treatment. At first the emphasis may be on exposure to rhyme, with the clinician reading a rhyming book as part of the session and then giving it to the child to take home to read with the family. Later, rhyming may be integrated into treatment discussions. For example, work on final consonant deletion of /t/ can also note that words rhyme, for example *eat*, *meat*, and *seat*. Or work on cluster/consonant sequence reduction can also include comments about rhyme, for example *nail* and *snail*, *pie* and *spy*. Once again, knowledge of phonetics, phonology, and phonotactics are important skills to help carry out this type of work.

ENGLISH-LANGUAGE LEARNERS AND SPEAKERS OF ENGLISH AS A SECOND LANGUAGE

This section addresses two primary areas of concern: preschool and school-aged children whose native language is not English, and adult ESL speakers. Depending on the child's degree of perceived English proficiency, a concern may be expressed that the child has a speech and language disorder, not just a dialect difference. In these cases, a speech-language pathologist is a primary player in assessment and must be careful to differentiate speech characteristics that may signal a difference, a disorder, or both. Both of the child's languages must be considered and assessed in determining if a disorder exists. If only dialectic differences appear to be involved, therapy is not necessary.

A different concern applies to adult ESL speakers, depending on their degree of English proficiency in vocabulary, syntax, and morphology. Sometimes these speakers encounter difficulty in being understood by native mainstream American English speakers. They may feel that their "accent" is interfering with their effectiveness in their job or career. In some cases, they are encouraged to seek services by their employers. Although these speakers are not considered to have a speech disorder, speech-language pathologists can and do offer elective services in accent reduction. A thorough understanding of English phonetics and phonemes in the ESL speaker's native language is crucial to effective work with these speakers.

ENGLISH LANGUAGE LEARNERS

As mentioned previously in this chapter and in Chapter 6, children and adults who are bilingual may have difficulty expressing themselves in English or being understood by monolingual American English speakers. It is not unusual for preschool and school-aged non–English-speaking and primarily Spanish-speaking children to be referred for speech-language evaluation. It is the responsibility of the speech-language pathologist to conduct a fair and accurate assessment in these cases. A detailed discussion is not within the scope of this book, but it is important that future speech-language pathologists, educators, and ESL teachers understand the basic considerations and knowledge necessary to accurately differentiate between bilingual children who do or do not have a speech or language disorder.

Contrary to what might be expected, research has shown that a child acquiring more than one language is not more likely to have a speech sound disorder. Instead, the bilingual child's phonological development tends to be commensurate with that of the monolingual child (Fabiano-Smith & Goldstein, 2010; Gildersleeve-Neumann & Wright, 2010; Goldstein & Washington, 2001; Goldstein, Fabiano, & Washington, 2005; Holm & Dodd, 2000). What does happen is that the languages influence each other (Goldstein, 2007; Goldstein & McLeod, 2012). Phonemes or allophones of one language may be substituted for those of another, for example. Final consonant usage in English might be initially limited to those consonants that occur in the final position of words in the first language (Cheng, 1987). In addition to language-specific influences, there are other influences on a bilingual child's development of English. These include length of exposure to English, language spoken in the home, the first language dialect, and the English speakers encountered by the child.

A detailed speech and language assessment is necessary for these children, just as it is for monolingual children. Culture-fair testing requires that a bilingual child be tested in the dominant language or in both languages (Goldstein, 2006). Very few tests are available for this type of work. If the speech-language pathologist is not bilingual, then a trained interpreter should be used to help conduct the testing (Kayser, 1995; Langdon & Cheng, 2002). In determining if there is a speech sound disorder, the speech-language pathologist must also be knowledgeable about any relevant research in the developing phonology of non-English languages as well as the characteristics of monolingual speakers of the child's first language (Goldstein & Iglesias, 2009).

Following a thorough speech assessment, the speech-language pathologist develops treatment goals and determines which treatment approach to use. These decisions help the practitioner decide which language to focus on. Two primary approaches have been suggested for treatment with bilingual children with speech sound disorders: **bilingual approach** and **cross-linguistic approach** (Kohnert & Derr, 2005; Kohnert, Yim, Nett, Kan, & Duran, 2005). The speech-language pathologist who uses a bilingual approach focuses on sounds or patterns common to both languages. With a cross-linguistic approach, more language-specific targets are emphasized. Within each type, phonetic and phonemic approaches that are used with English-speaking children may be adapted to bilingual children (Goldstein & Iglesias, 2013).

ACCENT REDUCTION

It is not unusual for adult ESL speakers to encounter difficulty communicating with native English speakers because of differences in pronunciation. The ESL speakers may not use English phonemes that do not occur in their native language or may substitute sounds from their first language into English. (Remember learning about characteristics often found in the speech of different ESL speakers in Chapter 6.) In addition, ESL speakers may pronounce all vowels as full vowels, rather than employing the stress reduction to /ə/ characteristic of native American English speakers. Thus, *television* may be produced as [t ɛ l ɛ v ɪ ʒ ɪ n] rather than [t ɛ l ə v ɪ ə ʒ ə n]. The result can be interference with the prosody of English, which also makes the speaker harder to understand. The regional English dialect also affects the speech characteristics of the ESL speaker.

Speech characteristics are only one of the considerations in offering work in accent reduction. The speech-language pathologist must consider the individual's language history, current pronunciation, life demands for clear English, and interest and motivation to change pronunciation. The way we speak is very much a part of our identity; changing our speech entails also changing our identity.

Although *accent reduction* is the term commonly used to refer to such work with ESL speakers, a better term might be *accent expansion*. The goal is to expand the speakers' speech awareness and speech skills to sound "more American" but not to totally change the way ESL speakers sound. ESL speakers may strive to be better understood in the work environment but may not wish to change for other communication settings. That is their prerogative. The primary concern is to help ESL speakers become effective communicators who are comfortable with their speaking ability.

VOICE AND DICTION TRAINING

This type of training is provided by clinicians who work with a variety of professionals who need to communicate more clearly and effectively, with ESL speakers, and sometimes with professional performers such as actors and actresses. Sometimes speech-language pathologists offer these services, but they may also be delivered by individuals specifically trained in accent, communication, and linguistics. Once again, knowledge of phonetics and phonology is extremely helpful for effective work in this area.

CONCLUSION

The importance of knowing the IPA and using phonetic transcription is not limited to speech-language pathologists. Linguists, ESL teachers, voice and diction coaches, and other professionals who work with oral speech often find it necessary to use the IPA. Phoneticians also make extensive use of the IPA across a variety of languages. The IPA provides a common "code" for different professionals to discuss speech and language concepts when different languages share the same or similar sounds. It is an invaluable tool for anyone who works with oral communication.

CONCEPT QUESTIONS

PART I

Are the following statements true or false?

_____ 1. Only speech-language pathologists need to know how to transcribe using the IPA.

_____ 2. Speech sound disorders consist of articulation disorders and phonological disorders.

_____ 3. Speech assessment procedures and analyses for adults are exactly like those used with children.

_____ 4. Phonological testing is not necessary for children with just one or two sounds in error.

_____ 5. Depending on a patient's age and language level, administration of a standardized articulation test may not be possible.

_____ 6. Speech sound assessment should include both word and conversational sampling.

_____ 7. Children who are bilingual should be tested in both languages.

_____ 8. Patients who speak English as a second language should be required to have therapy to make them better understood.

_____ 9. An interpreter may be necessary to help test bilingual children.

_____ 10. A patient who produces *Sue* as *shue* has a distortion error.

PART II: RECORDING SPEECH SOUND ERRORS

For the following speech sample, transcribe the error and indicate the position in which it occurs. The first example is completed for you.

Test Phoneme	Stimulus Word	Production	Error/Position(s)
/k/	**c**up	[t ʌ p]	
	ro**ck**et	[w ɑ t ə t]	
	ra**k**e	[w e t]	
			t/k (I, M, F)
/g/	**g**um	[d ʌ m]	
	wa**g**on	[w æ d ə n]	
	pi**g**	[p ɪ g]	
			_____
/ʧ/	**ch**air	[ʃ ɛ ə]	
	ma**tch**es	[m æ ʧ ə z]	
	wa**tch**	[w ɑ ʃ]	
			_____
/ʒ/	trea**s**ure	[t w ɛ ɚ]	
	gara**g**e	[g ə w ɑ d]	
			_____

PART III. IDENTIFICATION OF PHONOLOGICAL PATTERN USAGE

For the following speech sample, indicate which of the selected phonological processes/patterns are used in each word. Remember, you must account for all sound changes in each word. The first example has been completed for you.

Target Word	Transcription	Final Consonant Deletion	Stopping	Velar Fronting	Gliding
cup	[t ʌ]	X		X	
rocket	[w ɑ t ɪ]				
rake	[w eɪ]				
gum	[d ʌ]				
wagon	[w æ d ə]				
pig	[p ɪ]				
sun	[t ʌ]				
bicycle	[b aɪ t ɪ t ə]				
house	[h aʊ]				
shoe	[t u]				

What process occurred most often in this sample?

GLOSSARY

Abduction   The structures drawn apart from midline; for example, when the vocal folds are abducted, the glottis is open; adjective, abducted

Abutting consonants   Elements of a consonant sequence that cross a syllable boundary

Accent   (1) The stress applied to a syllable in a word (suprasegmental term); see **Word stress**; (2) the phonological characteristics of a dialect

Acoustic phonetics   The study of acoustic features of speech and their relationship to speech production and speech perception

Addition   Type of speech error in which a phoneme is added to a word

Adduction   The structures drawn together toward midline; for example, when the vocal folds are adducted, the glottis is closed; adjective, adducted

Affricate   A consonant produced by release of a stop into a fricative position as a single speech sound; English affricate consonants are /ʧ/ and /ʤ/

African-American vernacular English (AAVE)   A cultural dialect used by many, but not all, African Americans, depending on listeners and communicative situation

Allophone   Variations within a phoneme class; heard as one and the same phoneme

Alveolar flap/tap   The allophone of singleton /t/ and/or /d/ in the intervocalic position

Alveolar ridge   The prominent ridge behind maxillary incisors and cuspid (canine) teeth (adjective: alveolar)

Alveoli   Located in **alveolar sacs** (termination of alveolar ducts) in lungs; site of actual exchange of oxygen and carbon dioxide

Apex (of tongue)   The anterior end of the tongue

Appalachian English   The regional dialect used by speakers in the Appalachian region of the United States, now considered as a variant of Southern English

Approximants   Consonants produced by alterations of resonating cavities; two subdivisions: liquids and glides

Approximation   Position of closeness of speech organs; the vocal folds are approximated for phonation

Articulation   The shaping of outgoing breath stream into the sounds of speech

Articulation disorder   Consistent misarticulation of a phoneme or phonemes, related to motoric difficulty in producing speech sounds; see Phonetic Disorder

Articulation test   Test instrument designed to assess phoneme production in words and/or sentences to determine phoneme mastery; see Phonetic test

Arytenoid cartilages   Small, pyramidal-shaped cartilages that rest on top of the posterior portion of cricoid cartilage; they form movable, posterior attachments for the vocal folds

Asian/Pacific Islander-Influenced English   The English used by speakers whose first language is an Asian language; characteristics depend on Asian language of origin and a variety of other factors

Aspiration phase   The audible release of breath, as with the [p] in *pot*

Assimilation   (1) A change in a phoneme in place, manner, or voicing due to the effect of a neighboring sound; (2) conforming of one sound to the manner or place of articulation of a neighboring sound

Audition   Hearing

Back Vowels   Vowels produced with varying elevation of the posterior portion of the tongue relative to the palato-velar junction

Bilabial   Referring to consonants made with both lips, especially /p/, /b/, and /m/

Bilabial assimilation   A coarticulatory effect in which a non-bilabial consonant shifts to a bilabial consonant in the context of another bilabial in a word

Bilingual approach   Method of instruction for English language learners which uses both the native language and English

Bisyllabic   Referring to words consisting of two syllables

Blade (of tongue)   The part of the tongue dorsum immediately behind the tip; also known as the front of the tongue

Blends   A consonant sequence in which two or more consonants are contained in a syllable with no intervening vowel

Broad transcription   In the International Phonetic Alphabet (IPA), transcription not sensitive to allophonic variation, also known as phonemic transcription, enclosed in virgules (/ /)

Bronchiole   Smaller branch of bronchus

Bronchus (pl. bronchi)   A large air passage in the lungs; the primary, paired bronchi connect the trachea and the secondary bronchi

Centering Diphthongs   Diphthongs with /ɚ/ as the offglide portion

Central Vowels   Vowels produced with varying levels of elevation in central part of oral cavity.

Chain shifts (dialectic)   A change in vowel production characteristics that results in successive changes in other vowels; they affect vowel systems

Closed syllable   A syllable ending in a consonant, for example CVC (consonant–vowel–consonant) or VC (vowel–consonant)

Coarticulation   The influence of one speech sound upon the manner of production or place of articulation of a neighboring sound

Coda   In the context of a syllable, the consonants that follow the vowel nucleus

Code-switching   Alternating back and forth between two dialects, especially mainstream English and African-American vernacular English, but also occurs with regional dialects

Cognate   Consonants which share the same place and manner but differ in voicing

Consonant   A phoneme used marginally with a vowel to constitute a syllable; characterized by narrowing or blockage of the airstream

Consonant sequence   Two or more consonants contained with no intervening vowel; may be abutting consonants or blends.

Consonant sequence reduction   Loss of one more phonemes in a consonant sequence

Contiguous assimilation   A phoneme that changes place, manner, or voicing due to the influence of a phoneme immediately adjacent to it

Contrastive stress   A change in syllable stress in a bisyllabic word that affects the meaning

Cricoid cartilage   The ring-shaped base/most inferior cartilage of the larynx; arytenoid cartilages are positioned on top of its posterior expanded portion

Cultural dialect   A dialect associated with a particular cultural group, for example African-American vernacular English

Cycle   In phonation, vocal fold adduction → opening (puff of air released—vocal fold abduction); measured in hertz

De-accenting   A change in vowel identify (often to /ə/) in syllables that do not have a primary accent

Dental   Referring to the teeth; (inter)dental consonants are produced with the tongue tip against or between the teeth

Dentalization   The assimilation effect in which alveolar phonemes adjacent to a dental /θ/ or /ð/ shift to the dental place of articulation

Developmental phonology   The study of the acquisition of speech sounds in children and the rules governing their usage

Devoicing   The assimilation effect on glides and liquids in two-element pre-vocalic consonant sequences; a voiced phoneme becomes voiceless in this context

Diacritic markings   Special transcription modification markers, used to indicate allophonic variations

Dialect   A set of phonological, morphological, and syntactic characteristics of a particular way of speaking American English

Dialect deficit view   An outdated view that dialects vary in prestige and acceptability; not accepted by various professional organizations that study dialect

Dialect sociolinguistic view   The view that a dialect is a legitimate linguistic variation the serves a communicative function with a person's language community

Diaphragm   The primary muscle of inhalation; it is dome shaped, and separates the abdominal and thoracic cavities

Digraphs   An alphabetic letter combination representing a single phoneme; for example, *sh* represents the phoneme /ʃ/

Diphthongs   Vowels characterized by a change in tongue position during production, from a longer onglide position to a shorter offglide position; See also centering diphthongs and rising diphthongs.

Distinctive features   Binary acoustic and articulatory characteristics which can be used to distinguish both consonants and vowels

Distortion   A speech sound error in which a nonstandard speech sound replaces a standard speech sound

Dorsum (tongue)   The upper surface of the tongue

Ebonics   See **African-American vernacular English**

Egressive   Outgoing; refers to the airstream in exhalation

Elision   The omission of one or a few consonants as a result of coarticulation

Emphasis/sentence stress   The stress applied to a word in a phrase

English as a second language (ESL) speaker   Speaker of English who has learned English as another language after the native language; also referred to as English as Other Language speaker

Epenthesis   The addition of a sound or syllable to a word

Ethnic dialect   A dialect associated with a particular ethnic background

Etiology   Referring to the cause of a speech sound disorder

Exhalation   The expulsion of air from the lungs, which provides an outgoing airstream for speech; the second part of a respiratory cycle

Final consonant deletion   Refers to the omission of a speech sound or sounds occurring at the end of a word

Final position   Refers to speech sound or sounds at the end of a word; also known as postvocalic position

Formal standard English   A dialect characteristic of formal English grammar texts and English usage references, used most frequently in writing; cf. **Informal standard English**

Fricative   A consonant manner of articulation; a phoneme produced with audible friction as a result of narrowing of the vocal tract at some point; English fricative consonants are /f/, /v/, /θ/, /ð/, /s/, /z/, /ʃ/, /ʒ/, and /h/

Front Vowels   Vowels produced with the front or the blade of the tongue at varying heights in relation to the anterior palate

Fundamental frequency (F_o)   In reference to the voice, the rate at which the glottis opens and closes, measured in hertz (Hz); during phonation, it is heard by the listener as the pitch of the voice

Glide   A consonant manner of articulation, produced by an initial narrowing of the vocal tract followed by transition into the following vowel; English glides are /j/ and /w/

Gliding   A phonological pattern in which a liquid is replaced by a glide

Glottal stop   The abrupt release of air at the glottis in connected speech; transcription symbol /ʔ/

Glottis   The space between the vocal folds; may be open or closed (adjective: glottal)

Haplology   The omission of a whole syllable, typically occurring when two very similar syllables follow in close succession

Hard palate   Hard, bony portion of the roof of the mouth connecting posteriorly with the muscular soft palate

Harmonics   The overtones of fundamental frequency

Hearing screening   A brief audiologic test to determine if hearing is within normal limits for speech development

Hertz (Hz)   Unit of measure of the frequency of vibration or the number of vibratory cycles per second

High vowels   Vowels produced tongue position close to, but not touching the palate; include /i ɪ u ʊ/

Homorganic   Made in the same place/with the same articulator position

Hyoid bone   A bone that does not directly articulate (form a joint with) any other bone but that is held in position by muscles and connective tissues; the larynx is suspended from it (adjectival prefix: hyo-)

Incisors   Eight teeth (four maxillary, four mandibular) used for cutting; there are two central incisors and two lateral incisors per jaw

Independent analysis   A type of speech analysis in which all phonemes and words produced are analyzed regardless of the intended target sound

Informal standard English   A dialect based on general impressions of a standard within a speaker's community

Inhalation   The drawing of air into the lungs, the result of the action of the diaphragm and elastic forces; the first part of a respiratory cycle

Initial position   Refers to speech sound or sounds occurring at the beginning of a word; also referred to as prevocalic

Intelligibility   Refers to understandability of speech

Intensity   With regard to vocal fold vibration, the amount of displacement of folds; perceived as loudness

Intercostal muscles   The muscles of respiration attached to the ribs, involved in inhalation (external intercostals) and exhalation (internal intercostals)

Interdental   Referring to consonants made with the tongue placed between the teeth, for example /θ/ and /ð/

International Phonetic Alphabet (IPA)   A symbol system in which any phoneme used in a language or across languages has one, and only one, symbol

Intervocalic   Referring to the position of a consonant (C) singleton or sequence that occurs between two vowels (V), for example, VCV, VCCV

Intervocalic voicing   An assimilation effect in which a voiceless consonant in the intervocalic position takes on voicing due to the voicing of the vowels surrounding it

Intonation   Pitch variations within a phrase

Intonation contours   The pattern of pitch variations of intonation, including the degree, direction, and rate of pitch change

Intonational phrase   Two or more words characterized by an intonation contour

Juncture   The transition point between words and phrases

Labial   Referring to the lips; bilabial (both lips), labiodental (lips and teeth)

Labial assimilation   A coarticulatory effect in which a nonlabial consonant shifts to a labial consonant in the context of another labial consonant in a word

Labiodental   Referring to consonants produced with upper incisors contacting lower lip, for example /f/ and /v/

Language difference   Dialectic variation which is valid within its language community

Laryngo-/laryngeal   Referring to the larynx

Laryngopharynx   That portion of the pharynx surrounding the larynx

Larynx   The organ of phonation, containing vocal folds and attached by muscles to the hyoid bone

Lateral   A consonant phoneme in which the voiced airstream escapes around the sides of the tongue; the English lateral is /l/; also see **Liquid**

Lingua-/lingual   Referring to the tongue

Lingual frenum   The tissue connecting the front part of tongue to the floor of the oral cavity/mandible

Lingual septum   Internal midline of the tongue, composed of connective tissue

Liquid   Consonant phonemes produced with the tongue acting as an obstacle to the outgoing voiced breath stream; English liquids are /ɹ/ and /l/

Lisp   A problem in articulating the phoneme /s/

Loudness   Refers to perceived intensity of speech; related to degree of vocal fold displacement with greater intensity perceived as greater loudness

Low vowels   Vowels formed with tongue in low position, regardless of front-back location in the oral cavity

Mainstream English (ME)   A form of American English most commonly used in textbooks and in national broadcast media; also known as general American English or standard American English

Mandible   The lower jaw (adjective: mandibular)

Manner of articulation   The way the voiced or voiceless airstream is modified to produce different types of consonants, for example stops and fricatives

Maxilla   The upper jaw (adjective: maxillary)

Medial position   Speech sound or sounds occurringebetweenels; also termed intervocalic

Mergers (dialectic)   A factor that affects dialects; distinctions between two phonemes may be lost so that only one sound is used; it especially effects vowels

Mid vowels   Vowels produced with tongue elevation at mid height in the oral cavity, regardless of front-back position

Minimal pair   Words that differ by only one phoneme

Monophthong   Vowel produced with one, unchanging articulatory position

Morpheme   The smallest unit of phonological form(s) that signals a difference in meaning

Narrow transcription   In IPA, transcribing in phoneme symbols plus modifying markers to indicate variations in production, also known as phonetic transcription, enclosed in brackets ([ ])

Nasal   Referring to the nose or nasal cavity; consonant manner of articulation

Nasal assimilation   The result of coarticulation in which a nonnasal consonant becomes nasal due to the presence of another nasal consonant in the word

Nasal cavity   The nose, bounded by the nostrils and pharynx (anterior-posterior) and by the palate and base of the skull (inferior-superior)

Nasal consonant   Manner of articulation; consonants are produced with the lowering of the soft palate and closure within the oral cavity, allowing for a nasal airflow of the voiced breath stream; English nasals are /m/, /n/, and /ŋ/

Nasopharynx   The portion of the pharynx posterior to the nasal cavity

New England American English (NEE)   The regional dialect used by speakers in the northeastern United States

Noncontiguous assimilation   A consonant change in place, manner, or voicing caused by a nonadjacent consonant

Nonlinguistic speech aspects   The aspects of meaning beyond the phoneme level, including pitch, intonation, and tempo

Offglide   Shorter, second portion of a diphthong

Omission   Speech sound error in which a phoneme is deleted

Onglide   Longer, first portion of a diphthong

Onset   In a syllable, all consonants preceding the syllable nucleus; not a required element of a syllable

Open syllable   A syllable lacking a coda, ending in a vowel, for example CV, CCV

Oral   Adjective referring to the oral cavity

Oral cavity   The mouth, bounded by the lips and pharynx (anterior-posterior) and by the mandible and palate (inferior-superior)

Oropharynx   Portion of pharynx posterior to the oral cavity

Orthography   The commonly accepted spelling of language using alphabet letters

Palate (hard)   The hard, bony portion of the roof of the mouth, dividing the oral cavity from the nasal cavity (adjective: palatal)

Pause   A silent interval between phrases

Pharyngeal cavity (pharynx)   The throat; that part of the vocal tract bounded by the larynx and by the oral and nasal cavities; it has three subdivisions: laryngo-pharynx, oropharynx, and nasopharynx

Phonation   Vocal fold vibration in the larynx

Phoneme   An abstract class of speech sounds containing common elements and influencing the meaning of speech

Phonemic   Having the characteristic of a phoneme by virtue of influencing the meaning of speech

Phonemic accent   A change in the primary accent of a syllable changes the word's meaning

Phonemic transcription   See **broad transcription**

Phonemic treatment   Rule-based treatment method for phonological disorders

Phonetic disorder   Speech sound disorder associated with motoric difficulty in producing sounds; see articulation disorder

Phonetic transcription   See **narrow transcription**

Phonetic treatment   Treatment for speech sound disorders emphasizing production of individual speech sounds

Phonetics   The science devoted to the study of speech sounds of a language

Phonological awareness   Ability to analyze language into smaller components, e.g. sentences → words, words → syllables, words → individual sounds

Phonological processes   In normal and disordered speech, patterns that can affect sound production, including syllable structure processes and assimilation processes

Phonology   Study of how speech sounds are combined to create meaning

Phonotactics   Rules for combining sounds into syllables and words

Phrase   A continuous utterance bounded by silent intervals

Phrasing   Organizing flowing speech into phrases

Physiological phonetics   Branch of phonetics with emphasis on the physical structures and physiology of speech sound production

Pitch   The perception of fundamental frequency; faster frequency corresponds perceptually to higher pitch

Place of articulation   Refers to position of articulators in consonant formation

Postvocalic   Referring to the syllable or word position of a consonant or consonant sequence that follows a vowel

Prevocalic   Refers to consonant position at the beginning of a word or syllable

Primary accent   The syllable in a word that is produced with the greatest physiological force; may be perceived as being longer, louder, and higher in pitch

Progressive assimilation   The assimilatory effect in which the sound that changes is immediately adjacent to the sound causing the change

Prosody   The rhythm or "melody" of speech

Quality   Referring to voice, the distinctive sound resulting from a combination of a habitual range of fundamental frequency, blended with overtones amplified or subdued through resonation

Rate   The number of syllables or words per unit of time; see **Tempo**

Redundant   Having more information than is absolutely necessary for intelligibility

Regional dialect   A dialect associated with a particular geographic region of the United States

Regressive assimilation   An assimilation effect in which the phoneme that changes precedes the phoneme causing the change

Relational analysis   Type of speech sound analysis in which phonemes produced are compared to phonemes expected to determine possible presence of a speech sound disorder

Resonation   The process of modifying a sound by passing it through a cavity of air

Respiration   The process of moving airflow in and out of the lungs for breathing purposes and for speech

Retroflex   A bending backward of the tongue, especially applied to the tongue position for and retroflex /ɹ/

Rhotic   Referring to the positioning or influence of /ɹ/ or the vowels /ɝ/ and /ɚ/

Rhyme   The part of a syllable containing both a vowel nucleus and a coda

Rib cage   The bony framework encasing the lungs; movement involved in respiration

Rising diphthongs   Diphthongs which end in either the high front /ɪ/ position or high back /ʊ/ position

Secondary accent   A syllable accent level in multisyllabic words; the syllable is produced with less force than the syllable with the primary accent but with more force than the other, unaccented syllables in the word

Singleton consonant   Consonant not bounded by another consonant in a syllable or word

Soft palate   The soft muscular posterior one third of the roof of the mouth, attached to the hard palate; can be raised or lowered (adjective: velar)

Sonorant peak   A speech segment of maximum energy in a syllable, typically a vowel

Sonority   The relative loudness of speech sounds

Southern English (SE)   A regional dialect of speakers in the southern United States

Spanish-influenced English   The dialect(s) of English spoken by individuals whose native language is Spanish

Speech breathing   The quick inhalation and long, controlled exhalation that provides breath support for speech; cf. **Vegetative breathing**

Speech phrase   Continuous utterance bounded by "silent" intervals

Speech rhythm   A general term referring to the combined aspects of accent, emphasis, phrasing, intonation, and rate

Speech segments   Phonemes

Speech sound disorder   Failure to correctly produce the phonemes of a language; two types: articulation disorders and phonological disorders

Standard American English (SAE)   The American-English dialect characteristic of education and textbooks; also known as mainstream English (ME)

Stop   A consonant manner of articulation, in which a phoneme is produced with closure or stopping of the breath stream; air may or may not be released; English stops are /p/, /b/, /t/, /d/, /k/, and /g/

Stop phase   The first, necessary part of formation of a stop consonant in which air is compressed in the oral cavity; air release may or may not occur

Stopping   A phonological pattern in which a fricative or affricate is replaced by a stop

Stress   Pointing up or drawing special attention to a speech unit

Subglottal   Structures inferior to the glottis, for example the cricoid cartilage, trachea, and lungs

Subglottal pressure   In phonation, the buildup of air pressure beneath the approximated vocal folds

Sublaryngeal structures   The portions of the speech tract lying inferior to the laryngeal structures; consist of the lungs, bronchi, bronchioles, alveoli, and trachea; also known as the respiratory system

Substitution   Speech sound error in which a standard phoneme is replaced by another standard phoneme

Supraglottal structures   The structures lying superior to the glottis: the epiglottis, tongue, oral and nasal cavities

Suprasegmental features   The speech features over and above phoneme segments, especially aspects of speech rhythm

Syllabic consonant   A consonant that serves the function of a vowel as the nucleus of an unaccented syllable

Syllable   A cluster of coarticulated sounds with a single vowel or diphthong nucleus, with or without surrounding consonants

Syllable nucleus   The most prominent part of a syllable

Tempo   The suprasegmental aspect of speech, referring to speech timing or rate

Thyroid cartilage   The largest cartilage in the larynx, its halves are closed anteriorly and open posteriorly; anterior attachment point for vocal folds

Tongue   The primary organ of consonant and vowel articulation, consisting of both intrinsic and extrinsic muscles, capable of a large variety of movements (adjective: lingual)

Tongue apex   Anterior end of the tongue

Tongue dorsum   Upper surface of tongue

Tongue tip   The most anterior point of the tongue; used for articulation of many consonants

Trachea   The windpipe, composed of cartilaginous rings, connecting the larynx with the bronchi and lungs

Transliteration   Conversion of phonetic transcription into orthographic symbols

Trough   The portion of the syllable containing less energy, that is, the consonant(s)

Unaccented   Refers to the vowels in a multisyllabic word that are reduced to /ə/ as a result of de-stressing

Vegetative breathing   The breathing that is done for life support purposes; characterized by inhalation and exhalation of equal length

Velar assimilation   The type of assimilation in which a consonant shifts to a velar place of articulation due to the presence of another velar consonant in the word

Velopharyngeal port   The opening that connects the nasopharynx and the oropharynx

Velum   See **Soft Palate** (adjective: velar)

Vocal folds   The muscular shelves in the larynx, extending from the thyroid cartilage (anteriorly) to the arytenoid cartilages (posteriorly)

Voiced/voiceless   Refers to the presence/absence of vocal fold vibration; voiced sounds are produced with vocal fold vibration; voiceless sounds are produced without vocal fold vibration

Voicing   Refers to the presence of vocal fold vibration

Vowelization   Phonological pattern in which a postvocalic liquid is replaced by a vowel

Weak syllable deletion   A phonological pattern in which one or more syllables in a word is omitted

Word stress   The accent affecting a syllable within a word

APPENDIX A

CHAPTER EXERCISES

CHAPTER 1

After you have completed each exercise, you can check your answers against the answer key in Appendix C.

EXERCISE 1.1: DIGRAPHS: TWO LETTERS/ONE PHONEME

This exercise is designed to help you recognize single phonemes that are represented by digraphs in orthography. For each word in each row, mark the letters that constitute a digraph, representing a single phoneme. The first two rows emphasize consonant digraphs; the final two rows are for vowels only. For each set, the first word is marked for you as an example.

Consonants

<u>th</u>orn	wish	leather	chain	ring	photo	both
judge	other	laugh	sang	lock	bush	soothe

Vowels

b<u>oa</u>t	later	hoop	pouch	gain	nation	oiling
clown	bayou	bird	mouth	neigh	leash	found

EXERCISE 1.2: SAME LETTERS, DIFFERENT PHONEMES/SOUNDS

This exercise will help you listen for identical sounds across words with varied spellings. For this exercise, mark the one word in each line that has a phoneme that is different from the other five, even though the spelling is the same. Remember, the sound may be anywhere in the word. The first is completed for you in each set.

Consonants

chain	choose	<u>chord</u>	check	chill	child
sugar	lose	insure	conscience	reassure	blush
zinc	zoology	razor	brazier	daze	zap
Thomas	third	moth	thumb	earth	lath

Vowels

gown	wow	town	scowl	<u>pillow</u>	power
shoe	sloe	doe	hoed	toed	poet
mouse	lousy	mousse	loud	outside	pout
cart	tart	wart	karma	lark	farm

EXERCISE 1.3: SAME PHONEME, DIFFERENT LETTERS: CONSONANTS (FOUR WORDS)

Mark the four words that contain the same consonant phoneme, regardless of how each word is spelled. The first one is completed for you.

<u>fuzz</u>	<u>easy</u>	pleasure	<u>zone</u>	treasure	<u>rose</u>
mission	oceanic	anchored	sheep	backache	crèche
regal	hinge	jump	badge	night	engine
island	box	sound	pace	mercy	lose
carry	you	four	canyon	onion	cute
whose	hang	honesty	behind	whom	ache
rough	foreign	phonetics	of	graph	sleigh
grow	lozenge	again	begin	pig	large

EXERCISE 1.4: SAME PHONEME, DIFFERENT LETTERS: VOWELS (FOUR WORDS)

This exercise is designed to make you more aware of how the same phoneme can be spelled in many different ways. This time, mark the four words in each line that contain the same vowel phoneme, regardless of spelling/letters. The first one is completed for you.

<u>train</u>	<u>late</u>	<u>age</u>	sack	<u>crepe</u>	Saudi
beak	keep	deceive	meter	tread	credit
took	soup	flew	ruse	plume	mouse
pad	possible	palm	knock	jar	noise
pun	son	coupe	under	pouch	done
count	hood	should	cook	full	pool
hoe	boast	pot	shoe	cope	load
speak	priest	wisdom	sleek	friend	each

EXERCISE 1.5: SILENT LETTERS

Circle the letters for which there is no corresponding phoneme (e.g., silent letters). The first word in each group is completed for you.

Consonants

dum(b)	know	mnemonic	pneumonia	gnat	paradigm
knew	psalm	autumn	sign	sight	gnome

Vowels

lod(e)	stopped	entered	cage	rates	swine
bites	kicked	page	mine	asked	fanned

EXERCISE 1.6: TWO LETTERS, ONE PHONEME

This exercise is designed to help you identify these examples of "double letters." In each word, circle the two letters that correspond to only one phoneme.

Consonants

supper	cherry	barred	willing	passed	battle
shrugged	mall	betting	fell	tripped	missing

Vowels

goals	soon	soundless	beaten	bookcase	goulash
plywood	mournful	peaceful	braided	receive	sixteen

EXERCISE 1.7: IDENTIFYING MORPHEMES

This exercise is designed to help you identify morphemes. In each word, identify the number of morphemes by using slash marks, for example cow/boy, bat/s. If the word consists of only one morpheme, circle the whole word. The first two examples are completed for you.

beet/s	(last)	painful	machines	rusted	catnap	force
less	bigger	create	seeds	scrambled	stables	rehired
wishing	backfires	reasonable	littered	blinks	stream	retiring

CHAPTER 3

EXERCISE 3.1: RECOGNITION OF FRONT VOWELS

Listen to the recording or to your instructor's live-voice presentation of the following word lists. In each list, there is one common front vowel phoneme. After listening to each list, fill in the International Phonetic Alphabet (IPA symbol for the common phoneme in the space at the top of the lists.

List 1 / /	List 2 / /	List 3 / /	List 4 / /	List 5 / /	List 6 / /
lid	wrap	toothache	evil	bread	ale
hymn	plaid	stimulate	seam	ten	rail
gym	have	operate	bee	said	A-list
give	black	mediate	eat	guest	Monday
built	travel	meditate	these	leopard	baking
business	latch	renovate	ski	ebb	daylight

EXERCISE 3.2: DISCRIMINATION OF FRONT VOWELS

Listen to the recording or to your instructor's live voice presentation of the following word lists. In each list circle each word that contains the front vowel indicated at the top of the list.

List 1 /i/	List 2 /ɪ/	List 3 /e/	List 4 /ɛ/	List 5 /æ/	List 6 /eɪ/
eBay	myth	Kool-Aid	he	can	admire
when	kitchen	indicate	N	cane	payload
we	business	bear	head	calm	matter
find	itched	aggravate	well	apple	stray
brief	nylon	Patrick	end	knack	bandage
rein	gym	enemy	any	call	amaze
marine	litter	scarf	lean	half	calendar
style	sieve	renovate	speck	backed	radius
feline	lift	landscape	please	camera	tradition
demon	child	senator	eight	fade	fading

EXERCISE 3.3: FRONT VOWEL CONTRAST DRILLS

In Exercises 3.3 and 3.4 transcribe the front vowels in the words indicated. Be sure to follow the conventions for form in transcription. Because you will be transcribing from a live voice recording or speaker, use brackets [ ] rather than virgules to enclose your transcription, unless you instructor directs you otherwise.

List A: /i/–/ɪ/

1. lean-list _____
2. seep-sip _____
3. lift-leafed _____
4. pit-Pete _____
5. reed-rid _____
6. feet-fit _____
7. seen-sin _____
8. ship-sheep _____

List B: /ɪ/–/ɛ/

1. lean-Len _____
2. met-meat _____
3. said-seed _____
4. Chet-cheat _____
5. teen-ten _____
6. fell-feel _____
7. lead-led _____
8. beast-best _____

List C: /ɪ/–/ɛ/

1. knit-net _____
2. wet-wit _____
3. lit-let _____
4. beg-big _____
5. sit-set _____
6. den-din _____
7. bed-bid _____
8. will-well _____

List D: /ɛ/–/æ/

1. den-Dan _____
2. mess-mass _____
3. sad-said _____
4. Chet-chat _____
5. Ben-ban _____
6. pet-pat _____
7. fad-fed _____
8. tan-ten _____

List E: /ɛ/–/eɪ/

1. bet-bait _____
2. lace-less _____
3. whale-well _____
4. etch-H _____
5. fell-fail _____
6. debt-date _____
7. baste-best _____
8. shade-shed _____

EXERCISE 3.4: WORD TRANSCRIPTION FROM DICTATION: FRONT VOWELS

1. list _____
2. cap _____
3. dread _____
4. away _____
5. eggs _____
6. pitch _____
7. gasp _____
8. seek _____
9. jest _____
10. dim _____
11. match _____
12. land _____
13. yeast _____
14. skip _____
15. etch _____
16. in _____
17. seat _____
18. rack _____
19. rich _____
20. shade _____
21. dream _____
22. mist _____
23. van _____
24. debt _____
25. way _____
26. peanut _____
27. beech _____
28. catch _____
29. dent _____
30. date _____

EXERCISE 3.5: RECOGNITION OF BACK VOWELS

Exercises 3.5 and 3.6 require you to listen for, and identify or discriminate, the back vowels in words. Listen to the recording or to your instructor's live-voice presentation of each list in Exercise 3.5 and identify the one common back vowel phoneme. Fill in the IPA symbol for the common phoneme in the space at the top. In Exercise 3.6, circle the words containing the phoneme at the top of each list.

List 1 / /	List 2 / /	List 3 / /	List 4 / /	List 5 / /	List 6 / /
push	father	romantic	fruitful	owner	awning
should	palm	cooperate	whose	slow	audio
wool	knowledge	sailboat	crew	over	naught
book	cop	exponential	through	oak	saw
good	honest	introduce	canoe	pole	caught
wolf	bomb	oscilloscope	boot	croak	thought
full	opera	microphone	use	load	loss
puss	qualm	xylophone	loon	go	frog

EXERCISE 3.6: DISCRIMINATION OF BACK VOWELS

List 1 /u/	List 2 /ʊ/	List 3 /o/	List 4 /ɔ/	List 5 /ɑ/	List 6 /oʊ/
tomb	wool	obvious	naught	common	polar
stood	tool	voter	pawnshop	honor	south
look	pool	invocation	call	alms	locate
chewed	pull	location	shot	psalm	sew
cruiser	hooked	ostrich	hawk	father	few
blue	put	vocation	cot	gather	notice
doom	but	pottery	bawl	auto	police
soup	good	donation	ball	pawned	song
wood	full	moonlit	caught	sob	monster
cute	spook	momentous	got	oddity	gopher

EXERCISE 3.7: TRANSCRIPTION CONTRAST DRILLS

For Exercises 3.7 and 3.8, transcribe all the front vowels and back vowels contained in the word lists. Be sure to follow the conventions for form in transcription.

List A: /u/–/ʊ/

1. look-Luke _____
2. fool-full _____
3. who'd-hood _____
4. soot-suit _____
5. good-gooed _____
6. kook-cook _____
7. pool-pull _____
8. stood-stewed _____

List B: /ɑ/–/ɔ/

1. rah-raw _____
2. sought-sot _____
3. dawn-Don _____
4. caught-cot _____
5. hock-hawk _____
6. Lon-lawn _____
7. awed-odd _____
8. yon-yawn _____

List C: /oʊ/–/ɔ/

1. row-raw _____
2. law-low _____
3. cawed-code _____
4. owed-awed _____
5. loafed-loft _____
6. fall-foal _____
7. node-gnawed _____
8. lawn-loan _____

List D: /ɑ/–/æ/

1. sod-sad _____
2. lack-lock _____
3. sack-sock _____
4. Tom-tam _____
5. hat-hot _____
6. chop-chap _____
7. ban-Bonn _____
8. gash-gosh _____

EXERCISE 3.8: WORD TRANSCRIPTION: BACK AND FRONT VOWELS

1. tools _____
2. bookshelf _____
3. logbook _____
4. logic _____
5. popping _____
6. costly _____
7. eggnog _____
8. shot _____
9. castoff _____
10. pushing _____

11. chops _____
12. brooks _____
13. soot _____
14. smoothly _____
15. thought _____
16. ambush _____
17. fuse _____
18. soup _____
19. baboons _____
20. pawning _____

21. sleuth _____
22. shook _____
23. stewed _____
24. cheesecloth _____
25. tossing _____
26. choose _____
27. frost _____
28. pulled _____
29. shop _____
30. holly _____

EXERCISES 3.9–3.13: CENTRAL VOWELS

The first two exercises require you to identify the common central vowel among a list of words (Exercise 3.9) or discriminate central vowels from each other as well as other vowels (Exercise 3.10). Exercise 3.11 requires a transcription of minimal word pairs of central vowels as well as some of the back vowels. Finally, Exercise 3.12 emphasizes word transcription of central vowels but also includes all the vowels you have previously learned. Listen to the recording or to your instructor's live-voice presentation of words for transcription. Remember to enclose your transcriptions in brackets or you will not be following IPA standards.

EXERCISE 3.9: CENTRAL VOWEL RECOGNITION

List 1 / /	List 2 / /	List 3 / /	List 4 / /
burning	luck	computer	alone
fern	usher	urbane	pigeon
merchant	oven	over	fountain
firm	jumped	neighbor	alphabet
learning	other	better	Alabama
worded	under	terrain	away
myrtle	stump	batter	along
birth	cup	pertain	Indiana

EXERCISE 3.10: CENTRAL VOWEL DISCRIMINATION

List 1 /ʌ/	List 2 /ə/	List 3 /ɜ/	List 4 /ɚ/
lumber	banana	bird	other
once	lucky	pairs	pertain
could	umbrella	shirt	treasury
funny	atom	German	earnest
picture	aplomb	birthday	airy
none	Leah	colonel	arbor
unwind	elephant	merchant	loafers
mother	bundle	workman	nearer
funding	wool	car	chair
would	Dakota	under	wonder

EXERCISE 3.11: CENTRAL VOWEL CONTRAST DRILLS

List A: /ɝ/−/ʌ/

1. lurk-luck _____
2. bird-bud _____
3. shut-shirt _____
4. fun-fern _____
5. Turk-tuck _____
6. putt-pert _____
7. turf-tough _____
8. perk-puck _____

List B: /ʊ/−/ʌ/

1. book-buck _____
2. look-luck _____
3. cud-could _____
4. tuck-took _____
5. put-putt _____
6. shook-shuck _____
7. stud-stood _____
8. Huck-hook _____

List C: /ɔ/−/ʌ/

1. but-bought _____
2. long-lung _____
3. sung-song _____
4. cud-cawed _____
5. lost-lust _____
6. caught-cut _____
7. rung-wrong _____
8. done-dawn _____

EXERCISE 3.12: CENTRAL VOWEL COMPARISON DRILLS

The words in this exercise are designed to help you further distinguish among the stressed and unstressed versions of the central vowels. Listen to the recording or to your instructor's live-voice dictation to transcribe the words presented.

List A: /ɝ/−/ɚ/

1. rooster _____
2. mermaid _____
3. earthy _____
4. purse _____
5. author _____
6. birds _____
7. murdered _____
8. nursery _____
9. Saturn _____
10. beginner _____

List B: /ʌ/−/ə/

1. rhumba _____
2. Russian _____
3. aluminum _____
4. guppy _____
5. mushroom _____
6. accomplish _____
7. police _____
8. sunny _____
9. even _____
10. aloof _____

EXERCISE 3.13: TRANSCRIPTION: FRONT, BACK, AND CENTRAL VOWELS

Transcribe all the vowels you have learned in the words presented.

1. summer _____
2. worthy _____
3. lava _____
4. fender _____
5. worst _____
6. Abner _____
7. onion _____
8. blunder _____
9. church _____
10. meteor _____
11. earthling _____
12. buttery _____
13. search _____
14. neither _____
15. unlock _____
16. muskrat _____
17. honor _____
18. above _____
19. worsen _____
20. helicopter _____
21. vanilla _____
22. ginger _____
23. luscious _____
24. tuna _____
25. custom _____
26. wordy _____
27. tender _____
28. nursing _____
29. verse _____
30. touched _____

EXERCISES 3.14 AND 3.15: DIPHTHONG TRANSCRIPTION

These exercises focus on rising and centering diphthongs, respectively. Fill in the IPA symbol for the common phoneme in the / / space provided at the top of each word list.

EXERCISE 3.14: RECOGNITION OF RISING DIPHTHONGS

List 1 / /	List 2 / /	List 3 / /	List 4 / /	List 5 / /
skate	cope	house	oyster	mighty
major	Polish	count	noise	fine
sleigh	coat	crowd	foyer	sign
maniac	polar	loud	employ	China
caper	rose	down	moisture	tiger
danger	closing	pout	doily	riding

EXERCISE 3.15: RECOGNITION OF CENTERING DIPHTHONGS

List 1 / /	List 2 / /	List 3 / /[1]	List 4 / /	List 5 / /
market	ear	pure	foreman	wear
card	here	sure	chore	hare
heart	pier	cure	torn	share
carbon	steer	Murine	pouring	lair
scarred	cheer	curious	torso	barely
partake	mere	Puritan	corny	pear

EXERCISE 3.16: DISCRIMINATION OF RISING DIPHTHONGS

Exercises 3.16 and 3.17 will help you develop your ability to hear and discriminate the diphthongs from each other and from the monophthong vowels. In both exercises, circle the words that contain the phoneme at the top of the list.

List 1 /eɪ/	List 2 /oʊ/	List 3 /aʊ/	List 4 /ɔɪ/	List 5 /aɪ/
panic	hoping	count	poise	highly
prey	copy	foundry	porpoise	faithful
teak	doughnut	powder	hoist	kindness
eighty	loner	coach	mouth	bidding
katydid	long	bower	boyish	minded
payment	coast	Maude	pause	rhinoceros
matinee	thrown	pouch	avoidance	child
danger	beau	mountain	toys	children
wall	arrow	off	loiter	dynamite
highly	hopping	window	out	pain

EXERCISE 3.17: DISCRIMINATION OF CENTERING DIPHTHONGS

This exercise gives you practice in discriminating among the centering diphthongs. Circle the words that contain the phoneme at the top of the list.

---

[1] These words may contain /ʊɚ/ or /ɝ/, depending on the speaker and dialect.

List 1 /ɔɚ/	List 2 /ɪɚ/	List 3 /ɛɚ/	List 4 /ɑɚ/
court	bear	dear	hardest
boarded	fear	bear	Harry
lost	bird	airplane	partner
hoarse	deer	careful	Farsi
work	sheer	rare	gardener
border	near	warm	parsnip
torch	hearing	stairs	heartened
forest	gear	daring	ward
word	heart	fire	marvelous

EXERCISE 3.18: RISING DIPHTHONG CONTRAST DRILLS

This exercise contains drills contrasting the rising diphthongs as well as other, similar monophthong vowels. All vowels are included for transcription in **Exercise 3.19**. Listen to the recording or to your instructor's presentation of the words and transcribe them in the spaces indicated.

List A: /aʊ/–/aɪ/

1. mound mind _____
2. high how _____
3. nine noun _____
4. find found _____
5. signed sound _____
6. mouse mice _____
7. bite bout _____
8. down dine _____

List B: /aʊ/–/ɔɪ/

1. loud Lloyd _____
2. boys bows _____
3. towel toil _____
4. oil owl _____
5. joist joust _____
6. foul foil _____
7. vowel voile _____
8. coil cowl _____

List C: /ɔɪ/–/ɔ/

1. coil call _____
2. boil bawl _____
3. tall toil _____
4. loin lawn _____
5. jaw joy _____
6. foil fall _____
7. gnaws noise _____
8. awl oil _____

List D: /aʊ/–/ɔ/

1. out ought _____
2. mouse moss _____
3. fawned found _____
4. louse loss _____
5. bought bout _____
6. down dawn _____
7. cow caw _____
8. pound pawned _____

List E: /ʊ/–/aʊ/

1. could cowed _____
2. how'd hood _____
3. full fowl _____
4. pout put _____
5. wowed wood _____

EXERCISE 3.19: TRANSCRIPTION OF RISING DIPHTHONGS, FRONT, BACK, AND CENTRAL VOWELS

1. rhyme
2. chain
3. choice
4. high
5. rowdy
6. royalty
7. frown
8. training
11. cape
12. coins
13. point
14. stage
15. only
16. station
17. couch
18. open
21. frowning
22. myself
23. joined
24. denounced
25. amaze
26. nineteen
27. housing
28. approach

9. somehow   19. binder   29. surprise
10. polite   20. praise   30. founder

CHAPTER 4

For Exercises 4.1 to 4.3, the consonant exercises follow the same steps as the vowel exercises, beginning with vowel identification, discrimination, and then transcription.

EXERCISE 4.1: RECOGNITION OF STOP CONSONANTS

In each word list that follows, there is one common stop consonant. Listen to the instructional recording or to your instructor's reading of each word list. Fill in the IPA symbol for the common phoneme in the / / space.

List 1 / /	List 2 / /	List 3 / /	List 4 / /	List 5 / /	List 6 / /
clique	date	mattress	rabbit	guest	placed
park	today	taped	table	trigger	split
duck	waited	washed	tub	ghost	kept
cloud	saved	debt	broad	rogue	pound
ache	dressed	lettuce	number	sag	keeper
occur	address	yacht	pebble	eagle	happy
acre	breathed	court	lumber	anger	separate
okra	Adam	untie	umbrella	Pittsburgh	happy

EXERCISE 4.2: DISCRIMINATION OF STOP CONSONANTS

Listen to the words in each list as presented on the instructional recording or by your instructor. Circle the words that contain the stop consonant indicated at the top of each column.

List 1 /p/	List 2 /b/	List 3 /t/	List 4 /d/	List 5 /k/	List 6 /g/
apple	rabbit	doubt	adore	rice	rough
spring	mob	Thomas	jumped	baroque	again
psychic	thumb	laughed	medal	accord	higher
hopped	absolve	math	Wednesday	church	finger
telephone	bomb	liked	should	chasm	ghost
paper	urban	ptomaine	middle	accident	example
dipped	numb	nothing	hugged	liquid	bragged
upon	bright	antler	bored	tax	rogue
staph	elbow	wheat	stopped	extra	single

EXERCISE 4.3: WORD TRANSCRIPTION FROM SPELLING/DICTATION

1. paid _____
2. buggy _____
3. cub _____
4. god _____
5. candle _____
6. goody _____
7. gum _____
8. Gandalf _____

16. bigot _____
17. pawed _____
18. dirt _____
19. bought _____
20. bandana _____
21. cutter _____
22. baton _____
23. pit _____

9. toad _____   24. copy _____
10. teapot _____   25. get _____
11. dipped _____   26. gap _____
12. kite _____   27. goad _____
13. copay _____   28. biker _____
14. gab _____   29. cupcake _____
15. bad _____   30. decade _____

EXERCISE 4.4–4.10: FRICATIVES

For the following exercises, listen to the instructional recording or to your instructor's presentation. Remember to follow the guidelines for formation of fricative symbols found in Chapter 4.

EXERCISE 4.4: RECOGNITION OF FRICATIVES /f/ /v/ /θ/ /ð/

Fill in the fricative symbol common to each list in the space.

List 1 / /	List 2 / /	List 3 / /	List 4 / /
theirs	office	envy	third
weather	phonetics	of	thorn
neither	cough	heavy	pathway
southern	diphthong	leave	python
breathe	half	marvel	wreath
them	staff	vintage	with
bother	phase	move	moth
loathe	trough	pavement	anthem

EXERCISE 4.5: DISCRIMINATION OF FRICATIVE COGNATE PAIRS: /f/ /v/ /θ/ /ð/

Listen to the instructional recording or to your instructor's presentation of the following word lists. Circle the words containing the phoneme transcribed at the top of each list.

List 1 /f/	List 2 /v/	List 3 /θ/	List 4 /ð/
coffee	valet	these	these
elephant	confusion	booth	they'll
fifteen	vacuum	thigh	weather
prophet	driver	either	throw
half	offer	Thomas	bathe
Steven	halves	wreath	toothpaste
fault	of	anthem	motherly
infant	divide	south	heathen
leaves	river	thorny	soothe
farm	vase	myth	thyme

EXERCISE 4.6: TRANSCRIPTION OF VOWELS, STOPS, AND FRICATIVES: /f/ /v/ /θ/ /ð/

Listen to your instructional recording or to your instructor's presentation of the following words. Transcribe all the monophthongs, diphthongs, stops, and fricatives /f/ /v/ /θ/ /ð/ contained in the words.

1. foot _____
2. eleventh _____
3. theme _____
4. teeth _____
5. vivid _____
6. fatherhood _____
7. breathe _____
8. bath _____
9. fate _____
10. heathen _____

11. birthday _____
12. beaver _____
13. faith _____
14. fourth _____
15. victor _____
16. bather _____
17. thirty _____
18. huff _____
19. fifth _____
20. they've _____

EXERCISES 4.7–4.10: FRICATIVES

Exercises 4.7 to 4.10 emphasize the fricatives /s/, /z/, /ʃ/, /ʒ/, and /h/, followed by transcription of all vowels, stops, and fricatives in words. Remember to follow the guidelines for form and proportion of symbols; /s/, /z/, and /h/ resemble their lower case alphabetic counterparts.

EXERCISE 4.7: RECOGNITION OF FRICATIVES: /s/, /z/, /ʃ/, /ʒ/, /h/

Listen to the instructional recording or to your instructor's presentation, then fill in the fricative symbol common to each list in the space. The /ʃ/ resembles an elongated sigmoid, and the /ʒ/ resembles /z/ but with a partial loop added on the bottom.

List 1 / /	List 2 / /	List 3 / /	List 4 / /	List 5 / /
treasure	zebra	human	nice	seashore
barrage	scissors	reheat	social	shares
azure	roses	hash	police	partial
beige	ozone	behave	precious	machine
measured	zealous	hover	escape	portion
garage	please	hasty	mystery	sunshine
fusion	laser	hush	size	lashes
corsage	lies	unhurried	science	shoes

EXERCISE 4.8: DISCRIMINATION OF FRICATIVES: /s/, /z/, /ʃ/, /ʒ/, /h/

Listen to the following word lists on the instructional recording or as dictated by your instructor. Circle the words that contain the phoneme marked in the / / space at the top of each list.

List 1 /s/	List 2 /z/	List 3 /ʃ/	List 4 /ʒ/	List 5 /h/
racer	enzyme	insurance	treasure	with
mouse	misery	pressure	confusion	backhoe
icing	zigzag	occasion	ozone	hatch
escape	azure	confusion	beige	ache
casual	rose	caution	position	rehab
tons	closure	washed	leisure	halfway
previous	visible	tissue	casual	hawthorn
ensure	leisure	fresh	usual	halo
loose	breeze	messy	zookeeper	shoe

EXERCISE 4.9: WORD TRANSCRIPTION FROM SPELLING/DICTATION: /s/, /z/, /ʃ/, /ʒ/, /h/

In Exercises 4.9 and 4.10, listen to your instructor's presentation of the following words. Be sure to transcribe all vowels, stops, and fricatives in these words.

1. sash _____
2. zookeeper _____
3. hazard _____
4. seashell _____
5. azure _____
6. sheets _____
7. heather _____
8. pressure _____
9. pleasure _____
10. having _____

11. precious _____
12. hives _____
13. treasured _____
14. Persia _____
15. wish _____
16. ozone _____
17. easier _____
18. seizure _____
19. grazed _____
20. birdhouse _____

EXERCISE 4.10: TRANSCRIPTION OF VOWELS, STOPS, AND FRICATIVES

1. fastest _____
2. vacation _____
3. toothbrush _____
4. hover _____
5. corsage _____
6. themselves _____
7. shift _____
8. aspersion _____
9. birthplace _____
10. father _____

11. brotherhood _____
12. confusion _____
13. husband _____
14. garage _____
15. shoelace _____
16. frothy _____
17. phonate _____
18. mustache _____
19. explosion _____
20. Thursday _____

EXERCISES 4.11–4.13: AFFRICATES

These exercises are designed to help you recognize, discriminate, and transcribe the affricates. Remember that the symbol for /ʧ/ looks like a combination of /t/ and /ʃ/. The symbol for /ʤ/ looks like /d/ and /ʒ/ combined. Be careful to have the symbols touch or tied together by the narrow transcription symbol [⁀]. Otherwise, they will appear as separate stop and fricative, rather than one phoneme, an affricate.

EXERCISE 4.11: RECOGNITION OF AFFRICATES

Listen to the instructional recording or to your instructor's presentation of the word lists and fill in the affricate symbol common to each list in the / / space.

List 1 / /	List 2 / /	List 3 / /	List 4 / /
judge	choose	champion	jar
ridge	watching	cheese	fudge
jester	anchovy	picture	badge
adjourn	china	reach	angel
pledge	fracture	catcher	cage
jump	future	latch	gentle
agent	each	fetch	giant
lodge	enchant	chase	range

EXERCISE 4.12: DISCRIMINATION OF AFFRICATES

Listen to the recording or to your instructor's presentation of each of the following word lists. Circle the words that contain the affricate consonant transcribed at the top of the list.

List 1 /ʧ/	List 2 /ʤ/	List 3 /ʧ/	List 4 /ʤ/
scratch	large	chipmunk	jealous
choir	gopher	chorus	injure
natural	angel	backache	zoology
cheap	bungee	teacher	anger
jeep	jealous	chain	singer
capture	enjoy	charge	graduate
lecture	leisure	crèche	linger
kitchen	etching	pitch	reached
catcher	larger	cache	brazier
wager	crutch	patch	engine

EXERCISE 4.13: TRANSCRIPTION OF ALL PHONEMES

This exercise emphasizes words with /ʃ/, /ʒ/, /ʧ/, or /ʤ/, which can sometimes be confused. Transcribe all the vowels and consonants that you have learned up to now.

1. stitches _____
2. dodge _____
3. childhood _____
4. chopsticks _____
5. trudging _____
6. subject _____
7. lodger _____
8. chives _____
9. overture _____
10. Jacob _____
11. patchwork _____
12. bandage _____
13. adventure _____
14. speech _____
15. theology _____
16. badge _____
17. scratched _____
18. cheek _____
19. jerked _____
20. tangerine _____
21. chased _____
22. French fries _____
23. cheesecake _____
24. cabbage _____
25. stretched _____
26. grudge _____
27. ventured _____
28. passenger _____
29. challenge _____
30. change _____

EXERCISES 4.14–4.24: NASALS

For these exercises, listen to your instructional recording or to your instructor's presentation to recognize, discriminate, and transcribe the nasals in addition to the phonemes that you have already learned. Remember that /m/ and /n/ look like their lower case orthographic counterparts. /ŋ/ resembles /n/ with a tail added below the line.

EXERCISE 4.14: RECOGNITION OF NASALS: /m/, /n/, /ŋ/

Listen to the instructional recording or to your instructor's presentation of the following word lists. Fill in the nasal consonant symbol common to each list in the / / space.

List 1 / /	List 2 / /	List 3 / /
nice	singer	hymn
end	bring	enemy
noise	anger	autumn
green	long	most
soon	language	lemming
any	mining	empty
knee	hanger	lamp
mnemonic	bank	plum

EXERCISE 4.15: DISCRIMINATION OF NASALS: /m/, /n/, /ŋ/

Listen to the instructional recording or to your instructor's presentation of the word lists on the next page. Circle the words containing the phoneme transcribed at the top of each list.

List 1 /m/	List 2 /n/	List 3 /ŋ/
calm	hymn	anxious
infamous	knob	angle
diaphragm	gnash	hinge
shined	reign	donkey
summer	rank	branch
pneumonia	autumn	think
prism	gnat	song
mnemonic	bank	single
numb	cringe	longing
gnat	pneumonia	stranger

EXERCISE 4.16: TRANSCRIBING WORDS WITH SIMILAR SPELLINGS: /ŋ/, /ŋ k/, /ŋg/, /ndʒ/

Words such as *sing*, *finger*, and *stranger* are all spelled with the alphabet digraph *ng*, but the corresponding phonemes in these words are quite different: [s ɪ ŋ], [f ɪ ŋ g ɚ], and [s t ɹ e ndʒ ɚ], respectively. Listen to your instructor present these words or say them yourself and transcribe them. Listen carefully for the different phonemes, even though spelling is often similar.

1. stranger _____	11. lunge _____	21. danger _____
2. stronger _____	12. rungs _____	22. dangle _____
3. singer _____	13. ding _____	23. drank _____
4. finger _____	14. dinghy _____	24. Hank _____
5. hunger _____	15. bang _____	25. hang _____
6. hungry _____	16. banker _____	26. cringe _____
7. hanger _____	17. bling _____	27. crinkle _____
8. ranger _____	18. stingy _____	28. anger _____
9. sinker _____	19. sting _____	29. angel _____
10. linger _____	20. stinger _____	30. angry _____

EXERCISE 4.17: WORD TRANSCRIPTION FROM SPELLING/DICTATION: NASALS, AFFRICATES, STOPS, VOWELS, AND DIPHTHONGS

Listen to your instructional recording or to your instructor's presentation to recognize, discriminate, and transcribe the nasals in addition to the phonemes that you have already learned.

1. meter _____	16. himself _____
2. gang _____	17. everything _____
3. combing _____	18. sometimes _____
4. remove _____	19. cantor _____
5. chimney _____	20. slingshot _____
6. meant _____	21. stunning _____
7. infield _____	22. nation _____
8. taking _____	23. amend _____
9. mining _____	24. pneumatic _____
10. ones _____	25. smooth _____
11. drama _____	26. then _____
12. compete _____	27. longer _____
13. sanding _____	28. heading _____
14. smoking _____	29. motor _____
15. hangers _____	30. meaningful _____

EXERCISES 4.18–4.23: ORAL RESONANT CONSONANTS/LIQUIDS AND GLIDES

Exercises 4.18 and 4.19 are listening exercises to help you learn to recognize the sounds of glides and liquids and to discriminate these consonants from other, similar consonants. In Exercise 4.18, fill in the symbol for the phoneme that is characteristic of each word list. In Exercise 4.19, circle or underline the words containing the phoneme in the / / space at the top of each list.

EXERCISE 4.18: RECOGNITION OF LIQUIDS AND GLIDES

List 1 / /	List 2 / /	List 3 / /	List 4 / /
list	young	well	real
ally	foyer	lower	rewind
gold	music	sweep	royal
fuel	stallion	wind	train
swell	use	fewer	tomorrow
twelve	yoyo	would	rayon

EXERCISE 4.19: DISCRIMINATION OF LIQUIDS AND GLIDES

List 1 /w/	List 2 /j/	List 3 /l/	List 4 /ɹ/
reward	candy	gale	rhyme
memoirs	youthful	gulp	try
anywhere[1]	canyon	tulip	anchor

---

[1]May be produced as /ʍ/ by some speakers.

linguist	union	should	carrot
guide	booty	teller	bird
William	beauty	lilac	bread
watt	few	twelve	crowded
sword	yeast	would	rhythm
dwell	pewter	wall	Barry
shown	view	dearly	treasure

EXERCISE 4.20: TRANSCRIPTION: POSTVOCALIC /ɹ/ AND /ɚ/ DIPHTHONGS

This exercise is designed to help you practice consonant transcription using post-vocalic consonant /ɹ/ or /ɚ/-diphthongs to transcribe the same word. The r-consonant that follows a vowel (postvocalic ɹ) can be transcribed in one of two ways: as a consonant /ɹ/or as part of an /ɚ/-diphthong (see Chapter 3). Listen to the following words as recorded or as dictated by your instructor. Transcribe each word with consonant /ɹ/and then with the /ɚ/-diphthong. (The first two are done for you as examples.)

	/ɹ/	/ɚ/-diphthong
1. car	[k ɑ ɹ]	[kɑɚ]
2. bear	[b ɛ ɹ]	[bɛɚ]
3. torn	_____	_____
4. fierce	_____	_____
5. party	_____	_____
6. yearly	_____	_____
7. morning	_____	_____
8. partake	_____	_____
9. dared	_____	_____
10. cheer	_____	_____

EXERCISE 4.21: RHOTIC CONSONANTS AND VOWELS: RECOGNITION

This exercise will help you to distinguish the vowels /ɝ/and /ɚ/from the consonant singleton /r/. Listen to the instructional recording or to your instructor's presentation of the following word lists. Circle the words containing the phoneme indicated in the slash marks at the top of each list.

List 1 /ɹ/	List 2 /ɚ/	List 3 /ɝ/	List 4 /ɹ/
range	hammer	birch	trustee
earth	burden	standard	custard
butter	retry	crayon	broken
gray	dryer	turn	tearing
arrow	scary	murder	processor
prayer	understand	return	afraid
trailer	preacher	burn	courtesy
turn	overcoat	Barney	crowd
cream	mirthful	wordy	fur
frog	chair	corn	regal

EXERCISE 4.22: TRANSCRIPTION OF RHOTICS /ɹ/, /ɜ/, /ɚ/

This exercise helps you develop your ability to distinguish between rhotic vowels and the rhotic consonant. Listen to the instructional recording or to your instructor's presentation of the following word pairs, and transcribe them. The first pair is done for you as an example. (Note that postvocalic *r* is transcribed as consonant /ɹ/, rather than as different /ɚ/-diphthongs.)

1. curtain [kɝtən] _____   6. furnace _____
   carton [kɑɹtən] _____   fairness _____

2. hurry _____   7. firming _____
   Harry _____   farming _____

3. Carol _____   8. park _____
   curl _____   perk _____

4. furry _____   9. curb _____
   fairy _____   carob _____

5. hearts _____   10. worm _____
   hurts _____   warm _____

EXERCISE 4.23: TRANSCRIPTION CONTRASTS: CONSONANT /ɹ/ AND STRESSED VOWEL /ɜ/

Exercises 4.23 and 4.24 require you to transcribe glides and liquids as well as all the other consonants and vowels you have learned. You should listen to the instructional recording or to your instructor's presentation of the words in both exercises. Exercise 4.23 entails transcription of words with postvocalic /ɹ/ or the vowels /ɜ/ or /ɚ/.

1. car _____   11. bear _____
2. care _____   12. burr _____
3. core _____   13. bore _____
4. cur _____   14. hard _____
5. sheer _____   15. heard _____
6. shore _____   16. burn _____
7. sure _____   17. barn _____
8. hair _____   18. born _____
9. her _____   19. dare _____
10. bar _____   20. door _____

EXERCISE 4.24: TRANSCRIPTION OF ALL VOWELS AND CONSONANTS

1. lodging _____   11. William _____   21. youthful _____
2. witch _____   12. proud _____   22. yellow _____
3. radar _____   13. future _____   23. cubic _____
4. lilac _____   14. value _____   24. yarn _____
5. yield _____   15. rather _____   25. relay _____
6. frog _____   16. weakly _____   26. millions _____
7. freeway _____   17. cute _____   27. winter _____
8. water _____   18. laugh _____   28. sandwich _____
9. relative _____   19. wagered _____   29. woven _____
10. wishing _____   20. lacking _____   30. unused _____

CHAPTER 5

EXERCISE 5.1A,B: ASSIMILATORY CHANGES: PLACE

Exercise 5.1A,B has practice items for narrow transcription of devoicing and voicing of phonemes This exercise has four parts, all designed to help you integrate your knowledge regarding common assimilatory effects that can occur in connected speech. Exercise 5.1A focuses on the place change of dentalization. Remember that alveolar consonants /t d s z n l/ become dentalized if they occur next to an interdental /θ/ or /ð/: *one thing* [wʌnθɪŋ]. Exercise 5.1B contains examples of palatal assimilation. In phrases such as *Ridge Street*, the [s] often shifts to palatal [ʃ] as a result of assimilation: [rɪdʒʃtrit]. The first two examples have been completed for you in each exercise section. Remember to use the [ˌ], [°] and [ˌ] symbols (or [ɾ]) to note devoicing and voicing, respectively.

EXERCISE 5.1A: ASSIMILATORY CHANGES: DENTALIZATION

1. one thumb [wʌ n̪ θ ʌ m] _____
2. both ties [b oʊ θ t̪ aɪz] _____
3. code them _____
4. eighth star _____
5. with Tom _____
6. moth trap _____
7. bath soap _____
8. ride there _____
9. in there _____
10. cloth towel _____
11. lose them _____
12. south tower _____
13. on this _____
14. even though _____
15. fourth time _____
16. health text _____
17. want them _____
18. eat this _____
19. Miss Thornton _____
20. sees them _____

EXERCISE 5.1B: OTHER ASSIMILATORY PLACE SHIFTS

This exercise helps you learn to transcribe alveolar→palatal place shifts that can occur when an alveolar phoneme is immediately adjacent to a palatal phoneme such as /ʃ ʒ tʃ dʒ/. Listen to your instructor's presentation of these phrases or say them yourself. Then transcribe the coarticulated phrase that results. Notice that a change in duration can also accompany this change when a single phoneme results, so that the phoneme that results is of slightly longer duration.

1. place shift [p l eɪʃ ː ɪ f t] _____
2. miss Sheila _____
3. Pat's chalk _____
4. glass shop _____
5. Bench Street _____
6. bass shop _____
7. loose shelf _____
8. horse shoe _____

EXERCISES 5.2–5.4: NARROW TRANSCRIPTION

These exercises give you practice in recognizing and transcribing phonemes affected by assimilation. Exercise 5.2 is designed to help you recognize and transcribe changes in voicing. Remember that /l/, /ɹ/, /w/, and /j/ become devoiced (symbol [ˌ]) in prevocalic consonant sequences with voiceless consonants. Partial voicing of intervocalic /t/ and /h/ requires the use of the [ˌ] symbol. Or, if your instructor prefers, use [ɾ] for intervocalic /t/ changes. Exercise 5.3 has examples of assimilation nasality for you to recognize and transcribe. Finally, Exercise 5.4 requires you to use almost all the narrow transcription symbols that you have learned in this section, including dentalization, palatal assimilation, and assimilation nasality. You can listen to your instructor's presentation of these words or try saying them yourself. The first two examples have been completed for you.

EXERCISE 5.2: NARROW TRANSCRIPTION: CHANGES IN VOICING

1. plate [p ̥ l ̥ eɪ t]
2. three [θ ɹ ̥ i]
3. stagehand _____
4. pressure _____
5. bitter _____
6. behind _____
7. sleepy _____
8. club _____
9. frayed _____
10. rehearse _____
11. slumber _____
12. cluster _____
13. litter _____
14. cracker _____
15. row house _____
16. please _____
17. behave _____
18. crystal _____
19. motor _____
20. flu _____

EXERCISE 5.3: NARROW TRANSCRIPTION: NASAL ASSIMILATION

Transcribe the words characterized by nasal assimilation. Listen to your instructor's presentation of these words. The first two have been completed for you as examples.

1. banana [b ə n æ̃ n ə̃]
2. monk [m ʌ̃ ŋ k]
3. mention _____
4. framing _____
5. number _____
6. meaning _____
7. meantime _____
8. hammer _____
9. honey _____
10. mommy _____
11. known _____
12. monkey _____

EXERCISE 5.4: NARROW TRANSCRIPTION OF CHANGES IN PLACE, RESONANCE, AND VOICING

This exercise is designed to help you integrate the information on narrow transcription that you have learned so far. In these words, you should transcribe any applicable symbols for place and resonance changes. The first two have been completed for you.

1. nine things [n ãɪ n̪ θ ɪ ŋ z]
2. fourth meaning [f ɔ r θ m ĩ n ĩ ŋ]
3. plotting _____
4. mention them _____
5. tree house _____
6. mourned them _____
7. with Nan _____
8. morning anthem _____
9. Minnie Mouse _____
10. overhand _____
11. eat there _____
12. main theme _____

EXERCISE 5.5A,B: DURATION

Listen to your instructor's presentation as you practice recognizing and transcribing the occurrence of duration changes. For Exercise 5.5A, transcribe the phrases in IPA symbols, and use the [ː] symbol when applicable to indicate extended consonant duration. The first two are completed for you.

Example: bus stop [bʌsːtɑp]

EXERCISE 5.5A: NARROW TRANSCRIPTION: LENGTHENING IN PHRASES

1. bad dog [b æ dː ɑ g] _____
2. bar rail [bɑɹː el] _____
3. half full _____
4. some mice _____
5. call Linda _____

6. twelve vowels _____
7. ban nukes _____
8. same men _____
9. bathe them _____
10. his zippers _____

EXERCISE 5.5B: NARROW TRANSCRIPTION: SYLLABIC CONSONANTS

Listen to your instructor's presentation of the following words. Each word will be presented twice, once with an intervening vowel and once with a syllabic consonant. The order of presentation will be varied. Determine which word (of the pair) contains the syllabic consonant. Transcribe the words in IPA symbols, and use the [ˌ] symbol to indicate syllabic consonant use. The first two examples are completed for you.

1. cattle — [kaetʊl] — [kaet l̩]
2. mitten — [m ɪ t n̩] — [mɪten]
3. huddle — _____ — _____
4. frozen — _____ — _____
5. button — _____ — _____
6. soften — _____ — _____
7. bottle — _____ — _____
8. hassle — _____ — _____
9. topple — _____ — _____
10. cable — _____ — _____
11. ladle — _____ — _____
12. sniffle — _____ — _____
13. simple — _____ — _____
14. satin — _____ — _____
15. cotton — _____ — _____

EXERCISE 5.6A–D: ASPIRATION OF STOPS

Listen to your instructor's presentation of the following words. Each word will be produced twice, with aspiration varying on the postvocalic stop. Insert [ʰ] and [˺] diacritic markings as appropriate. The first two are done for you.

EXERCISE 5.6A: ASPIRATION OF SINGLETON STOPS

1. pop   [pʰɑp˺]   [pʰɑpʰ]
2. type   [tʰaɪpʰ]   [tʰaɪp˺]
3. hat   _____   _____
4. seat   _____   _____
5. peek   _____   _____
6. loop   _____   _____
7. fought   _____   _____
8. bait   _____   _____
9. cot   _____   _____
10. cope   _____   _____
11. soap   _____   _____
12. shock   _____   _____
13. set   _____   _____
14. wrote   _____   _____

EXERCISE 5.6B: NARROW TRANSCRIPTION OF PREVOCALIC /s/ + STOP SEQUENCES

This exercise is designed to help you apply the rules governing narrow transcription of voiceless stops in prevocalic consonant sequences. Review the rules on aspiration of stops in consonant sequences before you complete this exercise. The first two examples are completed for you.

1. stair [s t ˭ɛɹ]   6. sport _____
2. Spanish [sp˭ æ n ɪ ʃ]   7. scan _____
3. stern _____   8. spill _____
4. scoop _____   9. starch _____
5. scam _____   10. skill _____

EXERCISE 5.6C: NARROW TRANSCRIPTION OF INTERVOCALIC AND POSTVOCALIC STOP SEQUENCES

This exercise has examples of intervocalic stop + stop sequences and postvocalic fricative + stop, stop + stop, and nasal + stop sequences. Transcribe each word or phrase according to the rules given in Chapter 5.

1. kept [kʰɛ p˺tʰ]   13. into _____
2. hot car [h ɑ t˺kʰ ɑ ɹ]   14. sipped _____
3. laptop _____   15. coughed _____
4. daunt _____   16. that pair _____
5. lacked _____   17. kicked _____
6. limp _____   18. camp _____
7. sank _____   19. left _____
8. paste _____   20. missed _____
9. laughed _____ 21. necktie _____
10. leaked _____ 22. mashed _____
11. hot tub _____ 23. TicTac _____
12. that car _____ 24. wrecked _____

EXERCISE 5.6D: ASPIRATION OF STOPS: ALL ENVIRONMENTS

In this final exercise for aspiration of stops, you should apply all the rules that you have learned for narrow transcription up to this point.

1. span [s p ⌐ æ n] _____
2. cake [kʰ e kʰ] _____
3. back porch _____
4. hopped _____
5. payment _____
6. coat tails _____
7. spurt _____
8. stuck _____
9. last _____
10. pop-top _____
11. ant _____
12. skip _____
13. recover _____
14. popcorn _____
15. cusp _____
16. rent _____
17. take care _____
18. sent _____
19. laughed _____
20. spirit _____

EXERCISE 5.7A,B: SOUND OMISSIONS AND ADDITIONS

Sometimes the demands of connected speech lead to the loss of whole syllables, particularly unaccented ones. Such elision or omission is typically seen in the rapid coarticulation of expressions such as *meat and potatoes* as [mitnpəteɪtoz]. Exercise 5.7A is designed to help you listen for and transcribe occurrences of elision and haplology. Listen to your instructor's presentation of the phrases or say them yourself. Transcribe in IPA symbols each of the following words in two ways: first with *careful* pronunciation and second with natural, *casual* pronunciation typical of word production in connected speech. Pay special attention to the underlined syllables. The first example is done for you.

EXERCISE 5.7A: ELISION AND HAPLOLOGY

	Careful	**Casual**
1. veteran	[vɛtə˞ən]	[vɛtrən]
2. national	_____	_____
3. interest	_____	_____
4. chocolate	_____	_____
5. vegetable	_____	_____
6. federal	_____	_____
7. reasonable	_____	_____
8. favorite	_____	_____
9. separate	_____	_____
10. temperature	_____	_____

EXERCISE 5.7B: INTRUSIVE SOUNDS: /w/, /j/, /ʔ/

This exercise contains examples for transcription of epenthesis: /w/, /j/, or /ʔ/. They are grouped in one exercise because they often occur under similar circumstances. Transcribe the following phrases in IPA symbols, treating each group of words as a single speech utterance. In the first column, insert /w/ or /j/ as appropriate. You will need to listen to your instructor's presentation of these words. In the second column, insert a glottal stop. The first example is done for you.

	Intrusive Glide	**Glottal Stop**
1. be evil	[bijiv l̩]	[biʔiv l̩]
2. go out		
3. see it		
4. stay in		
5. how are		
6. sue us		
7. new ale		
8. tie up		
9. two eggs		
10. you all		
11. we each		
12. too easy		
13. he always		
14. who else		
15. may also		

EXERCISE 5.8: USE OF ALL NARROW TRANSCRIPTION SYMBOLS

This exercise contains examples of words with a variety of diacritic markings. Listen to your instructor's reading of the words or say them yourself. Use narrow transcription for each word. You will be most successful if you use both your listening skills and your knowledge of the conditions of use for the different symbols. The first two items have been completed for you as examples.

1. timer [tʰ aɪ m ɚ]
2. pity [pʰɪ t̬ i] or [pʰ ɪ ɾ i]
3. playhouse
4. slipped
5. trainer
6. blue hat
7. do it
8. top card
9. speak clearly
10. municipal
11. slept
12. planning
13. sleeting
14. hot time
15. sliced
16. three animals
17. see Ed
18. ninth batter
19. tell Lou
20. mumble
21. overhaul
22. spill less
23. one thimble
24. combing
25. future
26. both names
27. slimmer
28. spatter
29. find 'em
30. nine nets

EXERCISES 5.9–5.15: SUPRASEGMENTALS

EXERCISE 5.9: IDENTIFICATION OF CV STRUCTURE, ONSET/RHYME, AND OPEN/CLOSED SHAPE

This exercise is designed to help you identify structure of syllables according to CV, onset/rhyme, and open/closed shape. Transcribe each word; then fill in each column. The answers for the first item are completed for you.

Word	Transcription	CV Structure	Onset	Rhyme	Shape
1. bough	/baʊ/	CV	/b/	/aʊ/	Open
2. tree					
3. fix					
4. slant					
5. cubes					
6. blessed					
7. stretched					
8. sprints					
9. crests					
10. scrounge					

EXERCISE 5.10: DISCRIMINATION OF SYLLABLES

Underline the words that contain the number of syllables indicated at the top of each column. It may help to transcribe them. Remember that vowels are necessary to have a syllable. The first item is completed for you.

List A: 2 Syllables   **List B: 1 Syllable**   **List C: 5 Syllables**

List A: 2 Syllables	List B: 1 Syllable	List C: 5 Syllables
<u>accent</u>	<u>based</u>	<u>reactionary</u>
backed	snows	disability
boa	kicked	misarticulated
tearing	tasted	pronunciation
very	dried	inspiration
loaded	coded	analysis
splashed	drowned	laryngology
diphthongs	borne	velopharynx
kitten	little	maladjusted
aversion	branched	unreality

List D: 4 Syllables   **List E: 3 Syllables**

List D: 4 Syllables	List E: 3 Syllables
<u>dictionary</u>	<u>construction</u>
primarily	amazed
description	checkered
unaccented	syllable
substitute	nucleus
approximate	combination
consonants	primary
continuation	information
exhalation	coriander

EXERCISE 5.11: TRANSCRIPTION OF BISYLLABIC WORDS

In Exercises 5.11 and 5.12, listen to your instructor's presentation of the words or say them yourself. Transcribe each word and assign primary accent and secondary accent (if applicable). Remember that vowels that are completely distressed are heard as / ə /, regardless of the spelling of the word. The first item is completed for you for each exercise.

Word	Narrow Transcription		Word	Narrow Transcription
1. pontoon	[ˌpɑnˈtun]		11. gaily	
2. ladder			12. request	
3. language			13. heron	
4. debut			14. about	
5. panda			15. volume	
6. undone			16. employ	
7. cowboy			17. assign	
8. famous			18. riding	
9. presume			19. border	
10. pressure			20. observe	

EXERCISE 5.12: TRANSCRIPTION OF BISYLLABIC AND TRISYLLABIC WORDS

1. xylophone [ˈzaɪləˌfon]
2. muffler
3. mystery
4. accented
5. contain
6. generation
7. tasted
8. fortitude
9. porcupine
10. avatar
11. exclamation
12. television
13. biscuit
14. primrose
15. inspiration
16. substitute
17. description
18. nuclear
19. expert
20. politics

EXERCISE 5.13A–C: RECOGNIZING AND MARKING SENTENCE STRESS

This exercise set helps you identify and interpret examples of sentence stress (emphasis of a word/words within a phrase or sentence.) For parts A and B, match the question on the right with the result in the statement on the left. For Part C, indicate the stress (single underlining) to give specific meaning to each sentence. The first item in each exercise is completed for you as an example.

EXERCISE 5.13A: INTERPRETATION OF SENTENCE STRESS

 d 1. He saw one big red bird.
____ 2. He saw one big red bird.
____ 3. He saw one big red bird.
____ 4. He saw one big red bird.
____ 5. He saw one big red bird.
____ 6. He saw a big red bird.

a. Did he hear it or see it?
b. Was the big bird he saw red or blue?
c. What kind of animal did he see?
d. Who saw a big red bird?
e. Did he see a little red bird?
f. Did he see two big red birds?

EXERCISE 5.13B: INTERPRETATION OF SENTENCE STRESS: SENTENCE PAIRS

<u>b</u> I want <u>decaffeinated</u> coffee. a. I want coffee, not a soda.
<u>a</u> I want decaffeinated <u>coffee.</u> b. Make sure that the coffee is decaf.

____ I want the <u>red</u> apple. a. Not the yellow apple, the red one.
____ I want the red <u>apple.</u> b. Not the tomato, the apple.

____ She bought <u>five</u> books. a. Did she borrow the books?
____ She <u>bought</u> five books. b. That's a lot of books.

____ I'd like to see the <u>dessert</u> menu. a. I need to know what the selections are.
____ I'd like to see the dessert <u>menu.</u> b. I don't need the main menu.

____ I'll be there <u>tomorrow.</u> a. Don't expect me until then.
____ I'll be <u>there</u> tomorrow. b. I won't be here because I'll be out of town.

____ You want <u>me</u> to be the speaker? a. Don't you mean somebody else?
____ You want me to be the <u>speaker?</u> b. I'm much better at organizing than speaking.

EXERCISE 5.13C: MARKING SENTENCE STRESS

Underline the words most likely to be emphasized in each sentence to help a listener compare key words. The first example has been completed for you.

1. We <u>did</u> it, but we didn't <u>want</u> to.
2. They arrived, and then we arrived.
3. We drove home, but they walked home.
4. They went on a bus, and we went on a train.
5. A thesaurus is like a dictionary.
6. A penny saved is a penny earned.
7. We came early, and they came late.
8. I came, I saw, I conquered.
9. Do you need my help today or tomorrow?
10. He said yes, but he meant no.
11. I had fries, and she had onion rings.
12. I want the big one, not the little one.
13. Which is bigger, the left one or the right one?
14. His party is Friday, not Saturday.
15. His iPad has some great apps.

EXERCISE 5.14: MARKING PAUSES

This exercise has two transcriptions with pauses for each sentence. Only one of the transcriptions is correct. Mark the correct transcription. The first example has been completed for you.

_a_ 1. He wants butter, not margarine.

  a. [hiwantsbʌɾɚ] | [natmaɹdʒəɹə] ‖

  b. [hiwants] | [bʌɾɚnat] ‖ [maɹdʒəɹə] ‖

___ 2. When did they come, Tuesday or Wednesday?

  a. [wɛndɪd] | [ðekʌmtuzdeɪɔɹ] | [wɛnzdeɪ] ‖

  b. [wɛndɪdðekʌm] ‖ [tuzdeɪɔɹwɛnzdeɪ] ‖

___ 3. Can you be there or not?

  a. [kænjubiðɛɹ] | [ɔɹnat] ‖

  b. [kænju] | [biðɛɹɔɹ] | [nat] ‖

___ 4. Since the storm, it's been very cool.

  a. [sɪnsðəstɔɹm] | [ɪtsbɛn] | [vɛɹikul] ‖

  b. [sɪnsðəstɔɹm] | [ɪtsbɛnvɛɹikul] ‖

___ 5. Don't blame me! It's not my fault.

  a. [dontblem:i] ‖ [ɪtsnatmaɪfɔlt] ‖

  b. [dontblem:i] | [ɪts] | [natmaɪfɔlt] ‖

___ 6. That shirt is his, not mine.

  a. [ðætʃɝt] | [ɪzhɪznatmaɪn] ‖

  b. [ðætʃɝtɪzhɪz] | [natmaɪn] ‖

EXERCISE 5.15: TRANSLITERATION

Convert each transcribed utterance into orthographic symbols. Remember that in connected speech, sounds and words can change identity, be lost, become de-accented, etc. It will probably help if you say each utterance aloud.

 1. [wɛɹzigoʊʔn̩] _____

 2. [aɪdlaɪkəbɝgɚn̩fɹaɪz] _____

 3. [aɪsɔsəm:ɪlkn̩əfɹɪdʒ] _____

 4. [wɛnl̩ikəm] _____

 5. [wiʔeɪtmitn̩pəteɪtəzfɚdɪnɚ] _____

 6. [ɪthæpn̩danəfɔɹθədʒəlaɪ] _____

 7. [ɪz:ætənuhæt] _____

 8. [aɪwanʧətəkəmn̩saɪd] _____

 9. [huzikɪdn̩] _____

10. [haʊm̩aɪduʔn̩] _____

11. [wɛnzilivn̩] _____

12. [dɪdʒəwanfraɪzwɪðaet] _____

13. [bɪziæzəbi] _____

14. [wʌzikʌmn̩baɪtreɪnɚbʌs] _____

15. [aɪ w ɑ n ə p i t z ə w ɪ ð e v ɛ i θ ɪ ŋ] _____

16. [h u z ə n u g aɪ] _____

17. [ɑ ɹ j ə ʃ ɝ] _____

18. [aɪ m g ʌ n ə g ɛ ɾ ɛ r f ɝ s t] _____

19. [d ɪ ʤ ə i t j ɛ t] _____

20. [h i z ə n u t i ʃ ə] _____

CHAPTER 6

The three exercises for this chapter are designed to help you better understand the effects of regional dialects in relation to mainstream English (mainstream American English). Three regional dialects are emphasized and contrasted with ME: Eastern New England, inland North, and Southern. Use the information in the text and tables to complete the exercises. Refer especially to **Tables 6.2, 6.3,** and **6.4** then fill in the expected variation for each dialect. You may leave blank those items which are identical to mainstream American English pronunciation.

EXERCISE 6.1: REGIONAL DIALECT CONTRASTS

Word	Transcription	Eastern New England	Inland North	Southern
1. cent	[s ɛ n t]	_____	_____	_____
bend	[b ɛ n d]	_____	_____	_____
2. my	[m aɪ]	_____	_____	_____
hide	[h aɪ d]	_____	_____	_____
3. far	[f ɑ ɹ]	_____	_____	_____
better	[b ɛ ɾ ɚ]	_____	_____	_____
earth	[ɝ θ]	_____	_____	_____
4. haul	[h ɑ l]	_____	_____	_____
hall	[h ɑ l]	_____	_____	_____
collar	[k ɑ l ɚ]	_____	_____	_____
caller	[k ɑ l ɚ]	_____	_____	_____
5. red	[ɹ ɛ d]	_____	_____	_____
head	[h ɛ d]	_____	_____	_____
6. mid	[m ɪ d]	_____	_____	_____
bid	[b ɪ d]	_____	_____	_____

EXERCISE 6.2: AFRICAN-AMERICAN ENGLISH (AAE) DIALECT CONTRASTS

This exercise help you compare differences between ME and AAE. Fill in the probable AAE response in each space. Remember, not all the phonemes vary in pronunciation. As with regional dialects, there are both similarities and differences.

Word	ME	AAE
1. thumb	[θ ʌ m]	_____
wreath	[ɹ i θ]	_____
this	[ð ɪ s]	_____
weather	[w ɛ ð ɚ]	_____
2. ask	[æ s k]	_____
mask	[m æ s k]	_____
wolf	[w ʊ l f]	_____
meant	[m ɛ n t]	_____
3. less	[l ɛ s]	_____
bell	[b ɛ l]	_____
color	[k ʌ lɚ]	_____
4. awl	[ɔ l]	_____
oil	[ɔɪ l]	_____

EXERCISE 6.3: SPANISH-INFLUENCED ENGLISH (SIE) DIALECT CONTRASTS

This exercise helps you compare differences between ME and SIE. Fill in the probable SIE response in each space. Remember, not all the phonemes vary in pronunciation. As with regional dialects, there are both similarities and differences.

Word	ME	SIE
1. thumb	[θ ʌ m]	_____
earth	[ɝ θ]	_____
this	[ð ɪ s]	_____
bathe	[b e ð]	_____
2. lamb	[l æ m]	_____
yellow	[j ɛ l oʊ]	_____
bell	[b ɛ l]	_____
3. shed	[ʃ ɛ d]	_____
wash	[w ɑ ʃ]	_____
washing	[w ɑ ʃ ɪ ŋ]	_____
4. zoo	[z u]	_____
buzzing	[b ʌ z ɪ ŋ]	_____
nose	[n oʊ z]	_____
5. sun	[s ʌ n]	_____
passing	[p æ s ɪ ŋ]	_____
yes	[j ɛ s]	_____
school	[s k u l]	_____
spin	[s p ɪ n]	_____

CHAPTER 7

EXERCISE 7.1: ADULT SPEECH SAMPLE: TEST OF MINIMAL ARTICULATION COMPETENCE (TMAC), SENTENCE FORM

Transcribe the error, including the position in which it occurs. (The position can be indicated by I, M, F or 1, 2, 3 for initial, medial, and final position.) Then indicate the type of error (refer to **Table 7.2** for assistance). The first example has been completed for you.

Word	Response	Transcription and Position	Error Type
thumb	[s ʌ m]	s/θ (I)	Substitution
toothache	[t u s e k]		
feather	[f ɛ z ə]		
smooth	[ʃ m u z]		
shoe	[s u]		
dishes	[d ɪ s ə z]		
fish	[f ɪ s]		
lamp	[l̪ æ m p]		
balloon	[b ə l̪ u n]		
ball	[b ɔ l̪]		
rabbit	[ɹ æ b ə t]		
carrot	[k ɛ j ɪ t]		
star	[s t ɑ ə]		

EXERCISE 7.2: PEDIATRIC PATIENT SPEECH SAMPLE (GFTA-2)

This exercise contains sample responses from a 5-year-old child. The test used, the Goldman-Fristoe Test of Articulation-2 (GFTA-2) assesses more than one sound per word. Tested sounds are underlined. The first example is completed for you.

Word	Response	Transcription and Position	Error Type
house	[h aʊ ʃ]	ʃ/s (F)	Substitution
tree	[t w i]		
cup	[t ʌ p]		
spoon	[p u n]		
girl	[d ʊ l]		
shovel	[ʧ ʌ b ə l]		
zipper	[ʒ ɪ p ə]		
monkey	[m ʌ n t i]		
scissors	[ʃ ɪ d ə ʒ]		
plane	[p e n]		
rabbit	[w æ b ɪ t]		

EXERCISE 7.3: IDENTIFYING USAGE OF PHONOLOGICAL PATTERNS

This exercise contains sample responses from a 4-year-old child. The test used, the Hodson Assessment of Phonological Patterns (HAPP) is specifically designed to test for the use of phonological patterns. Unlike conventional articulation tests, you must account for every sound change in each of the words tested. Refer to Table 7.3 to help you in completing this exercise. The first two examples are completed for you.

Word	Response	Phoneme(s) Affected	Pattern
spoon	[p u]	/s/	ConSeqRed
		/n/	FinalConsDel
boats	[b o t]	/s/	ConSeqRed
fork	[p ɔ ə]	_____	_____
		_____	_____
chair	[t ɛ o]	_____	_____
		_____	_____
nose	[n oʊ]	_____	_____
screwdriver	[t u d aɪ]	_____	_____
		_____	_____
		_____	_____
		_____	_____
		_____	_____
thumb	[t ʌ]	_____	_____
		_____	_____
truck	[t ʌ]	_____	_____
		_____	_____

EXERCISE 7.4: INDEPENDENT ANALYSIS OF RESPONSES

This exercise contains responses from a 36-month-old child for independent analysis. Remember that in an independent analysis you note every sound the child produces, whether it is correct or not. Independent analysis examines both consonants and vowels as well as syllable structure. When you have completed the analysis, you should be able to supply the consonant, vowel, and syllable shape inventories at the end of the exercise.

Sounds Produced

Word	Transcription	Consonants (I) (M) (F)	Vowels	Syllable Structure
dog	[d ɑ]	/d/	ɑ	CV
cat	[t æ]	_____	_____	_____
star	[t ɑ]	_____	_____	_____
knife	[n ɑ p]	_____	_____	_____
fork	[p ɔ]	_____	_____	_____
deer	[d i]	_____	_____	_____
bubble	[b ʌ b ʌ]	_____	_____	_____
eyes	[ɑ t]	_____	_____	_____
nose	[n oʊ]	_____	_____	_____
mouth	[m ɑ]	_____	_____	_____

Summary:

Vowel Inventory: / /   Syllable Shapes:
Consonant Inventory: / /   (Initial)   V
                                (Medial)   VC
                                (Final)   CV
                                              CVC
                                              CVCV

ANSWER KEY: CHAPTER CONCEPT QUESTIONS

CHAPTER 1

PART I: CONCEPT INTEGRATION

1. True.
2. False. /t/ and /d/ are different phonemes, not different allophones.
3. True.
4. False. These are letters, not phonemes.
5. False. Phonemes outnumber alphabet letters.
6. True.
7. True.
8. False. The relationship between phonemes and alphabetic letters is not always consistent.
9. False. *Listen* /er/ s = three morphemes.
10. False. Phonetic transcription uses brackets; phonemic transcription uses / /.

PART II: SUPPLEMENTAL EXERCISES—LISTENING FOR PHONEMES

Consonant Exercises

1. Beginning sounds

a.	cobra	Canada	Kyle	chord	/k/
b.	first	phony	fairy	phase	/f/
c.	hope	who	hill	heather	/h/
d.	tone	Thomas	tie	table	/t/
e.	third	three	thirteen	thick	/θ/
f.	this	there	that	them	/ð/
g.	write	rain	wrought	rest	/ɹ/
h.	science	skirt	school	sci-fi	/s/

2. Ending sounds

a.	back	ache	sac	work	/k/
b.	cope	rope	hop	map	/p/
c.	boot	sight	eight	last	/t/
d.	less	bats	ice	box	/s/
e.	reach	such	patch	fetch	/ʧ/

f.	mines	rose	razz	ease	/z/
g.	rash	crèche	clash	seiche	/ʃ/
h.	far	pore	hair	dare	/ɹ/

3. Middle sounds

a.	danger	Roger	budgie	manager	/dʒ/
b.	singer	hanger	ringing	manganese	/ŋ/
c.	hugger	finger	hunger	ugly	/g/
d.	pressure	assure	Bashir	cashier	/ʃ/
e.	whistle	listener	dancing	relaxing	/s/
f.	razor	reason	reserve	observe	/z/
g.	measure	leisure	treasure	casual	/ʒ/
h.	backache	record	acre	bacon	/k/

Vowel Exercises

1. Beginning vowel sound

a.	able	atrium	eight	aim	/eɪ/
b.	every	ending	ember	etch	/ɛ/
c.	over	old	Oprah	ogee	/oʊ/
d.	on	aardvark	obelisk	ostrich	/ɑ/
e.	eel	east	even	eerie	/i/
f.	inner	if	is	Iliad	/ɪ/
g.	after	axe	afghan	aspirin	/æ/
h.	eyelid	Ivan	I'll	aisle	/aɪ/

2. Vowel sounds: any position

a.	turn	birch	work	earth	/ɝ/
b.	seam	least	reach	eagle	/i/
c.	fried	pie	bind	license	/aɪ/
d.	bait	age	lady	mane	/eɪ/
e.	apple	fact	patch	pasture	/æ/
f.	bend	edit	mellow	session	/ɛ/
g.	itch	singe	list	fill	/ɪ/
h.	done	fuss	upper	wonder	/ʌ/

Challenge Exercises

1. Counting phonemes

a/k/s <u>3</u> b/a/k/er <u>4</u> kn/o/t <u>3</u> s/q/u/ee/ze <u>5</u> s/ure <u>2</u> f/ir/s/t <u>4</u>

p/a/n/d/a <u>5</u> a/f/gh/a/n <u>5</u> k/a/r/a/t/e <u>6</u> r/e/c/ei/v/ed <u>6</u> p/ea/ch/y <u>4</u> wr/ea/th <u>3</u>

b/o/k/s/er <u>5</u> s/l/o/pe <u>4</u> c/ou/pe <u>3</u> q/u/e/s/t <u>5</u> b/o/n/d/i/ng <u>6</u> ho/n/e/s/t <u>5</u>

2. Phoneme reversal

Luke	<u>c oo l</u>	bag	<u>g a b</u>	dumb	<u>m u d</u>	rots	<u>s t a r</u>
stun	<u>n u t s</u>	niece	<u>s ee n</u>	knife	<u>f i ne</u>	licks	<u>s k i ll</u>
Mack	<u>c a m</u>	ouch	<u>ch ow</u>	caught	<u>t a lk</u>	zoo	<u>oo ze</u>
kneel	<u>N ea l</u>	gnome	<u>m oa n</u>	sigh	<u>ice</u>	bats	<u>s t a b</u>

CHAPTER 2

PART I: STRUCTURAL TERMS

1. Structures associated with terms:

   a. Bilabial: lips (both)

   b. Glottal: glottis

   c. Dental: teeth

   d. Velar: soft palate/velum

   e. Pharyngeal: pharynx/pharyngeal cavity

   f. Nasal: nasal cavity

   g. Alveolar: alveolar ridge

   h. Palatal: hard palate

2. Supralaryngeal structures:

   Lips, teeth, alveolar ridge, tongue, hard palate, velum, nasal cavity, oral cavity, nasopharynx, oropharynx, laryngopharynx

3. Sublaryngeal structures:

   Trachea, lungs, rib cage, diaphragm

4. Laryngeal structures and function/location:

   a. Larynx suspended from it   hyoid bone

   b. Protects larynx in swallowing   epiglottis

   c. Anterior attachment for vocal folds   thyroid cartilage

   d. Space between vocal folds   glottis

   e. Responsible for vocal fold abduction   arytenoid cartilages

   f. Most inferior laryngeal cartilage, attached to trachea cricoid cartilage

   g. Muscular tissue shelves in larynx   vocal folds

PART II: CONCEPT INTEGRATION

1. *Respiratory cycle pathway:*

   Diaphragm contracts + upward, and outward rib cage movement due to muscle action→ expansion of thoracic cavity

   Lungs expand (elastic properties)→air drawn into lungs

   Oxygen-carbon dioxide exchange in alveoli

   Actions of gravity (downward pull on ribs) + elastic properties of cartilage and lung tissue + muscle relaxation→exhalation via vocal tract

2. Frequency: rate of vibration/cycles per second, measured as Hertz and heard as pitch.

   Intensity: relative to vocal fold vibration, refers to extent of displacement of folds; heard as loudness

PART III: DIAGRAM OF THE VOCAL TRACT

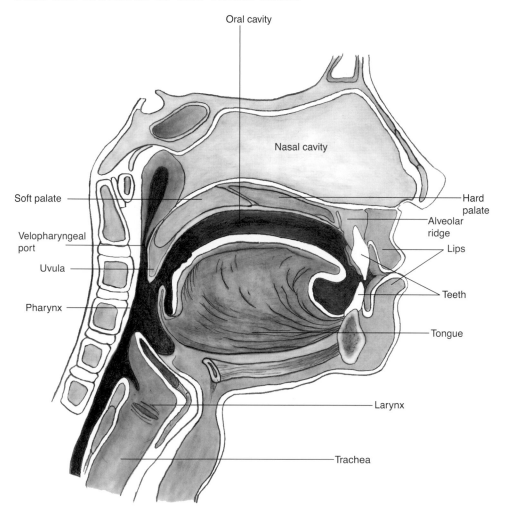

CHAPTER 3

PART I

1. True.

2. False. Consonants are characterized by constriction.

3. True.

4. True.

5. False. /ɑ/ is unrounded.

6. False. The vowel phonemes are /ə æ ə/.

7. False. The number of vowels determines the number of syllables; consonants are not necessary to have a syllable.

8. True.

9. True.

10. False. The high vowels include /i ɪ u ʊ/.

PART II

1. a.   /u ʊ o ɔ ɑ/
    b.   /æ ɛ e ɪ i/
    c.   /ɝ ɚ ʌ ə/
    d.   (1)   Rounded vowels
          (2)   Mid vowels
          (3)   Low vowels
          (4)   Tense vowels
          (5)   Lax vowels
          (6)   Front vowels
          (7)   Mid vowels

2. a.   /d θ ð ʃ ʤ n ɹ l/
    b.   /k ʃ ʤ h ŋ ɹ w j i æ u ɑ/
    c.   /f v s z ʃ ʒ ʤ/
    d.   /k h ŋ w u ɑ/
    e.   /m n ŋ/
    f.   /k ʃ ʒ ʤ i u/

CHAPTER 4

1.

			Position	Singleton/Sequence
a.	**ring**			
	r	/ɹ/	Prevocalic/initial	Singleton
	ng	/ŋ/	Postvocalic/final	Singleton
b.	**stove**			
	st	/st/	Prevocalic/initial	Sequence
	v	/v/	Postvocalic/final	Singleton
c.	**chicken**			
	ch	/ʧ/	Prevocalic/initial	Singleton
	k	/k/	Intervocalic/medial	Singleton
	n	/n/	Postvocalic/final	Singleton
d.	**basket**			
	b	/b/	Prevocalic/initial	Singleton
	sk	/sk/	Intervocalic/medial	Sequence
	t	/t/	Postvocalic/final	Singleton
e.	**telephone**			
	t	/t/	Prevocalic/initial	Singleton
	l	/l/	Intervocalic/medial	Singleton
	ph	/f/	Intervocalic/medial	Singleton
	n	/n/	Postvocalic/final	Singleton

2. a.   /m/
    b.   /t/
    c.   /ʃ/
    d.   /k/
    e.   /θ/

    f.   /j/
    g.   /f/
    h.   /ʧ/
    i.   /w/
    j.   /ð/
    k.   /g/
    l.   /ŋ/
    m.   /ʒ/
    n.   /v/
    o.   /b/
    p.   /l/
    q.   /p/
    r.   /h/
    s.   /n/
    t.   /d/
    u.   /ʤ/
    v.   /ɹ/

3. List the cognate for each of the following.
    a. /b/   b./s/   c. /ʧ/   d. /v/
    e. /d/   f./ʃ/   g. /ð/   h. /g/

4. List all the consonants included in each group described below.
    a.   /d z n l/
    b.   /ʃ ʒ ʧ ʤ j ɹ/
    c.   /b d g/
    d.   /f θ s ʃ h/
    e.   /m n ŋ/
    f.   /g ŋ/
    g.   /p b m w f v/
    h.   /ʤ/

5. a.   Alveolar
    b.   Palatal, voiced
    c.   Liquids, voiced
    d.   Palatal
    e.   Velar voiced
    f.   Alveolar
    g.   Voiced
    h.   Bilabial

CHAPTER 5

PART I

1. True.

2. False. Production of *think* as [θ ɪ ŋ k] is an example of an assimilatory change in place of articulation, not manner.

3. True.

4. True.

5. False. Postvocalic stops are not always audibly released.

6. False. *Eight owls* would be transcribed as [eɪ t aʊ l z]. Transcription is for eight towels.

7. True.

8. False. Statements and commands in English are characterized by falling intonation.

9. False. Secondary accent is not always present in a two syllabic word, e.g., under.

10. True.

PART II: DIACRITICS

1. a, b, c, e, f, g, and h are correct.

2. a, c, e, and f are correct.

3. a, b, and d are correct.

4. a: The second transcription is correct: /l/ devoicing, velar assimilation [n] →[ŋ], and audible aspiration of [kʰ] in the postvocalic consonant sequence.

   b: The third transcription is correct: devoicing of [l̥], postvocalic stop sequence with air held, [p̚] followed by audible release [tʰ].

   c: The first transcription is correct: nasalization on the vowels in the second and third syllables.

   d: The second transcription is correct: unreleased stop in sequence [sp̚] and nasalization of [ɪ].

   e: The third transcription is correct: dentalization of [s̪] and final consonant /z/, not /s/.

PART III: SPEECH RHYTHM AND SUPRASEGMENTAL FEATURES

1. suspect (verb)   [s ə s ˈp ɛ k̚ tʰ]   suspect (noun)   [ˈs ʌ s p ɛ k̚ tʰ]
   insult (verb)   [ɪ n ˈs ʌ l tʰ]   insult (noun)   [ˈɪ n s ə l tʰ]
   combine (noun)   [ˈkʰ ɑ m ˌb aɪ n]   combine (verb)   [ˈkʰ ə m ˈb aɪ n]
   reward   [ɹ i ˈw ɔ ɹ d]   cobra   [ˈkʰ oʊ b ɹ ə]

2. 1: e; 2: a; 3: b; 4: c; 5: d.

3. a. [aɪ d o n t b i l i v ɪ t] ‖ [aɪ g ɑ ɾ ə n eɪ] ‖
   b. [o m aɪ] | [ɪ t s t aɪ m t ə g oʊ] ‖
   c. [d ɪ d j u h ɹ ɹ ə b aʊ t̪ ð æ t] ‖ [aɪ d ɪ d n̩ t] ‖
   d. [ð e k e m ɪ n f ɝ s t] | [æ n d s ɛ k ə n d] | [ɹ ɪ s p ɛ k t ə v l i] ‖
   e. [p l i z b ɹ ɪ ŋ m i j ə p ɛ n] | [s ə m p eɪ p ɚ] | [æ n ə d ɪ k ʃ ə n ɛ ɹ i] ‖

4. a. Rising
   b. Falling
   c. Rising
   d. Rising
   e. Rising

CHAPTER 6

PART I

1. True.

2. True.

3. False. Various professional organizations view dialects as equivalent, but not all Americans do.

4. True.

5. True.

6. True.

7. False. Even when the same vowels are affected, they do not always change in the same way.

8. True.

9. True.

10. True.

PART II: REGIONAL DIALECTS

a. Southern English
b. Eastern New England English
c. Southern English
d. Southern English
e. Inland Northern English

PART III: AFRICAN-AMERICAN ENGLISH

a. [m ɪ n]   e. [f ɝ ə s]
b. [ʌ d ə] or [ʌ v ə]   f. [ʃ ɛ f]
c. [h ɝ s ɛ f]   g. [b ɝ f d eɪ]
d. [d ɛ s]   h. [θ oʊ]

PART IV: SPANISH-INFLUENCED ENGLISH

a. [b e ɪ ɹ i]   e. [ɛ s k ɛ ɹ]
    [ʧ a b l]   [ɛ s k ɛ ɹ i]
b. [b ɹ i d]   f. [k oʊ l]
    [t i s] or [t i t]   [l oʊ]
c. [ʃ u s]   g. [ʧ i n]
    [d u s]   [ʃ i n]
d. [h u i ʃ]   h. [t i n] or [s i n]
    [h u i n]   [s i n]

CHAPTER 7

PART I

1. False. A variety of professionals find use of the IPA helpful.

2. True.

3. False. The use of picture cards is inappropriate with adults.

4. True.

5. True.

6. True.

7. True.

8. False. A dialect is not a disorder. Accent reduction is optional and must be desired by the speaker.

9. True.

10. False. s/ʃ is a substitution (one standard speech sound replaces another standard speech sound).

PART II: RECORDING SPEECH SOUND ERRORS

/k/: t/k (I, M, F)
/g/: d/g (I, M)
/ʧ/: ʃ/ʧ (I, F)
/ʒ/: -/ʒ (M) d/ʒ (F)

PART III: IDENTIFICATION OF PHONOLOGICAL PATTERN USAGE

Target Word	Transcription	Final Consonant Deletion	Stopping	Velar Fronting	Gliding
cup	[t ʌ]	X		X	
rocket	[w ɑ t ɪ]	X		X	X
rake	[w eɪ]	X			X
gum	[d ʌ]	X		X	
wagon	[w æ d ə]	X		X	
pig	[p ɪ]	X			
sun	[t ʌ]	X	X		
bicycle	[b aɪ t ɪ t ə]	X	X	X	
house	[h aʊ]	X			
shoe	[t u]		X		

What process occurred most often in this sample? Final consonant deletion.

ANSWER KEY: CHAPTER EXERCISES

CHAPTER 1

EXERCISE 1.1: DIGRAPHS: TWO LETTERS/ONE PHONEME

Consonants

thorn	wish	leather	chain	ring	photo	both
judge	other	laugh	sang	lock	bush	soothe

Vowels

boat	later	hoop	pouch	gain	nation	oiling
clown	bayou	bird	mouth	neigh	leash	found

EXERCISE 1.2: SAME LETTERS, DIFFERENT PHONEMES/SOUNDS

Consonants

chain	choose	chord	check	chill	child
sugar	lose	insure	conscience	reassure	blush
zinc	zoology	razor	brazier	daze	zap
Thomas	third	moth	thumb	earth	lath

Vowels

gown	wow	town	scowl	pillow	power
shoe	sloe	doe	hoed	toed	poet
mouse	lousy	mousse	loud	outside	pout
cart	tart	wart	karma	lark	farm

EXERCISE 1.3: SAME PHONEME, DIFFERENT LETTERS: CONSONANTS

fuzz	easy	pleasure	zone	treasure	rose
mission	oceanic	anchored	sheep	backache	crèche
regal	hinge	jump	badge	night	engine
island	box	sound	pace	mercy	lose
carry	you	four	canyon	onion	cute
whose	hang	honesty	behind	whom	ache
rough	foreign	phonetics	of	graph	sleigh
grow	lozenge	again	begin	pig	large

EXERCISE 1.4: SAME PHONEME, DIFFERENT LETTERS: VOWELS

train	late	age	sack	crepe	Saudi
beak	keep	deceive	meter	tread	credit
took	soup	flew	ruse	plume	mouse
pad	possible	palm	knock	jar	noise
pun	son	coupe	under	pouch	done
count	hood	should	cook	full	pool
hoe	boast	pot	shoe	cope	load
speak	priest	wisdom	sleek	friend	each

EXERCISE 1.5: SILENT LETTERS

Consonants

dum(b)　(k)now　(m)nemonic　(p)neumonia　(g)nat　paradi(g)m
(k)new　(p)salm　autum(n)　si(g)n　si(gh)t　(g)nome

Vowels

lod(e)　stopp(e)d　enter(e)d　cag(e)　rat(e)s　swin(e)
bit(e)s　kick(e)d　pag(e)　min(e)　ask(e)d　fann(e)d

EXERCISE 1.6: TWO LETTERS, ONE PHONEME

Consonants

su(pp)er　che(rr)y　ba(rr)ed　wi(ll)i(ng)　pa(ss)ed　ba(tt)le
shru(gg)ed　ma(ll)　be(tt)ing　fe(ll)　tri(pp)ed　mi(ss)i(ng)

Vowels

g(oa)ls　s(oo)n　s(ou)ndless　b(ea)ten　b(oo)kcase　g(ou)lash
plyw(oo)d　m(ou)rnful　p(ea)ceful　br(ai)ded　rec(ei)ve　sixt(ee)n

EXERCISE 1.7: IDENTIFYING MORPHEMES

beet/s　(last)　pain/ful　machine/s　rust/ed　cat/nap　(force)
(less)　bigg/er　(create)　seed/s　scramble/d　stable/s　re/hir/ed
wish/ing　back/fire/s　reason/able　litter/ed　blink/s　(stream)　re/tir/ing

CHAPTER 3

EXERCISE 3.1: RECOGNITION OF FRONT VOWELS

List 1 /ɪ/　**List 2** /æ/　**List 3** /e/　**List 4** /i/　**List 5** /ɛ/　**List 6** /eɪ/

EXERCISE 3.2: DISCRIMINATION OF FRONT VOWELS

List 1 /i/　Ebay　we　brief　marine　feline　demon
List 2 /ɪ/　myth　kitchen　business　itched　gym　litter　sieve　lift
List 3 /e/　Kool-Aid　indicate　aggravate　renovate　landscape
List 4 /ɛ/　N　head　well　end　any　speck
List 5 /æ/　can　apple　knack　half　backed　camera
List 6 /eɪ/　payload　stray　amaze　radius　fading

EXERCISE 3.3: FRONT VOWEL CONTRAST DRILLS

List A: /i/−/ɪ/   **List B: /i/−/ɛ/**   **List C: /ɪ/−/ɛ/**

1. [i] [ɪ]   1. [i] [ɛ]   1. [ɪ] [ɛ]
2. [i] [ɪ]   2. [ɛ] [i]   2. [ɛ] [ɪ]
3. [ɪ] [i]   3. [ɛ] [i]   3. [ɪ] [ɛ]
4. [ɪ] [i]   4. [ɛ] [i]   4. [ɛ] [ɪ]
5. [i] [ɪ]   5. [i] [ɛ]   5. [ɪ] [ɛ]
6. [i] [ɪ]   6. [ɛ] [i]   6. [ɛ] [ɪ]
7. [i] [ɪ]   7. [i] [ɛ]   7. [ɛ] [ɪ]
8. [ɪ] [i]   8. [i] [ɛ]   8. [ɪ] [ɛ]

List D: /ɛ/−/æ/   **List E: /ɛ/−/eɪ/**

1. [ɛ] [æ]   1. [ɛ] [eɪ]
2. [ɛ] [æ]   2. [eɪ] [ɛ]
3. [æ] [ɛ]   3. [eɪ] [ɛ]
4. [ɛ] [æ]   4. [ɛ] [eɪ]
5. [ɛ] [æ]   5. [ɛ] [eɪ]
6. [ɛ] [æ]   6. [ɛ] [eɪ]
7. [æ] [ɛ]   7. [eɪ] [ɛ]
8. [æ] [ɛ]   8. [eɪ] [ɛ]

EXERCISE 3.4: WORD TRANSCRIPTION FROM DICTATION: FRONT VOWELS

1. [ɪ]	11. [æ]	21. [i]
2. [ae]	12. [æ]	22. [ɪ]
3. [ɛ]	13. [i]	23. [æ]
4. [eɪ]	14. [ɪ]	24. [ɛ]
5. [ɛ]	15. [ɛ]	25. [eɪ]
6. [ɪ]	16. [ɪ]	26. [i]
7. [æ]	17. [ɪ]	27. [i]
8. [i]	18. [æ]	28. [æ]
9. [ɛ]	19. [ɪ]	29. [ɛ]
10. [ɪ]	20. [eɪ]	30. [eɪ]

EXERCISE 3.5: RECOGNITION OF BACK VOWELS

List 1 /ʊ/   **List 2** /ɑ/   **List 3** /o/   **List 4** /u/   **List 5** /oʊ/   **List 6** /ɔ/

EXERCISE 3.6: DISCRIMINATION OF BACK VOWELS

List 1 /u/   tomb   chewed   cruiser   blue   doom   soup   cute
List 2 /ʊ/   wool   pull   hooked   put   good   full
List 3 /o/   invocation   location   vocation   donation   momentous
List 4 /ɔ/   naught   pawnshop   call   hawk   bawl   ball   caught
List 5 /ɑ/   common   honor   alms   psalm   father   sob   oddity
List 6 /oʊ/   polar   locate   sew   notice   gopher

EXERCISE 3.7: TRANSCRIPTION CONTRAST DRILLS

List A: /u/−/ʊ/   **List B: /ɑ/−/ɔ/**   **List C: /oʊ/−/ɔ/**   **List D: /ɑ/−/æ/**

1. [ʊ] [u]	1. [ɑ] [ɔ]	1. [oʊ] [ɔ]	1. [ɑ] [æ]
2. [u] [ʊ]	2. [ɔ] [ɑ]	2. [ɔ] [oʊ]	2. [æ][ɑ]
3. [u][ʊ]	3. [ɔ] [ɑ]	3. [ɔ] [oʊ]	3. [æ][ɑ]
4. [ʊ][u]	4. [ɔ] [ɑ]	4. [oʊ] [ɔ]	4. [ɑ] [æ]
5. [ʊ] [u]	5. [ɑ] [ɔ]	5. [oʊ][ɔ]	5. [æ] [ɑ]
6. [u] [ʊ]	6. [ɑ] [ɔ]	6. [ɔ][oʊ]	6. [ɑ] [æ]
7. [u] [ʊ]	7. [ɔ] [ɑ]	7. [oʊ] [ɔ]	7. [æ] [ɑ]
8. [ʊ] [u]	8. [ɑ] [ɔ]	8. [ɔ][oʊ]	8. [æ] [ɑ]

EXERCISE 3.8: WORD TRANSCRIPTION: BACK AND FRONT VOWELS

1. [u]	11. [ɑ]	21. [u]
2. [ʊ ɛ]	12. [ʊ]	22. [ʊ]
3. [ɔ ʊ]	13. [ʊ]	23. [u]
4. [ɑ ɪ]	14. [u i]	24. [i ɔ]
5. [ɑ ɪ]	15. [ɔ]	25. [ɔ ɪ]
6. [ɔ i]	16. [æ ʊ]	26. [u]
7. [ɛ ɑ]	17. [u]	27. [ɔ]
8. [ɑ]	18. [u]	28. [ʊ]
9. [æ ɔ]	19. [æ u]	29. [ɑ]
10. [ʊ ɪ]	20. [ɔ ɪ]	30. [ɑ i]

EXERCISE 3.9: CENTRAL VOWEL RECOGNITION

List 1 /ɝ/   **List 2 /ʌ/**   **List 3 /ɚ/**   **List 4 /ə/**

EXERCISE 3.10: CENTRAL VOWEL DISCRIMINATION

List 1 /ʌ/   lumber   once   funny   none   mother   funding
List 2 /ə/   banana   umbrella   atom   aplomb   Leah   elephant   Dakota
List 3 /ɝ/   bird   shirt   German   birthday   colonel   merchant   workman
List 4 /ɚ/   other   pertain   treasury   arbor   loafers   nearer   wonder

EXERCISE 3.11: CENTRAL VOWEL CONTRAST DRILLS

List A: /ɝ/−/ʌ/   **List B: /ʊ/−/ʌ/**   **List C: /ʌ/−/ɔ/**

1. [ɝ] [ʌ]	1. [ʊ] [ʌ]	1. [ʌ] [ɔ]
2. [ɝ] [ʌ]	2. [ʊ] [ʌ]	2. [ɔ] [ʌ]
3. [ʌ] [ɝ]	3. [ʌ] [ʊ]	3. [ʌ] [ɔ]
4. [ʌ] [ɝ]	4. [ʌ] [ʊ]	4. [ʌ] [ɔ]
5. [ɝ] [ʌ]	5. [ʊ] [ʌ]	5. [ɔ] [ʌ]
6. [ʌ] [ɝ]	6. [ʊ] [ʌ]	6. [ɔ] [ʌ]
7. [ɝ] [ʌ]	7. [ʌ] [ʊ]	7. [ʌ] [ɔ]
8. [ɝ] [ʌ]	8. [ʌ] [ʊ]	8. [ʌ] [ɔ]

EXERCISE 3.12: CENTRAL VOWEL COMPARISON DRILLS

List A: /ɝ/–/ɚ/   **List B: /ʌ/–/ə/**

List A	List B
1. [u ɚ]	1. [ʌ ə]
2. [ɝ e]	2. [ʌ ə]
3. [ɝ i]	3. [ə u ɪ ə]
4. [ɝ]	4. [ʌ i]
5. [ɔ ɚ]	5. [ʌ u]
6. [ɝ]	6. [ə ɑ ɪ]
7. [ɝ ɚ]	7. [ə i]
8. [ɝ ɚ i]	8. [ʌ i]
9. [æ ɚ]	9. [i ə]
10. [i ɪ ɚ]	10. [ə u]

EXERCISE 3.13 TRANSCRIPTION: FRONT, BACK, AND CENTRAL VOWELS

1. [ʌ ɚ]	11. [ɝ ɪ]	21. [ə ɪ ə]
2. [ɝ i]	12. [ʌ ɚ i]	22. [ɪ ɚ]
3. [ɑ ə]	13. [ɝ]	23. [ʌ ə]
4. [ɛ ɚ]	14. [i ɚ]	24. [u ə]
5. [ɝ]	15. [ə ɑ]	25. [ʌ ə]
6. [æ ɚ]	16. [ʌ æ]	26. [ɝ i]
7. [ʌ ə]	17. [ɑ ɚ]	27. [ɛ ɚ]
8. [ʌ ɚ]	18. [ə ʌ]	28. [ɝ ɪ]
9. [ɝ]	19. [ɝ ə]	29. [ɝ]
10. [i i ɚ]	20. [ɛ ə ɑ ɚ]	30. [ʌ]

EXERCISE 3.14: RECOGNITION OF RISING DIPHTHONGS

List 1 /eɪ/   **List 2** /oʊ/   **List 3** /aʊ/   **List 4** /ɔɪ/   **List 5** /aɪ/

EXERCISE 3.15: RECOGNITION OF CENTERING DIPHTHONGS

List 1 /ɑɚ/   **List 2** /ɪɚ/   **List 3** /ʊɚ/   **List 4** /ɔɚ/   **List 5** /ɛɚ/

EXERCISE 3.16: DISCRIMINATION OF RISING DIPHTHONGS

List 1 /eɪ/   prey   eighty   katydid   payment   matinee   danger
List 2 /oʊ/   hoping   donut   loner   coast   thrown   beau   arrow
List 3 /aʊ/   count   foundry   powder   bower   pouch
List 4 /ɔɪ/   poise   hoist   boyish   avoidance   toys   loiter
List 5 /aɪ/   highly   kindness   inded   rhinoceros   child   dynamite

EXERCISE 3.17: DISCRIMINATION OF CENTERING DIPHTHONGS

List 1 /ɔɚ/   courtship   boarded   hoarse   border   torch   forest
List 2 /ɪɚ/   fear   dear   sheer   near   hearing   gear
List 3 /ɛɚ/   bear   airplane   careful   rare   stairs   daring
List 4 /ɑɚ/   hardest   partner   Farsi   gardener   heartened   marvelous

EXERCISE 3.18: RISING DIPHTHONG CONTRAST DRILLS

List A: /aʊ/−/ɔɪ/   **List B: /aʊ/−/ɔɪ/**   **List C: /ɔɪ/−/ɔ/**

List A	List B	List C
1. [aʊ] [aɪ]	1. [aʊ] [ɔɪ]	1. [ɔɪ] [ɔ]
2. [aɪ] [aʊ]	2. [ɔɪ] [aʊ]	2. [ɔɪ] [ɔ]
3. [aɪ] [aʊ]	3. [aʊ] [ɔɪ]	3. [ɔ] [ɔɪ]
4. [aɪ] [aʊ]	4. [ɔɪ] [aʊ]	4. [ɔɪ] [ɔ]
5. [aɪ] [aʊ]	5. [ɔɪ] [aʊ]	5. [ɔ] [ɔɪ]
6. [aɪ] [aʊ]	6. [aʊ] [ɔɪ]	6. [ɔɪ] [ɔ]
7. [aʊ] [aɪ]	7. [aʊ] [ɔɪ]	7. [ɔ] [ɔɪ]
8. [aʊ] [aɪ]	8. [ɔɪ] [aʊ]	8. [ɔ] [ɔɪ]

List D: /aʊ/−/ɔ/   **List E: /ʊ/−/aʊ/**

List D	List E
1. [aʊ] [ɔ]	1. [ʊ] [aʊ]
2. [aʊ] [ɔ]	2. [aʊ] [ʊ]
3. [ɔ] [aʊ]	3. [ʊ] [aʊ]
4. [aʊ] [ɔ]	4. [aʊ] [ʊ]
5. [ɔ] [aʊ]	5. [aʊ] [ʊ]
6. [aʊ] [ɔ]	
7. [aʊ] [ɔ]	
8. [aʊ] [ɔ]	

EXERCISE 3.19: TRANSCRIPTION OF RISING DIPHTHONGS, FRONT, BACK, AND CENTRAL VOWELS

1. [aɪ]	11. [eɪ]	21. [aʊ ɪ]
2. [eɪ]	12. [ɔɪ]	22. [aɪ ɛ]
3. [ɔɪ]	13. [ɔɪ]	23. [ɔɪ]
4. [aɪ]	14. [eɪ]	24. [i aʊ]
5. [aʊ i]	15. [oʊ i]	25. [ə eɪ]
6. [ɔɪ ə i]	16. [eɪ ə]	26. [aɪ i]
7. [aʊ]	17. [aʊ]	27. [aʊ ɪ]
8. [eɪ ɪ]	18. [oʊ ə]	28. [ə oʊ]
9. [ʌ aʊ]	19. [aɪ ɚ]	29. [ɚ aɪ]
10. [ə aɪ]	20. [eɪ]	30. [aʊ ɚ]

CHAPTER 4

EXERCISE 4.1: RECOGNITION OF STOP CONSONANTS

List 1 /k/   **List 2** /d/   **List 3** /t/   **List 4** /b/   **List 5** /g/   **List 6** /p/

EXERCISE 4.2: DISCRIMINATION OF STOP CONSONANTS

List 1: /p/   apple   spring   hopped   paper   upon
List 2: /b/   rabbit   mob   absolve   bomb   bright   elbow
List 3: /t/   doubt   Thomas   laughed   liked   ptomaine   antler   wheat
List 4: /d/   adore   medal   wednesday   should   middle   hugged   bored
List 5: /k/   baroque   accord   chasm   accident   liquid   tax   extra
List 6: /g/   again   finger   ghost   example   bragged   rogue   single

EXERCISE 4.3: WORD TRANSCRIPTION FROM SPELLING/DICTATION

1. [p eɪ d]
2. [b ʌ ɡ i]
3. [k ʌ b]
4. [ɡ ɑ d]
5. [k æ d ə]
6. [ɡ ʊ d i]
7. [ɡ ʌ]
8. [ɡ æ d ɑ]
9. [t oʊ d]
10. [t i p ɑ t]

11. [d ɪ p t]
12. [k aɪ t]
13. [k oʊ p eɪ]
14. [ɡ æ b]
15. [b æ d]
16. [b ɪ ɡ ə t]
17. [p ɔ d]
18. [d ɝ t]
19. [b ɔ t]
20. [b æ d æ ə]

21. [k ʌ t ɚ]
22. [b ə t ɑ]
23. [p ɪ t]
24. [k ɑ p i]
25. [ɡ ɛ t]
26. [ɡ æ p]
27. [ɡ oʊ d]
28. [b aɪ k ɚ]
29. [k ʌ p k e k]
30. [d ɛ k e d]

EXERCISE 4.4: RECOGNITION OF FRICATIVES: /f/ /v/ /θ/ /ð/

List 1 /ð/   **List 2** /f/   **List 3** /v/   **List 4** /θ/

EXERCISE 4.5 DISCRIMINATION OF FRICATIVE COGNATE PAIRS: /f/ /v/ /θ/ /ð/

List 1 /f/   coffee   elephant   fifteen   prophet   half   fault   infant   farm
List 2 /v/   valet   vacuum   driver   halves   of   divide   river   vase
List 3 /θ/   booth   thigh   wreath   anthem   south   thorny   myth
List 4 /ð/   these   they'll   weather   bathe   motherly   heathen[1]   soothe

EXERCISE 4.6: TRANSCRIPTION OF VOWELS, STOPS, AND FRICATIVES: /f/ /v/ /θ/ /ð/

1. [f ʊ t]
2. [i ɛ v ə θ]
3. [θ i]
4. [t i θ]
5. [v ɪ v ɪ d][1]
6. [f ɑ ð ɚ h ʊ d]
7. [b i ð]
8. [b æ θ]
9. [f eɪ t]
10. [h i ð ə]

11. [b ɝ θ d eɪ]
12. [b i v ɚ]
13. [f eɪ θ]
14. [f ɔ θ]
15. [v ɪ k t ɚ]
16. [b eɪ ð ɚ]
17. [θ ɝ t i]
18. [h ʌ f]
19. [f ɪ f θ]
20. [ð eɪ v]

EXERCISE 4.7: RECOGNITION OF FRICATIVES: /s/, /z/, /ʃ/, /ʒ/, /h/

List 1 /ʒ/   **List 2** /z/   **List 3** /h/   **List 4** /s/   **List 5** /ʃ/

---

[1]Second vowel may be produced as /ə/.

EXERCISE 4.8: DISCRIMINATION OF FRICATIVES: /s/, /z/, /ʃ/, /ʒ/, /h/

List 1 /s/   racer   mouse   icing   escape   previous   loose
List 2 /z/   enzyme   misery   zigzag   rose   visible   breeze
List 3 /ʃ/   insurance   pressure   caution   washed   tissue   fresh
List 4 /ʒ/   treasure   confusion   beige   leisure   casual   usual
List 5 /h/   backhoe   hatch   rehab   halfway   hawthorn   halo

EXERCISE 4.9: WORD TRANSCRIPTION FROM SPELLING/DICTATION: /s/, /z/, /ʃ/, /ʒ/, /h/

1. [s æ ʃ]
2. [z u k i p ɚ]
3. [h æ z ɚ d]
4. [s i ʃ ɛ]
5. [æ ʒ ɚ]
6. [ʃ i t s]
7. [h ɛ ð ɚ]
8. [p ɛ ʃ ɚ]
9. [p ɛ ʒ ɚ]
10. [h æ v ɪ]
11. [p ɛ ʃ ə s]
12. [h a ɪ v s]
13. [t ɛ ʒ ɚ d]
14. [p ɝ ʒ ə]
15. [ɪ ʃ]
16. [o ʊ z o]
17. [i z i ɚ]
18. [s i ʒ ɚ]
19. [g eɪ z d]
20. [b ɚ d h aʊ s]

EXERCISE 4.10: TRANSCRIPTION OF VOWELS, STOPS, AND FRICATIVES

1. [f æs t əs t]
2. [v e k eɪ ʃ ə]
3. [t u θ b ə ʃ]
4. [h ʌvɚ]
5. [k ɔ s ɑʒ]
6. [ð ɛ s ɛv z]
7. [ʃ ɪ f t]
8. [æ s p ɚ ʒ ə]
9. [b ɝ θ e s]
10. [f ɑ ð ɚ]
11. [b ʌ ðɚ h ʊd]
12. [k ə f u ʒ ə]
13. [h ʌ z b əd]
14. [g ə ɑ ʒ]
15. [ʃ u e s]
16. [f ɔ θ i]
17. [f o e t]
18. [ʌ s t æ ʃ]
19. [ɛ k s p o ʒ ə]
20. [θ ɚ z d eɪ]

EXERCISE 4.11: RECOGNITION OF AFFRICATES

List 1 /ʤ/   **List 2** /ʧ/   **List 3** /ʧ/   **List 4** /ʤ/

EXERCISE 4.12: DISCRIMINATION OF AFFRICATES

List 1 /ʧ/   scratch   natural   cheap   capture   lecture   kitchen   catcher
List 2 /ʤ/   large   angel   bungee   jealous   enjoy   larger
List 3 /ʧ/   chipmunk   teacher   chain   charge   pitch   patch
List 4 /ʤ/   jealous   injure   zoology   graduate   engine

EXERCISE 4.13: TRANSCRIPTION OF ALL PHONEMES

1. [s t ɪ ʧ ɛ z][1]
2. [d ɑ ʤ]
3. [ʧ aɪ d h ʊ d]
4. [ʧ ɑ p s t ɪ k s]
5. [t ʌ ʤ ɪ]
6. [s ʌ b ʤ ɛ k t]
7. [ɑ ʤ ɚ]
8. [ʧ aɪ v z]
9. [oʊ v ɚ ʧ ɚ]
10. [ʤ eɪ k ə b]

11. [p æ ʧ ɚ k]
12. [b æ d ɪ ʤ][1]
13. [æ d v ɛ ʧ ə]
14. [s p i ʧ]
15. [θ i ɑ ə ʤ i]
16. [b æ ʤ]
17. [s k æ ʧ t]
18. [ʧ i k]
19. [ʤ ɚ k t]
20. [t æ ʤ ɚ i][2]

21. [ʧ eɪ s t]
22. [f ɛ ʧ f aɪ z]
23. [ʧ i z k e k]
24. [k æ b ɪ ʤ][1]
25. [s t ɛ ʧ t]
26. [g ʌ ʤ]
27. [v ɛ ʧ ɚ d]
28. [p æ s ɛ ʤ ɚ][1]
29. [ʧ æ ə ʤ]
30. [ʧ eɪ ʤ]

EXERCISE 4.14: RECOGNITION OF NASALS: /m/, /n/, /ŋ/

List 1 /n/   **List 2** /ŋ/   **List 3** /m/

EXERCISE 4.15: DISCRIMINATION OF NASALS: /m/, /n/, /ŋ/

List 1 /m/   calm   infamous   diaphragm   summer   pneumonia   prism
mnemonic   numb

List 2 /n/   knob   gnash   reign   gnat   cringe   pneumonia

List 3 /ŋ/   anxious   angle   donkey   think   song   single   longing

EXERCISE 4.16: TRANSCRIBING WORDS WITH SIMILAR SPELLINGS: /ŋ/, /ŋ k/, /ŋg /, /nʤ/

1. [s t eɪ n ʤ ɚ]
2. [s t ɔ ŋ ɚ]
3. [s ɪ ŋ ɚ]
4. [f ɪ ŋ g ɚ]
5. [h ʌ ŋ ɚ]
6. [h ʌ ŋ g i]
7. [h æ ŋ ɚ]
8. [eɪ n ʤ ɚ]
9. [s ɪ ŋ k ɚ]
10. [ɪ ŋ g ɚ]

11. [ʌ n ʤ]
12. [ʌ ŋ z]
13. [d ɪ ŋ]
14. [d ɪ ŋ i]
15. [b æ ŋ]
16. [b æ ŋ k ɚ]
17. [b l ɪ ŋ]
18. [s t ɪ n ʤ i]
19. [s t ɪ ŋ]
20. [s t ɪ ŋ ɚ]

21. [d eɪ n ʤ ɚ]
22. [d æ ŋ g ɚ]
23. [d æ ŋ k]
24. [h æ ŋ k]
25. [h æ ŋ]
26. [k ɪ n ʤ]
27. [k ɪ ŋ k ɚ]
28. [æ ŋ g ɚ]
29. [e n ʤ ə]
30. [æ ŋ g i]

---

[1]Second vowel may be produced as /ə/, depending on dialect.

[2]May also be produced and transcribed as [t æ n ʤ ə ɹ i n].

EXERCISE 4.17: WORD TRANSCRIPTION FROM SPELLING/DICTATION: NASALS, AFFRICATES, STOPS, VOWELS, AND DIPHTHONGS

1. [m i t ɚ]
2. [g æ ŋ]
3. [k oʊ m ɪ ŋ]
4. [r i m u v]
5. [ʧ ɪ m n i]
6. [m ɛ n t]
7. [ɪ n f i d]
8. [t eɪ k ɪ ŋ]
9. [m aɪ n ɪ ŋ]
10. [ʌ n z]

11. [d ɑ m ə]
12. [k ə m p i t]
13. [s æ n d ɪ ŋ]
14. [s m oʊ k ɪ ŋ]
15. [h ae ŋ ɚ z]
16. [h ɪ m s ɛ f]
17. [ɛ v i θ ɪ ŋ]
18. [s ʌ m t aɪ m z]
19. [k æ n t ɚ]
20. [s ɪ ŋ ʃ ɑ t]

21. [s t ʌ n ɪ ŋ]
22. [n eɪ ʃ ə n]
23. [ə m ɛ n d]
24. [n u m æ t ɪ k][1]
25. [s m u ð]
26. [ð ɛ n]
27. [ɔ ŋ g ɚ]
28. [h ɛ d ɪ ŋ]
29. [m oʊ t ɚ]
30. [m i n ɪ ŋ f ʊ][1]

EXERCISE 4.18: RECOGNITION OF LIQUIDS AND GLIDES

List 1 /l/   **List 2** /j/   **List 3** /w/   **List 4** /ɹ/

EXERCISE 4.19: DISCRIMINATION OF LIQUIDS AND GLIDES

List 1 /w/   reward   memoirs   anywhere[2]   linguist   William   watt   dwell
List 2 /j/   youthful   canyon   union   beauty   few   yeast   pewter   view
List 3 /l/   gale   gulp   tulip   teller   lilac   twelve   wall   dearly
List 4 /ɹ/   rhyme   try   carrot   bread   crowded   rhythm   Barry   treasure

EXERCISE 4.20: TRANSCRIPTION OF POSTVOCALIC /ɹ/ AND /ɚ/ DIPHTHONGS

1. car   [k ɑ ɹ]   [k ɑɚ]
2. bear   [b ɛ ɹ]   [b ɛɚ]
3. torn   [t ɔ ɹ n]   [t ɔɚ n]
4. fierce   [f ɪ ɹ s]   [f ɪɚ s]
5. party   [p ɑ ɹ t i]   [p ɑɚ t i]
6. yearly   [j ɪ ɹ l i]   [j ɪɚ l i]
7. morning   [m ɔ ɹ n ɪ ŋ] [m ɔɚ n ɪ ŋ]
8. partake   [p ɑ ɹ t eɪ k] [p ɑɚ t eɪ k]
9. dared   [d ɛ ɹ d]   [d ɛɚ d]
10. cheer   [ʧ ɪ ɹ]   [ʧ ɪɚ]

EXERCISE 4.21: RHOTIC CONSONANTS AND VOWELS: RECOGNITION

List 1 /ɹ/   range   gray   arrow   prayer   trailer   cream   frog
List 2 /ɚ/   hammer   dryer   understand   preacher   overcoat
List 3 /ɝ/   birch   turn   murder   return   burn   wordy
List 4 /ɹ/   trustee   broken   tearing   processor   afraid   crowd   regal

---

[1]Last vowel may be [ə] in some dialects.

[2][ʍ] may replace [w].

EXERCISE 4.22: TRANSCRIPTION OF RHOTICS /ɹ/, /ɝ/, /ɚ/

1. [k ɝ t ə n]   6. [f ɝ n ə s]
   [ka ɹ t ə n]   [f ɛ ɹ n ə s]

2. [h ɝ i]   7. [f ɝ m ɪ ŋ]
   [h ɛ ɹ i]   [f a ɹ m ɪ ŋ]

3. [k ɛ ɹ ə l]   8. [p a ɹ k]
   [k ɝ l]   [p ɝ k]

4. [f ɝ i]   9. [k ɝ b]
   [f ɛ ɹ i]   [k ɛ ɹ ə b]

5. [h a ɹ t s]   10. [w ɝ m]
   [h ɝ t s]   [w ɔ ɹ m]

EXERCISE 4.23: TRANSCRIPTION CONTRASTS: CONSONANT /ɹ/ AND STRESSED VOWEL /ɝ/

1. [k a ɹ]   11. [b ɛ ɹ]
2. [k ɛ ɹ]   12. [b ɝ]
3. [k ɔ ɹ]   13. [b ɔ ɹ]
4. [k ɝ]   14. [h a ɹ d]
5. [ʃ ɪ ɹ]   15. [h ɝ d]
6. [ʃ ɔ ɹ]   16. [b ɝ n]
7. [ʃ ɝ]   17. [b a ɹ n]
8. [h ɛ ɹ]   18. [b ɔ ɹ n]
9. [h ɝ]   19. [d ɛ ɹ]
10. [b a ɹ]   20. [d ɔ ɹ]

EXERCISE 4.24: TRANSCRIPTION OF ALL VOWELS AND CONSONANTS

1. [l a dʒ ɪ ŋ]   11. [w ɪ l j ə m]   21. [j u θ f ə l]
2. [w ɪ ʧ]   12. [p ɹ aʊ d]   22. [j e l oʊ]
3. [ɹ eɪ d a ɹ]   13. [f j u ʧ ɚ]   23. [k j u b ɪ k]
4. [l aɪ l æ k]   14. [v æ l j u]   24. [j a ɹ n]
5. [j i l d]   15. [ɹ æ ð ɚ]   25. [ɹ i l eɪ]
6. [f ɹ ɔ g]   16. [w i k l i]   26. [m ɪ l j ə n z]
7. [f ɹ i w eɪ]   17. [k j u t]   27. [w ɪ n t ɚ]
8. [w a t ɚ]   18. [l æ f]   28. [s æ n d w ɪ ʧ]
9. [r ɛ l ə t ɪ v]   19. [w eɪ dʒ ɚ d]   29. [w oʊ v ə n]
10. [w ɪ ʃ ɪ ŋ]   20. [l æ k ɪ ŋ]   30. [ə n j u z d]

CHAPTER 5

EXERCISE 5.1A,B: ASSIMILATORY CHANGES: PLACE

EXERCISE 5.1A: ASSIMILATORY CHANGES: DENTALIZATION

1. [w ʌ n̪ θ ɝ d]
2. [b o θ t̪ aɪ z]
3. [k o d̪ ð ɛ m]
4. [e t̪ θ s̪ t̪ a ɹ]
5. [w ɪ θ t̪ a m]
6. [m ɔ θ t̪ ɹ æ p]
7. [b æ θ s̪ o p]
8. [r aɪ d̪ ð ɛ ɹ]
9. [ɪ n̪ ð ɛ ɹ]
10. [k l ɔ θ t̪ aʊ w ə l]
11. [l u z̪ ð ɛ m]
12. [s aʊ θ t̪ aʊ w ɚ]
13. [a n̪ ð ɪ s]
14. [i v ə n̪ ð oʊ]
15. [f ɔ ɹ θ t̪ aɪ m]
16. [h ɛ l̪ θ ɛ k s t]
17. [w a n̪ t̪ ð ɛ m]
18. [i t ð̪ ɪ s]
19. [m ɪ s̪ θ ɔ ɹ n t ə n]
20. [s i z̪ ð ɛ m]

EXERCISE 5.1B: OTHER ASSIMILATORY PLACE SHIFTS

1. [p l e ʃ ː ɪ f t]
2. [m ɪ ʃː i l ə]
3. [p æ ʧ ʧː ɑ k]
4. [g l æ ʃː ɑ p]
5. [b ɛ n ʧ ʃ t r i t]
6. [b æ ʃː ɑ p]
7. [l u ʃː ɛ l f]
8. [h ɔ ɹ ʃː u]

EXERCISE 5.2: NARROW TRANSCRIPTION: CHANGES IN VOICING

1. [p l̥ eɪ t]
2. [θ ɾ̥ i]
3. [s t e ʤ h̩ æ n d]
4. [p ɹ̥ ɛ ʃ ɚ]
5. [b ɪ t̬ ɚ] or [b ɪ ɾ ɚ]
6. [b i h̩ aɪ n d]
7. [s l̥ i p i]
8. [k l̥ ʌ b]
9. [f ɹ̥ eɪ d]
10. [r i h̩ ɝ s]
11. [s l̥ ʌ m b ɚ]
12. [k l̥ ʌ s t ɚ]
13. [l ɪ t̬ ɚ] or) [l ɪ ɾ ɚ]
14. [k ɹ̥ æ k ɚ]
15. [r o h̩ aʊ s]
16. [p l̥ i z]
17. [b i h̩ e v]
18. [k ɹ̥ ɪ s t ə l]
19. [m o t̬ ɚ] or [m o ɾ ɚ]
20. [f l̥ u]

EXERCISE 5.3: NARROW TRANSCRIPTION: NASAL ASSIMILATION

1. [b ə n æ̃ n ɔ̃]
2. [m ʌ̃ ŋ k]
3. [m ɛ̃ n ʃ ə n]
4. [f r e m ɪ̃ ŋ]
5. [n ʌ̃ m b ɚ]
6. [m ɪ̃ n ɪ̃ ŋ]
7. [m ɪ̃ n t aɪ m]
8. [h æ m ɔ̃]
9. [h ʌ n ɪ̃]
10. [m ɑ̃ m ɪ̃]
11. [n õʊ n]
12. [m ʌ̃ ŋ k i]

EXERCISE 5.4: NARROW TRANSCRIPTION OF CHANGES IN PLACE, RESONANCE, AND VOICING

1. [n a͜ɪ ŋ̟ θ ɪ ŋ z]
2. [f ɔ ɹ̪ θ m ĩ n ĩ ŋ]
3. [p l̪ a ʈ ɪ ŋ] or [p l a ɾ ɪ ŋ]
4. [m ɛ̃ ʃ ə ŋ̪ ð ɛ m]
5. [t ɹ̥ i ḫ a͜ʊ s]
6. [m ɔ̃ r ŋ̟ ḑ ð ɛ m]
7. [w ɪ θ ŋ̟ æ̃ n]
8. [m ɔ ɹ n ĩ ŋ æ̃ ŋ̟ θ ə m]
9. [m ĩ n ĩ m a͜ʊ s]
10. [o ɣ ɚ ḫ æ n d]
11. [i t̪ ð ɛ ɹ]
12. [m ɛ̃ ŋ̟ θ i m]

EXERCISE 5.5A,B: DURATION

EXERCISE 5.5A: NARROW TRANSCRIPTION: LENGTHENING IN PHRASES

1. [b o ʊ θ : ʌ m z]
2. [b a ɹ : e l]
3. [h æ f : ʊl]
4. [s ʌ m : a͜ɪ s]
5. [k ɔ l : ɪ n d ə]
6. [t w ɛ v : a͜ʊ l z]
7. [b æ n : u k s]
8. [s e m : ɛ n]
9. [b e ð̩ : ɛ m]
10. [h ɪ z : ɪ p ɚ z]

EXERCISE 5.5B: NARROW TRANSCRIPTION: SYLLABIC CONSONANTS

1. [k æ t ʊ l]   [k æ t l̩]
2. [m ɪ t n̩]   [m ɪ t ə n]
3. [h ʌ d l̩]   [h ʌ d ʊ l]
4. [f ɹ o ʊ z ə n]   [f ɹ o ʊ z n̩]
5. [b ʌ t ə n]   [b ʌ t n̩]
6. [s ɔ f ə n]   [s ɔ f n̩]
7. [b a t ə l]   [b a t l̩]
8. [h æ s l̩]   [h æ s ʊ l]
9. [t a p l̩]   [t a p ʊ l]
10. [k e͜ɪ b ə l]   [k e͜ɪ b l̩]
11. [l e͜ɪ d l̩]   [l e͜ɪ d ə l]
12. [s n ɪ f l̩]   [s n ɪ f ʊ l]
13. [s ɪ m p l̩]   [s ɪ m p ʊ l]
14. [s æ t ə n]   [s æ t n̩]
15. [k a t n̩]   [k a t ə n]

EXERCISES 5.6A–D: ASPIRATION OF STOPS

EXERCISE 5.6A: ASPIRATION OF SINGLETON STOPS

1. [pʰ a p˺]   [pʰ a pʰ]
2. [tʰ a͜ɪ pʰ]   [tʰ a͜ɪ p˺]
3. [h ae t˺]   [h ae tʰ]
4. [s i tʰ]   [s i t˺]
5. [pʰ i k˺]   [pʰ i kʰ]
6. [l u p˺]   [l u pʰ]
7. [f ɔ t˺]   [f ɔ tʰ]
8. [b e͜ɪ tʰ]   [b e͜ɪ t˺]
9. [kʰ a t˺]   [kʰ a tʰ]
10. [kʰ o pʰ]   [kʰ o p˺]
11. [s o pʰ]   [s o p˺]
12. [ʃ a k˺]   [ʃ a kʰ]
13. [s ɛ tʰ]   [s ɛ t˺]
14. [ɹ o t˺]   [ɹ o tʰ]

EXERCISE 5.6B: NARROW TRANSCRIPTION OF PREVOCALIC /s/ + STOP SEQUENCES

1. [s t⁼ ɛ ɹ]
2. [s p⁼ æ n ɪ ʃ]
3. [s t⁼ ɝ n]
4. [s k⁼ u p⁼]
5. [s k⁼ æ m]
6. [s p⁼ ɔ ɹ t⁼]
7. [s k⁼ æ n]
8. [s p⁼ ɪ l]
9. [s t⁼ ɑ ɹ ʧ]
10. [s k⁼ ɪ l]

EXERCISE 5.6C: NARROW TRANSCRIPTION OF INTERVOCALIC AND POSTVOCALIC STOP SEQUENCES

1. [kʰɛ p⁼ tʰ]
2. [h ɑ t⁼kʰ ɑ ɹ]
3. [l æ p⁼tʰ ɑ p⁼]
4. [d ɔ n tʰ]
5. [l æ k⁼t ʰ]
6. [l ɪ m p ʰ]
7. [s æ ŋ kʰ]
8. [pʰ e s t ʰ]
9. [l æ f tʰ]
10. [l i k⁼tʰ]
11. [h ɑ t⁼: ʰʌ b]
12. [ð æ t kʰ ɑ ɹ]
13. [ɪ n tʰ u]
14. [s ɪ p⁼tʰ]
15. [kʰ ɔ f tʰ]
16. [ð æ t⁼pʰ ɛ ɹ]
17. [kʰ ɪ k⁼tʰ]
18. [kʰ æ m pʰ]
19. [l ɛ f t]
20. [m ɪ s tʰ]
21. [n ɛ k⁼tʰaɪ]
22. [m æʃ tʰ]
23. [tʰɪ k⁼tʰ ækʰ]
24. [ɹ ɛ k⁼tʰ]

EXERCISE 5.6D: ASPIRATION OF STOPS: ALL ENVIRONMENTS

1. [s p⁼ æ ṇ]
2. [k ʰ a m ə̃ ṇ] or [k ʰ a m ṇ]
3. [b æ k⁼pʰ ɔ ɹ ʧ]
4. [h a p⁼tʰ]
5. [pʰ e m ə̃ ṇ tʰ] or [pʰ e m ṇ tʰ]
6. [kʰ o t⁼: ʰe l z]
7. [s p⁼ ɝtʰ]
8. [s t⁼ ʌ kʰ]
9. [l æ s tʰ]
10. [pʰ a p⁼tʰ a p⁼]
11. [æ ṇ tʰ]
12. [s k⁼ ɪ p⁼]
13. [ɹ i kʰ ʌ v ɚ]
14. [pʰa p⁼kʰ ɔ ɹ ṇ]
15. [kʰʌ s pʰ]
16. [ɹ ɛ ṇ t ʰ]
17. [tʰ e k⁼: ʰ ɛ ɹ]
18. [s ɛ ṇ tʰ]
19. [l æ f tʰ]
20. [s p⁼ ɪ ɹ ə t⁼]

EXERCISES 5.7A,B: SOUND OMISSIONS AND ADDITIONS

EXERCISE 5.7A: ELISION AND HAPLOLOGY

1. [v ɛ t ɚ ə n]   [v ɛ t ɹ ə n]
2. [n æ ʃ ə n ḷ]   [n ae ʃ n ḷ]
3. [ɪ n t ɚ ə s t]   [ɪ n t ɹ ə s t]
4. [ʧ a k ə l ɛ t]   [ʧ a k l ə t]
5. [v ɛʤ ə t ə b ḷ]   [v ɛʤ t ə b ḷ]
6. [f ɛ d ɚ ʊ l]   [f ɛ d r ə l]
7. [r i z ə n ə b ə l]   [r i z n ə b ḷ]
8. [f e ɪ v ə ɹ ɪ t]   [f e ɪ v ɹ ə t]
9. [s ɛ p ɚ ə t]   [s ɛ p ɹ ə t]
10. [t ɛ m p ɚ ə ʧ ɚ]   [t ɛ m p ɹ ə ʧ ɚ]

EXERCISE 5.7B: INTRUSIVE SOUNDS: /w/, /j/, /ʔ/

1. [b i j i v l̩]   [b i ʔ i v l̩]
2. [g o w aʊ t]   [g o ʔ aʊ t]
3. [s i j ɪ t]   [s i ʔ ɪ t]
4. [s t eɪ j ɪ n]   [s t eɪ ʔ ɪ n]
5. [h aʊ w a ɹ]   [h aʊ ʔ a ɹ]
6. [s u w ʌ s]   [s u ʔ ʌ s]
7. [n u w e l]   [nu ʔ e l]
8. [t aɪ j ʌ p]   [t aɪ ʔ ʌ p]
9. [t u w ɛ g z]   [t u ʔ ɛ gz]
10. [j u w ɔ l]   [j u ʔ ɔ l]
11. [w i j i ʧ]   [w i ʔ i ʧ]
12. [t u w i z i]   [t u ʔ i z i]
13. [h i j ɔ l w e z]   [h i ʔ ɔ l w e z]
14. [h u w ɛ l s]   [h u ʔ ɛ l s]
15. [m e j ɔ l soʊ]   [m e ʔ ɔ l s oʊ]

EXERCISE 5.8: USE OF ALL NARROW TRANSCRIPTION SYMBOLS

1. [tʰ aɪ m ɚ̃]
2. [pʰ ɪ t̪ i] or [pʰ ɪ ɾ i]
3. [p l̥ e h aʊ s]
4. [s l̥ ɪ p˺ tʰ]
5. [t ̪ e n ɚ]
6. [b l u h̪ æ t˺]
7. [d u w ɪ t˺] or [d u ɾ ɪ t˺]
8. [tʰ a p˺ kʰ a ɹ d]
9. [s p˭ i k: l ɪ ɹ l i]
10. [m j u n ɪ s ə p l̩]
11. [s l̥ ɛ p˺ tʰ]
12. [p l̥ æ n ĩ ŋ]
13. [s l̥ i t̪ ɪ ŋ] or [s l̥ i ɾ ɪ ŋ]
14. [h ɑ t:ʰ aɪ m]
15. [s l̥ aɪ s tʰ]
16. [θ ɹ i æ n ɚ̃ m l̩ z]
17. [s i j ɛ d] or [s i ʔ ɛ d]
18. [n ãɪ ŋ̊ θ bæ t̪ ɚ] or [n ãɪ ŋ̊ θ bæ ɾ ɚ]
19. [tʰ ɛ l: u]
20. [m ʌ̃ m b l̩]
21. [o v ɚ h̪ ɔ l]
22. [s p˭ i l: ɛ s]
23. [w ʌ ŋ̊ θ ɪ m b l̩]
24. [kʰ o m ĩ ŋ]
25. [f j u ʧ ɚ]
26. [b o θ ŋ̊ ẽ m z]
27. [s l̥ ɪ m ɚ̃]
28. [s p˭ æ t̪ ɚ] or [s p˭ æ ɾ ɚ]
29. [f aɪ n d m̩]
30. [n ãɪ n: ɛ t s]

EXERCISE 5.9: IDENTIFICATION OF CV STRUCTURE, ONSET/RHYME, AND OPEN/CLOSED SHAPE

Word	Transcription	CV Structure	Onset	Rhyme	Open/Closed
1. bough	/baʊ/	CV	/b/	/aʊ/	Open
2. tree	/tɹi/	CCV	/tɹ/	/i/	Open
3. fix	/fɪks/	CVCC	/f/	/ɪks/	Closed
4. slant	/slænt/	CCVCC	/sl/	/ænt/	Closed
5. cubes	/kjubz/	CCVCC	/kj/	/ubz/	Closed
6. blessed	/blɛst/	CCVCC	/bl/	/ɛst/	Closed
7. stretched	/stɹɛʧt/	CCCVCC	/stɹ/	/ɛʧt/	Closed
8. sprints	/spɹɪnts/	CCCVCCC	/spɹ/	/ɪnts/	Closed
9. crests	/kɹɛsts/	CCVCCC	/kɹ/	/ɛsts/	Closed
10. scrounge	/skɹaʊndʒ/	CCCVCC	/skɹ/	/aʊndʒ/	Closed

EXERCISE 5.10: DISCRIMINATION OF SYLLABLES

List A: 2 Syllables	List B: 1 Syllable	List C: 5 Syllables
<u>accent</u>	<u>based</u>	<u>reactionary</u>
backed	<u>snows</u>	<u>disability</u>
<u>boa</u>	<u>kicked</u>	misarticulated
<u>tearing</u>	tasted	<u>pronunciation</u>
<u>very</u>	<u>dried</u>	inspiration
<u>loaded</u>	<u>coded</u>	analysis
splashed	<u>drowned</u>	<u>laryngology</u>
<u>diphthongs</u>	<u>borne</u>	velopharynx
<u>kitten</u>	little	maladjusted
aversion	<u>branched</u>	<u>unreality</u>

List D: 4 Syllables	List E: 3 Syllables
<u>dictionary</u>	<u>construction</u>
<u>primarily</u>	combination
description	checkered
<u>unaccented</u>	<u>syllable</u>
substitute	<u>nucleus</u>
<u>approximate</u>	amazed
consonants	<u>primary</u>
continuation	information
<u>exhalation</u>	coriander

EXERCISE 5.11: TRANSCRIPTION OF BISYLLABIC WORDS

	Narrow Transcription		Narrow Transcription
1.	[ˌpɑnˈtun]	11.	[ɡeli]
2.	[ˈlædɚ]	12.	[ˌɹiˈkwɛst]
3.	[ˈlæŋɡˌwɪdʒ]	13.	[ˈhɛɹən]
4.	[ˌdeˈbju]	14.	[əˈbaʊt]
5.	[ˈpændə]	15.	[ˈvɑlˌjum]
6.	[ənˈdʌn]	16.	[ˌɛmˈplɔɪ]
7.	[ˈkaʊˌbɔɪ]	17.	[əˈsaɪn]
8.	[ˈfeməs]	18.	[ˈɹaɪdɪŋ]
9.	[ˌpɹiˈzum]	19.	[ˈbɔɹdɚ]
10.	[ˈpɹɛʃɚ]	20.	[əbˈzɚv]

EXERCISE 5.12: TRANSCRIPTION OF BISYLLABIC AND TRISYLLABIC WORDS

1. [ˈzaɪləˌfon]
2. [ˈmʌflɚ]
3. [ˈmɪstɚˌi]
4. [ˈækˌsɛntəd]
5. [kənˈteɪn]
6. [ˌdʒɛnəˈɹeɪʃən]
7. [ˈteɪstəd]
8. [ˈfɔɹtəˌtud]
9. [ˈpɔɹkjəˌpaɪn]
10. [ˈævəˌtaɹ]
11. [ˌɛkskləˈmeʃən]
12. [ˈtɛləˌvɪʒən]
13. [ˈbɪskət]
14. [ˈpɹɪmˌɹoz]
15. [ˌɪnspəˈɹeɪʃən]
16. [ˈsʌbstəˌtut]
17. [ˌdɪˈskɹɪpʃən]
18. [ˈnuˌklijɚ]
19. [ˈɛkspɚt]
20. [ˈpɑləˌtɪks]

EXERCISE 5.13: RECOGNIZING AND MARKING SENTENCE STRESS

EXERCISE 5.13A: INTERPRETATION OF SENTENCE STRESS

1: d; 2: a; 3: f; 4: e; 5: b; 6: c.

EXERCISE 5.13B: INTERPRETATION OF SENTENCE STRESS: SENTENCE PAIRS

_b_ I want decaffeinated <u>coffee</u>.   a. I want coffee, not a soda.
_a_ I want <u>decaffeinated</u> coffee.   b. Make sure that the coffee is decaf.

_a_ I want the <u>red</u> apple.   a. Not the yellow apple, the red one.
_b_ I want the red <u>apple</u>.   b. Not the tomato, the apple.

_b_ She bought <u>five</u> books.   a. Did she borrow the books?
_a_ She <u>bought</u> five books.   b. That's a lot of books.

_b_ I'd like to see the dessert <u>menu</u>.   a. I need to know what the selections are.
_a_ I'd like to see the <u>dessert</u> menu.   b. I don't need the main menu.

_a_ I'll be there <u>tomorrow</u>.   a. Don't expect me until then.
_b_ I'll be <u>there</u> tomorrow.   b. I won't be here because I'll be out of town.

_a_ You want <u>me</u> to be the speaker?   a. Don't you mean somebody else?
_b_ You want me to be the <u>speaker</u>?   b. I'm much better at organizing than

EXERCISE 5.13C: MARKING SENTENCE STRESS

1. We <u>did</u> it, but we didn't <u>want</u> to.
2. <u>They</u> arrived, and then <u>we</u> arrived.
3. We <u>drove</u> home, but they <u>walked</u> home.
4. <u>They</u> went on a <u>bus</u>, and <u>we</u> went on a <u>train</u>.
5. A <u>thesaurus</u> is like a <u>dictionary</u>.
6. A penny <u>saved</u> is a penny <u>earned</u>.
7. <u>We</u> came <u>early</u>, and <u>they</u> came <u>late</u>.
8. I <u>came</u>, I <u>saw</u>, I <u>conquered</u>.
9. Do you need my help <u>today</u> or <u>tomorrow</u>?
10. He <u>said</u> yes, but he <u>meant</u> no.

11. I had fries, and she had onion rings.

12. I want the big one, not the little one.

13. Which is bigger, the left one or the right one?

14. His party is Friday, not Saturday.

15. His iPad has some great apps.

EXERCISE 5.14: MARKING PAUSES

__a__ 1. He wants butter, not margarine.
   a. [hiwantsbʌɾə] | [natmɑɹdʒəɹə] ‖
   b. [hiwants] | [bʌɾənat] ‖ [mɑɹdʒəɹə] ‖

__b__ 2. When did they come, Tuesday or Wednesday?
   a. [wɛndɪd] | [ðekʌmtuzdeɪɔɹ] | [wɛnzdeɪ] ‖
   b. [wɛndɪdðekʌm] ‖ [tuzdeɪɔɹwɛnzdeɪ] ‖

__a__ 3. Can you be there or not?
   a. [kænjubiðɛɹ] | [ɔɹnat] ‖
   b. [kænju] | [biðɛɹɔɹ] | [nat] ‖

__b__ 4. Since the storm, it's been very cool.
   a. [sɪnsðəstɔɹm] | [ɪtsbɛn] | [vɛɹikul] ‖
   b. [sɪnsðəstɔɹm] | [ɪtsbɛnvɛɹikul]‖

__a__ 5. Don't blame me! It's not my fault.
   a. [dontblem:i] ‖ [ɪtsnatmaɪfɔlt] ‖
   b. [dontblem:i] | [ɪts] | [natmaɪfɔlt] ‖

__b__ 6. That shirt is his, not mine.
   a. [ðætʃɝt] | [ɪzhɪznatmaɪn] ‖
   b. [ðætʃɝtɪzhɪz] | [natmaɪn] ‖

EXERCISE 5.15: TRANSLITERATION

1. Where's he going?

2. I'd like a burger and fries.

3. I saw some milk in the fridge

4. When will he come?

5. We ate meat and potatoes for dinner.

6. It happened on the Fourth of July.

7. Is that a new hat?

8. I want you to come inside.

9. Who's he kidding?

10. How am I doing?

11. When is he leaving?

12. Did you want fries with that?

13. busy as a bee

14. Was he coming by train or bus?

15.   I want a pizza with everything.

16.   Who's the new guy?

17.   Are you sure?

18.   I'm gonna get there first.

19.   Did you eat yet?

20.   He's the new teacher.

CHAPTER 6

EXERCISE 6.1: REGIONAL DIALECT CONTRASTS

Word	Transcription	Eastern New England	Inland North	Southern
1. cent	[s ɛ n t]	[s ɛ n t]	[s ɛ n t]	[s ɪ n t]
bend	[b ɛ n d]	[b ɛ n d]	[b ɛ n d]	[b ɪ n d]
2. my	[m aɪ]	[m aɪ]	[m aɪ]	[m a:] or [m ɑ:]
hide	[h aɪ d]	[h aɪ d]	[h aɪ d]	[h a:d or [h ɑ:d]
3. far	[f ɑ ɹ]	[f ɑ ə]	[f ɑ ɹ]	[f ɑ ɹ] or [f ɑ ə]
better	[b ɛ ɾ ɚ]	[b ɛ ɾ ə]	[b ɛ ɾ ɚ]	[b ɛ ɾ ɚ] or [b ɛ ɾ ə]
earth	[ɝ θ]	[ɜ θ]	[ɝ θ]	[ɝ θ] or [ɜ θ]
4. haul	[h ɑ l]	[h a l]	[h ɔ l]	[h ɑ l]
hall	[h ɑ l]	[h a l]	[h ɑ l]	[h ɑ l]
collar	[k ɑ l ɚ]	[k a l ə]	[k ɑ l ɚ]	[k ɑ l ɚ] or [k ɑ l ə]
caller	[k ɑ l ɚ]	[k a l ɚ]	[k ɔ l ɚ]	[k ɑ l ɚ] or [k ɑ l]
5. red	[ɹ ɛ d]	[ɹ ɛ d]	[ɹ ɛ d] or [ɹ ʌ d]	[ɹ ɛ d] or [ɹ e d]
head	[h ɛ d]	[h ɛ d]	[h ɛ̯ d] or [h ʌ d]	[h ɛ̯ d] or [h e d]
6. mid	[m ɪ d]	[m ɪ d]	[m ɪ̯ d] or [m ʌ d]	[m ɪ̯ d] or [m i d]
bid	[b ɪ d]	[b ɪ d]	[b ɪ̯ d] or [b ʌ d]	[b ɪ̯ d] or [b i d]

EXERCISE 6.2: AFRICAN-AMERICAN ENGLISH (AAE) DIALECT CONTRASTS

Word	ME	AAE
1. thumb	[θ ʌ m]	[θ ʌ m] or [θ ʌ̃]
wreath	[ɹ i θ]	[ɹ i f]
this	[ð ɪ s]	[d ɪ s]
weather	[w ɛ ð ɚ]	[w ɛ d ə] or [w ɛ v ə]
2. ask	[æ s k]	[æ k s]
mask	[m æ s k]	[m æ s]
wolf	[w ʊ l f]	[w ʊ f]
meant	[m ɛ n t]	[m ɪ n]
3. less	[l ɛ s]	[l ɛ s]
bell	[b ɛ l]	[b ɛ ə]
color	[k ʌ l ɚ]	[k ʌ l ə]
4. awl	[ɔ l]	[ɔ l]
oil	[ɔɪ l]	[ɔ l]

EXERCISE 6.3: SPANISH-INFLUENCED ENGLISH (SIE) DIALECT CONTRASTS

Word	ME	SIE
1. thumb	[θ ʌ m]	[t ɑ] or [s ɑ]
earth	[ɝ θ]	[ɛ ɹ t] or [ɛ ɹ s]
this	[ð ɪ s]	[d i s]
bathe	[b e ð]	[b eɪ d]
2. lamb	[l æ m]	[l ɛ]
yellow	[j ɛ l oʊ]	[ʤ eɪ l oʊ] or [ʤ æ l oʊ]
bell	[b ɛ l]	[b eɪ l] or [b æ l]
3. shed	[ʃ ɛ d]	[ʧ eɪ d] or [ʧ æ d]
wash	[w ɑ ʃ]	[hu ɑ ʧ]
washing	[w ɑ ʃ ɪ ŋ]	[hu ɑ ʧi n] or [hu ɑ s i n]
4. zoo	[z u]	[s ʊ]
buzzing	[b ʌ z ɪ ŋ]	[b ɑ s i n]
nose	[n oʊ z]	[n o s]
5. sun	[s ʌ n]	[s ɑ n]
passing	[p æ s ɪ ŋ]	[p ɛ s i n]
yes	[j ɛ s]	[ʤ eɪ s] or [ʤ æ s]
school	[s k u l]	[ɛ s k ʊ l]

CHAPTER 7

EXERCISE 7.1: ADULT SPEECH SAMPLE: TEST OF MINIMAL ARTICULATION COMPETENCE (TMAC), SENTENCE FORM

Word	Response	Transcription and Position	Error Type
<u>th</u>umb	[s ʌ m]	s/θ (I)	Substitution
too<u>th</u>ache	[t u s e k]	s/θ (M)	Substitution
fea<u>th</u>er	[f ɛ z ə]	z/ð (M)	Substitution
smoo<u>th</u>	[ʃ m u z]	ʃ/s (I)	Substitution
		z/ð (F)	Substitution
shoe	[s u]	s/ʃ (I)	Substitution
dishes	[d ɪ s ə z]	s/ʃ (M)	Substitution
fish	[f ɪ s]	s/ʃ (F)	Substitution
lamp	[ɬ æ m p]	ɬ/l (I)	Distortion
balloon	[b ə ɬ u n]	ɬ/l (M)	Distortion
ball	[b ɔ ɬ]	ɬ/l (F)	Distortion
rabbit	[ɻ æ b ə t]	ɻ/ɹ (I)	Distortion
carrot	[k ɛ j ɪ t]	j/ɹ (M)	Substitution
star	[s t ɑ ə]	ə/ɹ (F)	Substitution

EXERCISE 7.2: PEDIATRIC PATIENT SPEECH SAMPLE (GFTA-2)

Word	Response	Transcription and Position	Error Type
house	[h aʊ ʃ]	ʃ/s (F)	Substitution
tree	[t w i]	tw/tɹ (I)	Substitution
cup	[t ʌ p]	t/k (I)	Substitution
spoon	[p u n]	p/sp (I)	Omission
girl	[d ʊ l]	d/g (I)	Substitution
wagon	[w æ d ə n]	d/g (M)	Substitution
shovel	[ʧ ʌ b ə l]	ʧ/ʃ (I)	Substitution
		b/v (M)	Substitution
zipper	[ʒ ɪ p ə]	ʒ/z (I)	Substitution
monkey	[m ʌ n t i]	n/ŋ (2)	Substitution
scissors	[ʃ ɪ d ə ʒ]	ʃ/s (I)	Substitution
		d/z (M)	Substitution
plane	[p e n]	p/pl (I)	Omission
rabbit	[w æ b ɪ t]	w/ɹ (I)	Substitution

EXERCISE 7.3: IDENTIFYING USAGE OF PHONOLOGICAL PATTERNS

Word	Response	Phoneme(s) Affected	Pattern
spoon	[p u]	/s/	ConSeqRed
		/n/	FinalConsDel
boats	[b o t]	/s/	ConSeqRed
fork	[p ɔ ə]	/f/	Stopping
		/ɹ/	Vowelization
		/k/	Final ConsDel
chair	[t ɛ o]	/ʧ/	Stopping
		/ɹ/	Vowelization
nose	[n oʊ]	/z/	Final ConsDel
screwdriver	[t u d aɪ]	/s/	ConSeqRed
		/k/	Velar Fronting
		/ɹ/	ConSeqRed
		/v ɚ/	WeakSylDel
thumb	[t ʌ]	/θ/	Stopping
		/m/	FinConsDel
truck	[t ʌ]	/ɹ/	ConSeqRed
		/k/	FinConsDel

EXERCISE 7.4: INDEPENDENT ANALYSIS OF RESPONSES

Sounds Produced

Word	Transcription	Consonants (I) (M) (F)			Vowels	Syllable Structure
dog	[d ɑ]	/d/			/ɑ/	CV
cat	[t æ]	/t/			/æ/	CV
star	[t ɑ]	/t/			/ɑ/	CV
knife	[n ɑ p]	/n/		/p/	/ɑ/	CVC
fork	[p ɔ]	/p/			/ɔ/	CV
deer	[d i]	/d/			/i/	CV
bubble	[b ʌ b ʌ]	/b/	/b/		/ʌ/	CVCV
eyes	[ɑ t]			/t/	/ɑ/	VC
nose	[n oʊ]	/n/			/oʊ/	CV
mouth	[m ɑ]	/m/			/ɑ/	CV

Summary:

			Syllable Shapes:	
Vowel Inventory:	/ɑ æ ɔ i ʌoʊ/			
Consonant Inventory:	/d t b p m n/	(Initial)	V	0
	/b/	(Medial)	VC	1
	/p t/	(Final)	CV	7
			CVC	1
			CVCV	1

APPENDIX D

REFERENCES

American Dialect Society. (2001). *Purposes.* [On-line]: Available: www.americandialect .org.

American Speech-Language-Hearing Association. (1983). Social dialects. *ASHA, 25*(9), 23–24

American Speech-Language-Hearing Association. (2003). American English dialects.[Technical report]. Available: www.asha.org/policy

Anthony, J. L., Aghara, R. G., Dunkelberger, M. J., Anthony, T. I., Williams, J.M., & Zhang, Z. (2011). What factors place children with speech sound disorders at risk for reading problems? *American Journal of Speech-Language Pathology, 20*(2), 146–160

Apel, K., & Lawrence, J. (2011). Contributions of morphological awareness skills to word-level reading and spelling in first-grade children with and without speech sound disorder. *Journal of Speech, Language, and Hearing Research, 54*(5), 1312–1327

Arlt, P. B., & Goodban, M. T. A comparative study of articulation acquisition as based on a study of 240 normals, aged three to six. *Language, Speech, and Hearing Services in Schools, 7*, 173–180

Battle, D. E. (2002). *Communication disorders in multicultural populations* (3rd ed.) Woburn, MA: Butterworth-Heinemann

Bauman-Waengler, J. (2009). *Articulatory and phonological impairments: a clinical focus* (3rd ed.). Boston: Pearson Education

Bauman-Waengler, J. (2012). *Articulatory and phonological impairments: a clinical focus* (4th ed.). Boston: Allyn & Bacon

Bernhardt, B., & Stemberger, J. P. (1998). *Handbook of phonological development: from the perspective of constraint-based nonlinear phonology.* San Diego: Academic Press

Bernthal, J., Bankson, N. J., & Flipsen, P. (2013). *Articulation and phonological disorders: speech sound disorders in children* (7th ed.). Boston: Pearson Education

Bird, J., Bishop, D. V., & Freeman, N. H. (1995). Phonological awareness and literacy development in children with expressive phonological impairments. *Journal of Speech, Language, and Hearing Research, 38*(2), 446–46

Blache, S. E. (1978). *The acquisition of distinctive features.* Baltimore, MD: University Park Press

Black, J. (1949). Natural frequency, duration, and intensity of vowels in reading. *Journal of Speech and Hearing Disorders, 14*, 216–221

Bleile, K. M. (2006). *The late eight.* San Diego: Plural Publishing

Boberg, C. (2001). The phonological status of western New England. *American Speech, 76*(1), 3–29

Boberg, C., & Strassel, S. (2000). Short-a in Cincinnati: A change in progress. *Journal of English Linguistics, 28,* 108–126

Boliek, C. A., Hixon, T. J., Watson, P. J., & Jones, P. B. (2009). Refinement of speech breathing in healthy 4- to 6-year-old children. *Journal of Speech, Language, and Hearing Research, 52*(4), 990–1007

Buck, S., Maynard, D., Garn-Nunn, P. G., & Seyfried, D. (1996). Appalachian English speakers and naive listeners: Potential for listener bias and communication interference. *Journal of the Speech-Language-Hearing Association of Virginia, 36,* 24–33

Bunton, K. (2008). Speech versus nonspeech: different tasks, different neural organization. *Seminars in Speech and Language, 29*(4), 267–275

Calvert, D. (1986). *Descriptive phonetics.* New York: Thieme

Calvert, D., Garn-Nunn, P. G., & Lynn, J. M. (2004). *Descriptive phonetics* (3rd ed.). New York: Thieme

Carver, C. (1987). *American regional dialects.* Ann Arbor: University of Michigan Press

Catts, H. W., Fey, M. E., Tomblin, J. B., & Zhang, X. (2002). A longitudinal investigation of reading outcomes in children with language impairments. *Journal of Speech, Language, and Hearing Research, 45*(6), 1142–1157

Cheng, L. R. L. (1987). *Assessing Asian language performance: guidelines for evaluating limited-English-proficient students.* Rockville, MD: Aspen

Cheng, L. R. L. (1991). *Assessing Asian language performance: guidelines for evaluating limited-English-proficient students* (2nd ed.). Oceanside, CA: Academic Communication Associates

Cheng, L. R. L. (1994). Asian-Pacific Students and the Learning of English. In J. E. Bernthal & N.W Bankson (Eds.), *Child phonology: characteristics, assessment, and intervention with special populations.* Boston: Allyn & Bacon

Cheng, L. R. L. (1999). Moving beyond accent: Social and cultural realities of living with many tongues. *Topics in Language Disorders, 19*(4), 1–10

Chomsky, N., & Halle, M. (1968). *The sound pattern of English.* New York: Harper & Row

Connaghan, K. P., Moore, C. A., & Higashakawa, M. (2004). Respiratory kinematics during vocalization and nonspeech respiration in children from 9 to 48 months. *Journal of Speech, Language, and Hearing Research, 47*(1), 70–84

Curzan, A., & Emmons, K., Eds. (2004). *Studies in the history of the English language,* vol II. Berlin: Walter de Gruyer

Dodd, B. (1995). Children's acquisition of phonology. In B. Dodd (Ed.), *Differential Diagnosis and Treatment of Children with Speech Disorders* (pp. 21–48). San Diego: Singular Publishing

Duckworth, M., Allen, G., Hardcastle, W., & Ball, M. J. (1990). Extensions to the International Phonetic Alphabet for the transcription of atypical speech. *Clinical Linguistics and Phonetics, 4,* 273–280

Elbert, N., & Gierut, J. (1986). *Handbook of clinical phonology: approaches to assessment and treatment.* San Diego: College-Hill Press

Fabiano-Smith, L., & Goldstein, B. A. (2010). Phonological acquisition in bilingual Spanish-English speaking children. *Journal of Speech, Language, and Hearing Research, 53*(1), 160–178

Fairbanks, G., House, A., & Stevens, E. (1950). An experimental study in vowel intensities. *Journal of the Acoustical Society of America, 22,* 457–459

Fang, X., & Ping-an, H. (1992). Mandarin phonetic inventory. http://www.asha.org/...practice/multicultural/MandarinPhonemicInventory.pdf

Farr, M. (1991). Dialects, culture, and teaching the English language arts. In J. Flood, J. M. Jenson, D. Lap, & J. Squire (Eds.). *Handbook of Research on Teaching the English Language Arts.* New York: McMillan

Flipsen, P. (2006). Measuring the intelligibility of conversational speech in children. *Clinical Linguistics and Phonetics, 20*(4), 303–312

Foy, J. G., & Mann, V. (2001). Does strength of phonological representations predict phonological awareness? *Applied Psycholinguistics, 22,* 301–325

Gierut, J. A. (1990). Differential learning of phonological oppositions. *Journal of Speech, Language, and Hearing Research, 33*(3), 540–549

Gierut, J. A. (1992). The conditions and course of clinically induced phonological change. *Journal of Speech, Language, and Hearing Research, 35*(5), 1049–1063

Gierut, J. A. (2001). Complexity in phonological treatment: Clinical factors. *Language, Speech, and Hearing Services in Schools, 32,* 229–241

Gildersleeve-Neumann, C. E., & Wright, K. L. (2010). English speech acquisition in 3- to 5-year-old children learning Russian and English. *Language, Speech, and Hearing Services in Schools, 41*(4), 429–444

Goldman, R., & Fristoe, M. (2000). *Goldman-Fristoe Test of Articulation-2.* Circle Pines, MN: American Guidance Service

Goldstein, B. (2006). Clinical implications of research on language development and disorders in bilingual children. *Topics in Language Disorders, 26,* 318–344

Goldstein, B. A. (2007). Phonological skills in Puerto Rican and Mexican Spanish-speaking children with phonological disorders. *Clinical Linguistics and Phonetics, 21*(2), 93–109, American Guidance Service

Goldstein, B., Fabiano, L., & Washington, P. (2005). Phonological skills in predominantly English, predominantly Spanish, and Spanish-English speaking children. *Language, Speech, and Hearing Services in Schools, 36,* 201–218

Goldstein, B. A., & Iglesias, A. (2009). Language and dialectal variations. In J. E. Bernthal, N. W. Bankson, & P. Flipsen (Eds.), *Articulation and phonological disorders: speech sound disorders in children* (7th ed., pp. 331–357). Boston: Pearson Education

Goldstein, B. A., & Iglesias, A. (2013). Language and dialectal variations. In J. E. Bernthal, N. W. Bankson, & P. Flipsen (Eds.), *Articulation and phonological disorders: speech sound disorders in children* (7th ed., pp. 326–354). Saddle River, NJ: Allyn Bacon

Goldstein, B., & McLeod, S. (2012). Typical and atypical multilingual speech acquisition. In S. McLeod & B. Goldstein (Eds.), *Multilingual aspects of speech sound disorders* (pp. 84–100). Clevedon, UK: Multilingual Matters

Goldstein, B., & Washington, P. (2001). An initial investigation of phonological patterns in 4-year-old typically developing Spanish-English bilingual children. *Language, Speech, and Hearing Services in Schools, 10,* 153–164

Graddol, D., Leith, D., & Swann, J., eds. (1996). *English: history, diversity, and change.* New York: Routledge

Green, J. R., Moore, C. A., & Reilly, K. J. (2002). The sequential development of jaw and lip control for speech. *Journal of Speech, Language, and Hearing Research, 45*(1), 66–79

Grunwell, P. (1982). *Clinical phonology.* Rockville, MD: Aspen

Haelsig, P. C., & Madison, C. L. (1986). A study of phonological processes exhibited by 3-, 4-and 5-year-old children. *Language, Speech, and Hearing Services in Schools, 47,* 107–114

Hodson, B. W. (1994). Helping children become intelligible, literate, and articulate: The role of phonology. *Topics in Language Disorders, 14*(2), 1–16

Hodson, B. W., & Edwards, M. (2002). *Perspectives in applied phonology.* Gaithersburg, MS: Aspen Publications

Hodson, B. W., & Paden, E. P. (1981). Phonological processes which characterize unintelligible and intelligible speech in early childhood. *Journal of Speech and Hearing Disorders, 46,* 369–373

Hodson, B. W., & Paden, E. P. (1991). *Targetting intelligible speech: a phonological approach to remediation* (2nd ed.). Austin, TX: ProEd

Holm, A., & Dodd, B. (2000). A longitudinal study of the phonological development of two Cantonese-English bilingual children. *Applied Psycholinguistics, 20,* 349–376

Howell, J., & Dean, E. (1991). *Treating phonological disorders in children: Metaphon— theory to practice.* San Diego: Singular Publishing

Hwa-Froelich, D., Hodson, B., & Edwards, H. (2002). Characteristics of Vietnamese phonology. *American Journal of Speech-Language Pathology, 11,* 264–273

Ingram, D. (1976). *Phonological disability in children.* London: Edward Arnold

International Phonetic Association. (2002). *The International Phonetic Association.* Online. Available: www.arts.gla.ac.uk/IPA/ipa.html

Kamhi, A. G., Pollack, K. E., & Harris, J. L. (1996). *Communication development and disorders in African American children.* Baltimore: Paul H. Brookes

Kayser, H. (1995). Interpreters. In H. Kayser (Ed.), *Bilingual speech-language pathology: an Hispanic focus* (pp. 207–221). San Diego, CA: Singular Publishing

Kohnert, K., & Derr, A. (2005). Language intervention with bilingual children. In B. Goldstein (Ed.), *Bilingual language development and disorders in Spanish-English speakers* (pp. 311–342). Baltimore, MD: Paul H. Brookes

Kohnert, K., Yim, D., Nett, K., Kan, P. F., & Duran, L. (2005). Intervention with linguistically diversepreschool children: A focus on developing home languages. *Language, Speech, and Hearing Services in Schools, 36,* 252–263

Kurath, H. (1949). *Word geography of the eastern United States.* Ann Arbor: University of Michigan Press

Kurath, H., Hanley, M., Bloch, B., & Lowman, G. S. (1943). *The linguistic atlas of New England.* Providence: Brown University Press

Kurath, H., & McDavid, R. I. (1961). *The pronunciation of English in the Atlantic states: based upon the collections of the linguistic atlas of the Eastern United States.* Ann Arbor: University of Michigan Press

Labov, W. (1991). The three dialects of English. In P. Eckert (Ed.), *New ways of analyzing sound change* (pp. 1–44). San Diego, CA: Academic Press

Labov, W. (1994). *Principles of linguistic change, Vol I: internal factors.* Oxford: Basil Blackwell

Labov, W. (2001). *Principles of linguistic change, Vol II: social factors*. Oxford: Wiley/Blackwell;

Labov, W. (2010). *Principles of linguistic change, Vol III: cognitive and cultural factors*. Oxford: Wiley/Blackwell

Labov, W., Ash, S., & Boberg, C. (2006). *The atlas of North American English*. Berlin: Mouton de Gruyter

Langdon, H., & Cheng, L. R. L. (2002). *Collaborating with interpreters and translators*. Eau Claire, WI: Thinking Publications

Larrivee, L., & Catts, H. W. (1999). Early reading achievement in children with expressive phonological disorder. *American Journal of Speech-Language Pathology, 8*(2), 118–128

Lehiste, L., & Peterson, G. (1959). Vowel amplitude and phonemic stress in American English. *Journal of the Acoustical Society of America, 31*, 428–435

Liberman, A., Cooper, F., Harris, K., & MacNeilage, P. (1963). Motor theory of speech perception. In *Stockholm Speech Communication Seminar, Vol II, Paper D3*. Stockholm, Sweden: Speech Transmission Laboratory, Royal Institute of Technology

Lof, G. (2008). Evidence-driven speech sound intervention: alternatives to nonspeech motor exercises. Presented at the ASHA Convention, Chicago

Lowe, R. J., Knutson, P. J., & Monsen, M. A. (1985). Incidence of fronting in preschool children. *Language, Speech, and Hearing Services in Schools, 16*, 119–123

Mann, V. A., & Foy, J. G. (2007). Speech development patterns and phonological awareness in preschool children. *Annals of Dyslexia, 57*(1), 51–74

Massey, D. S., & Lundy, G. (2001). Use of Black English and racial discrimination in urban housing markets: New methods and findings. *Urban Affairs Review, 36*, 452–469 http://uar.sagepub.com/content/36/4/452

McDonald, E. T. (1964). *Articulation testing and treatment: a sensory motor approach*. Pittsburgh, PA: Stanwix House

Merriam-Webster. (2012). *Online Dictionary*. Merriam-Webster, m-w.com

Mines, M. A., Hanson, B. F., & Shoup, J. E. (1978). Frequency of occurrence of phonemes in conversational English. *Language and Speech, 21*(3), 221–241

Montgomery, J. (1999). Accents and dialects: Creating a national professional statement. *Topics in Language Disorders, 19*(4), 78–88

Moore, C. A., Caulfield, T. J., & Green, J. R. (2001). Relative kinematics of the rib cage and abdomen during speech and nonspeech behaviors of 15-month-old children. *Journal of Speech, Language, and Hearing Research, 44*(1), 80–94

Nathan, L., Stackhouse, J., Goulandris, N., & Snowling, M. J. (2004). The development of early literacy skills among children with speech difficulties: a test of the critical age hypothesis. *Journal of Speech, Language, and Hearing Research, 47*(2), 377–391

National Council of Teachers of English. (2001). Position statements. [On-line]: Available: *www.ncte.org/positions*.

Ohde, R., & Sharf, D. (1992). *Phonetic analysis of normal and abnormal speech*. New York: Merrill

Otomo, K., & Stoel-Gammon, C. (1992). The acquisition of unrounded vowels in English. *Journal of Speech, Language, and Hearing Research, 35*(3), 604–616

Parham, D. F., Buder, E. H., Oller, D. K., & Boliek, C. A. (2011). Syllable-related breathing in infants in the second year of life. *Journal of Speech, Language, and Hearing Research, 54*(4), 1039–1050

Pascoe, M., Stackhouse, J., & Wells, B. P. (2006). *Persisting speech difficulties in children: children's speech and literacy difficulties.* Hoboken, NJ: John Wiley & Sons

Perez, E. (1994). Phonological differences among speakers of Spanish-influenced English. In J. E. Bernthal & N. W. Bankson (Eds.), *Child phonology: characteristics, assessment, and intervention with special populations* (pp. 245–254). New York: Thieme

Porter, J. H., & Hodson, B. W. (2001). Collaborating to obtain phonological acquisition data for local schools. *Language, Speech, and Hearing Services in Schools, 32,* 165–171

Prather, E. M., Hedrick, D. L., & Kern, C. A. (1975). Articulation development in children aged two to four years. *Journal of Speech and Hearing Disorders, 40*(2), 179–191

Purnell, T., Idsardi, W., & Baugh, J. (1999). Perceptual and phonetic experiments on American English dialect identification. *Journal of Language and Social Psychology, 18,* 10–30

Reilly, K. J., & Moore, C. A. (2009). Respiratory movement patterns during vocalizations at 7 and 11 months of age. *Journal of Speech, Language, and Hearing Research, 52*(1), 223–239

Rosenthal, M. S. (1974). The magic boxes: Preschool children's attitudes toward black and standard English. *Florida FL Reporter,* 55–93

Rvachew, S., Ohberg, A., Grawburg, M., & Heyding, J. (2003). Phonological awareness and phonemic perception in 4-year-old children with delayed expressive phonology skills. *American Journal of Speech-Language Pathology, 12*(4), 463–471

Sander, E. K. (1972). When are speech sounds learned? *Journal of Speech and Hearing Disorders, 37*(1), 55–63

Schuele, C. M. (2004). The impact of developmental speech and language impairments on the acquisition of literacy skills. *Mental Retardation and Developmental Disabilities Research Review, 10*(3), 176–183

Secord, W. A. (1981). *Test of Minimal Articulation Competence (T-MAC).* Columbus, OH: Merrill

Secord, W. (1989). The traditional approach to treatment. In N. Creaghead, P. Newman, and W. Secord (Eds.). *Assessment and remediation of articulatory and phonological disorders.* Columbus, OH: Merrill;

Shriberg, L., & Kent, R. (1982). *Clinical phonetics* (1st ed.). Boston: Pearson Education

Shriberg, L., & Kent, R. (2013). *Clinical phonetics* (4th ed.). Boston: Pearson Education

Small, L. (2005). *Fundamentals of phonetics: a practical guide for students* (2nd ed.). Upper Saddle River, NJ: Pearson Education

Small, L. H. (2012). *Fundamentals of phonetics: a practical guide for students.* Upper Saddle River, NJ: Pearson Education

Smit, A. (2003a). *Articulation and phonology resource guide.* New York: Thomson-Delmar Learning

Smit, A. (2003b). *Articulation and phonology resource guide for school-age children and adults.* New York: Thomson-Delmar Learning

Smit, A. B., Hand, L., Freilinger, J. J., Bernthal, J. E., & Bird, A. (1990). The Iowa articulation norms project and its Nebraska replication. *Journal of Speech and Hearing Disorders, 55*(4), 779–798

Snowling, M., Bishop, D. V., & Stothard, S. E. (2000). Is preschool language impairment a risk factor for dyslexia in adolescence? *Journal of Child Psychologu and Psychiatry, 41*(5), 587–600

So, L., & Dodd, B. (1997). Cantonese phonetic inventory. http://www.asha.org/ .../practice/multicultural/CantonesePhonemicInventory.pdf

Spiteri, E., Konopka, G., & Coppola, G., Bomar, J., Oldhan, M., Ou, J., Vernes, S. C., Fisher, S. E., Ren, B., & Geschwind, D. H. (2007). Identification of the transcriptional targets of *FOXP2P*, a gene linked to speech and language, in developing human brain. *Journal of Human Genetics, 31*(6), 1144–1157

Stackhouse, J. (1992). Promoting reading and spelling skills through speech therapy. In P. Fletcher & D. Hall (Eds.), *Specific speech and language disorders in children* (pp. 194–203). London: Whurr 194–203

Stackhouse, J., & Snowling, M. (1992). Barriers to literacy development in two cases of developmental verbal dyspraxia. *Cognitive Neuropsychology, 9,* 273–299

Stockman, I. (1996). Phonological development and disorders in African-American children. In A. Kamhi, K. Pollack, & J. Harris (Eds.), *Communication development and disorders in African-American children* (pp. 117–154). Baltimore: Brookes

Stoel-Gammon, C. (1985). Phonetic inventories, 15-24 months: a longitudinal study. *Journal of Speech, and Hearing Research, 28*(4), 505–512

Stoel-Gammon, C. (1987). Phonological skills of two-year-olds. *Language, Speech, and Hearing Services in Schools, 18,* 323–329

Stoel-Gammon, C., & Dunn, C. (1985). *Normal and disordered phonology in children.* Baltimore: University Park Press

Templin, M. (1957). Certain language skills in children. *Institute of Child Welfare Monograph Series 26.* Minneapolis, MN: University of Minnesota

Terrell, S. L., & Terrell, F. (1983). Effects of speaking Black English upon employment opportunities. ASHA 25(6):27–29

VanKeulen, J. E., Weddington, G. T., & DeBose, C. E. (1998). *Speech, language, learning, and the African American child.* Boston: Allyn & Bacon

Van Riper, C., & Erickson, R. (1996). *Speech correction: an introduction to speech pathology and audiology* (9th ed.). Englewood Cliffs, NJ: Prentice-Hall

Watson, M. M., & Scukanec, G. P. (1997a). Phonological changes in the speech of two-year olds: A longitudinal investigation. *Infant-Toddler Intervention, 7,* 67–77

Watson, M. M., & Scukanec, G. P. (1997b). Profiling the phonological abilities of 2-year-olds: A longitudinal investigation. *Child Language Teaching and Therapy, 13,* 3–14

Weiner, F. (1981). Treatment of phonological disability using the method of meaningful minimal contrast: Two case studies. *Journal of Speech and Hearing Disorders, 46*(1), 97–103

Williams, A. L. (2000a). Multiple oppositions: Case studies of variables in phonological intervention. *American Journal of Speech-Language Pathology, 9,* 289–299

Williams, A. L. (2000b). Multiple oppositions: Theoretical foundations for an alternative contrastive intervention approach. *American Journal of Speech-Language Pathology, 9,* 282–288

Williams, A. L. (2003). Target selection and treatment outcomes. *Perspectives on Language Learning and Education, 10*(1), 12–16

Williams, W., & Wolfram, W. (1977). *Social dialects: differences vs. disorders.* Rockville, MD: American Speech-Language-Hearing Association

Wilson, E. M., Green, J. R., Yunusova, Y. Y., & Moore, C. A. (2008). Task specificity in early oral motor development. *Special Education and Communication Disorders Faculty Publications.* Paper 38. http://digitalcommons.unl.edu/specedfacpub/38

Winitz, H. (1975). *From syllable to conversation.* Baltimore: University Park Press

Winitz, H., ed. (1984). *Treating articulation disorders: for clinicians by clinicians.* Baltimore: University Park Press

Wolfram, W. (1991). *Dialects and American English.* Englewood Cliffs, NJ: Prentice-Hall

Wolfram, W. (1994). The phonology of a sociocultural society: The case of African American vernacular English. In J. E. Bernthal & N. W Bankson (Eds.), *Child phonology: characteristics, assessment, and intervention with special populations* (pp. 227–244). New York: Thieme

Wolfram, W., Adger, C. T., & Christian, D. (1999). *Dialects in schools and communities.* Mahwah, NJ: Lawrence Erlbaum Associates

Wolfram, W., & Fasold, R. W. (1974). *The study of social dialects in American English.* Englewood Cliffs, NJ: Prentice-Hall

Wolfram, W., & Schilling-Estes, N. (2006). *American English: dialects and variation* (2nd ed.). Malden/Oxford: Blackwell

INDEX

Italic page numbers refer to information in figures and tables.

A

Accent
    defined, 101, 117
    levels of, 101–102
    phonemic, *104,* 104–105
    secondary, effect on pronunciation shifts, 104–105, *105*
    speech rhythm and, 101–105
Accent expansion/reduction, 145, 146
Acoustic phonetics. *See also* Speech sounds
    of consonants, 56–83
    defined, 6
Addition, 97–98, 137
    defined, 136
African-American vernacular English (AAEV), *125,* 125–126, *126*
Allophones, defined, 6
Alphabetic letters, differentiated from phonemes, 3–5, *4*
Alphabets, differences in, 1–2
Alveolar ducts, anatomy of, 18
Alveolar ridge
    anatomy of, *13,* 14
    in consonant production, 23–24
Alveolar sacs, anatomy of, 18
Alveolar tap, 91
Alveoli, anatomy of, 18
American Dialect Society, 117
American English
    accent/word stress in, 101–105
    affricative consonants, 73–75
    back vowels, 37–42, *38*
    central vowels, 43–47
    consonants, 56–85
    dialects. *See* Dialects
    fricative consonants, 56, 64–73
    front vowels, 33, 36
    nasal consonants, 76–78
    stop consonants, 59–64
Appalachian English dialect, 115–116
Applied phonetics, 135–148

English as a second language (ESL) speakers, 145, 146, 147
    English-language learners, 145–146
    speech sound disorders, 135–144
    voice and diction training, 147
Articulation
    of consonants, 15, 23–24, 56, 58–83
    defined, 23
    disorders of, 135
        analysis of, 140–143
        assessment of, 136–137, *137*
        treatment of, 143
    manner of, 28, 56
    place of, 28, 56
        effect of assimilation on, *89,* 89–92
    in speech process, 11
    supralaryngeal structures in, 12–15, *13*
Arytenoid cartilage, anatomy of, 16, *17, 18*
Asian languages, intonation in, 108–109
Asian-Pacific Islands/Asian English, 81, 129–132, *130*
Aspiration (plosive) phase, in stop consonant articulation, 58, 93–94, *94*
Assimilation processes
    bilabial, 89
    contiguous, 88
    diacritic markings in, 87
    effect on place of articulation, *89,* 89–92
    labial, 90
    narrow transcription of, 89, *89*
    nasal, 92, *92*
    noncontiguous, 88
    progressive, 88
    regressive, 88, 89
    resonance/nasality, 92
Atlas of North American English, 116, 118–119
Audition, 11
Auditory/ear training, 143

B

Bilingual approach, in speech sound disorders treatment, 146
Bilingual children, speech sound disorders in, 132–133, 145–146
Bisyllable words, stress (accent) assignment in, 102, *103*
Black English, 125. *See also* African-American vernacular English (AAVE)
Bold type, emphasis using, 105
Breathing. *See also* Respiration
    speech, 20–21
    vegetative, 20
British English, 83, 101, 105
Bronchi, anatomy of, 18, *19*
Bronchioles, anatomy of, 18

C

Childhood apraxia of speech (CAS), 144
Chinese languages, intonation in, 108–109, 130, *131*
Chomsky, Noam, 28
Coarticulation, relationship to assimilation, 86–88, 89, 112
Connected speech, 86–114
    contextual influences
        aspiration stops, 58, 93–94, *94*
        assimilation, 87–92
        coarticulation, 86–87, 89, 112
        place of articulation, *89,* 89–92
    defined, 86
    phonological processes in
        addition/epenthesis, 97–98
        changes in phoneme duration, 94–96, 100–101
        omissions/elision/haplology, 96–97
        syllable consonants, 95–96
    rhythmic/suprasegmental features of, 99–112
        accent, 101–105
        emphasis, 105
        intonation, 108–111
        phrasing, 106–108
        rate, 111
        syllables, 99–101, *100*
Consonants, 56–85
    abutting, 57
    acoustic phonetics of, 56–83
    affricative, 56, 73–75
    in African-American English, 125–126, *126, 127*
    age of acquisition, 142, *142*
    alveolar, 14, 15
    approximant/oral resonant, 78–83, 556
    articulatory processes for, 15, 23–24, 27, 56
    bilabial, 12, 24
    blends, 57
    classification, 27–30, *28,* 56
    cognate pairs, 56
    defined, 56
    dental, 12
    devoiced, 88
    differentiated from vowels, 26–30
    duration, 94, 95–96
    final, 6–7
    fricative, 56, 64–73
    glides, 56, 78–83
    glottal, 56
    homorganic, 105
    interdental, 12
    International Phonetic Alphabet (IPA) symbols for, *3*
    intervocalic, 56–57, 93
    labial, 12, 56
    labiodental, 12
    liquid, 47–48, 56, 78–83, 88
    nasal, 14, 15, 23, 56, 76–78
    nonresonant, 23–24
    palatal, 14
    postvocalic, 56–57, 93
        deletion of, 135, 138, *138, 139*
    prevocalic, 56–57, 93
    sequences, 56–57, *57*
    singleton, 56–57, *57*
    in Spanish-influenced English, 129, *129*
    stop, 56, 59–64
        aspiration of, 58, 93–94, *94*
        intervocalic, 93
        intrusive, 97, 98
        prevocalic, 93
    in syllable formation, 26, 95–96
    velar, 14, 15
    voiced/voiceless, 28, 56
Cricoid cartilage, anatomy of, 16, *16, 17, 18*
Cross-linguistic approach, to speech sound disorders treatment, 146

Cross-sectional studies, of speech sound acquisition, 142, *142*
Cultural/ethnic dialects, 117, 124–132

D

De-emphasis, in speech, 105
Dentalization, 89
Dentition
    effect on fricative consonant articulation, 69–70
    role in speech production, 12
Developmental phonology, defined, 6–7
Diacritic markings, *88*
    for accents, 102, *102*
    allophonic differences in, 6
    for aspiration of stops, 93, *94*
    for assimilation, 87
    defined, 87
    for dentalization, 89
    for partial loss of voicing, 91
Dialects, 1, 115–134. *See also* English as second language (ESL); *specific dialects, e.g.,* African-American vernacular English (AAEV)
    back vowels, 42, 43
    code switching in, 118, 125
    cultural/ethnic, 117, 124–132
    defined, 116–117
    evolution of, 118–119
    regional, 117, 119–124, *120*
        chain shifts in, 119–124, *120, 121–122*
        mergers in, 119–124
        research about, 118–119
        sociolinguistic/deficit theory of, 117–118
Diaphragm
    anatomy of, 18
    in speech production, 20
Diction training, 147
Diphthong vowels, 26
    centering, 47–48, *48,* 50, 54
    defined, 31
    off-glide/on-glide, 31, 47, 48, 49, 50, 52
    rising, *48,* 49–54
    syllable pronunciation and, 47
    tongue height/placement for, *48, 48–53*
    transcription of, 47–48, 49, 51

Distinctive feature classification, of phonemes, 28–30, *29*
Distortion, *136, 137*
Dorsum (lingual), 14
Duration
    of consonants, 94, 95–96
    of syllables, 100–101
    of vowels, 94–95

E

Ebonics, 125. *See also* African-American vernacular English (AAVE)
Elision, 96–97
Emphasis, in speech, 105
English as second language (ESL)
    accent expansion/reduction training and, 145, 146
    fricative consonants, 66, 67, 68, 71
    intonation, 111
    lack of fluency, 98–99
    voiceless stops, 94
English language. *See also* American English; British English
    origin, 4
    orthographic inconsistencies, *4,* 4–5
English language learners, speech sound disorders in, 132–133, 145–46
Epenthesis, 97–98
Exhalation, in speech production, 20

F

Falling intonation, 108, *109*
Final consonant, deletion of. *See* Consonants, postvocalic, deletion of
Fundamental frequency, 21–23

G

General American English (GAE), 116. *See also* American English; Mainstream American English
Glossing, 140
Glottal stops, 97–98
Glottis
    anatomy of, 16
    in phonation, 21, 22

H

Halle, Morris, 28
Haplology, 97, *97*
Hard palate, anatomy of, *13,* 14

Harmonics, 22
Hearing screenings, 144
Hertz frequency, of fundamental frequency, 21
Hispanic English, 66, 71, 117, *128,* 128–129, *129*
Hyoid bone, anatomy of, 16, *16*

I

Incisors, role in speech production, 12
Independent analysis, of speech sound disorders, 141, *141*
Inhalation, in speech production, 20, 107
Intelligibility, 143
Intensity (loudness), of voice, 22
Intercostal muscles
    anatomy of, 18
    in speech production, 20
Interdental phonemes, 89
International Phonetic Alphabet (IPA), 2–3, *2–3. See also* Diacritic markings
    back vowel symbols, 37–43
    central vowel symbols, 44–46
    front vowel symbols, 32–37
    speech sound disorder symbols, 136, *137*
    transcriptional variations in, 6
Intonation, 21, 108–111, *109*
    in Asian languages, 108–109
    contours in, 108–111, *109*

J

Japanese language, intonation in, 108–109
Junctions, in speech rhythm, 100–101

K

Korean language, 130, 131–132

L

Laryngopharynx, anatomy of, 15
Larynx
    anatomy of, *16, 17*
    in phonation, 21
    in resonation, 22–23
    in speech production, *16*
Lingual frenum, 14–15
Lingual septum, 14
Linguistic Society of America, 117
Lips
    in coarticulation, 86
    in vowel production, 31

Liquid consonants, 47–48, 56, 78–83, 88
Lisp, 12, 69–70, 135

M

Mainstream American English, 116, 117. *See also* American English
Mandible
    anatomy of, *13,* 14
    in speech sound articulation, 15
Maxilla, anatomy of, *13,* 14
Medial consonants. *See* Consonants, intervocalic
Melody, 99. *See also* Rhythm, in speech
Midland dialect regions, *120,* 123–124
Minimal pairs, defined, 7, 57
Monophthong vowels, 26
    central, 30–31, 37–43, 45
    front, 30–37
Morphemes, defined, 7

N

Nasal cavity, anatomy of, *13,* 12, 15, *19*
Nasality, effect of assimilation on, 92, *92*
Nasopharynx, anatomy of, 15
New England English (NEE) dialect, 34, 37, 83, *120,* 122–123
Nonnative English speakers. *See* English as second language (ESL)
Northern Cities Chain Shift, 119, *121, 122*

O

Omission, 96–97, 136
Oral cavity, anatomy of, *13,* 12
Oral mechanism examination, 144
Oropharynx, anatomy of, 15
Orthography
    defined, 1
    English orthographic inconsistencies in, *4,* 4–5

P

Palate
    anatomy of, *13,* 14
    in consonant production, 23–24
Pharyngeal cavity, anatomy of, *13,* 12, 15
Phonation
    anatomical structures in, 16, 21–22
    in speech process, 11

Phonemes. *See also* Consonants; Vowels
  age of acquisition, 142, *142*
  allophones, 6
  defined, 2, 86
  differentiated from alphabetic letters,
      3–5, *4*
  distinctive feature classification of,
      28–30, *29*
  lateral, 81
  orthographic symbols for, 2–3
  voiced/voiceless, 16
Phonetics. *See also* Acoustic phonetics;
      Physiologic phonetics
  defined, 5–6
Phonological awareness, 144
Phonological disorders, 6–7, 135
  analysis of, 140–143
  assessment of, 136, *138,* 138–140,
      139, 144
  treatment of, 143–144
Phonologists, 6
Phonology, defined, 6
Phonotactics, defined, 7
Phrasing. *See* Speech phrases
Physiologic phonetics. *See also* Speech
      mechanism
  defined, 6
Pitch
  fundamental frequency of, 21
  intonation and, 108–111
Production training, 143
Prosody, 99, 112. *See also* Rhythm, in
      speech

R

Rate, of speech, 111
  rapid speech, sound omissions in, 96–97
Regional dialects, 117, 119–124, *120*
Relational analysis, of speech sound
      disorders, 140–141, 142
Resonance, assimilation and, 92, *92*
Resonation, 11, 22–23
Respiration
  exhalations and inhalations in, 20
  in speech production, 11, 18, *19,* 20–21
Rhotic diphthongs/vowels, 46, 83
Rhyming, 144
Rhythm, in speech
  accent, 101–105
  intonation, 108–111, *109*

  phrasing, 106–107
  rate/tempo, 111
  syllables in, 99–101, *100*
Rib cage, anatomy of, 18, *19*
Rising intonation, 108, *109*
Rule-based speech disorders. *See*
      Phonological disorders

S

Segmental speech components, 86, 99.
      See also Phonemes
Semivowels. *See* Consonants, glide
Sociolinguistic theory, of dialects, 117
Soft palate (velum), anatomy of, 13, 14
Sonority, of speech, 99
Southern English (SE) dialect, 34, 83, 119,
      120
  Southern Cities Chain Shift in, 119,
      121–122, 123
Spanish-influenced English (SIE), 66, 71,
      117, *128,* 128–129, *129*
Spanish language, 83, 101
Speech mechanism, 11–25
  examination of, 144
  larynx in, 17, 16
  subglottal structures in, 17, 16, *17*
  sublaryngeal structures in, 18, *19*
  supraglottal structures in, 12–15, *13, 16*
Speech phrases, 106–108
Speech processes, 21–24
Speech sound disorders, 135–144
  accent in, 101–102
  analysis of, 140–143
  assessment of, 136–143, 146
  in English as second language (ESL)
      learners, 132–133, 145–146
  etiology of, 143–144
  treatment of, 143–144, 146
Speech sounds. *See also* Phonemes
  International Phonetic Alphabet (IPA)
      symbols for, 2–3, *2–3*
  relationship to spelling, 4
Standard American English (SAE), 116.
      See also American English
Stopping, as a phonological process, 135
Stress, in speech. *See also* Accent
  sentence/phrasal stress, 105–108
Stressed/unstressed syllables, 43–44, 47
Stress-timed languages, 101
Subglottal pressure, 21–22

Sublaryngeal structures, in speech, 18, *19*
Substitution, 136, *137*
Supraglottal structures, in speech, 12–15, *13, 16*
Suprasegmental speech features, 99–112
    accent, 101–105
    defined, 87
    syllables, 99–101, *100*
Suprasegmental speech functions
    emphasis, 105–106
    rate/tempo, 111
Syllables
    accented/deaccented, 101–105
    age of acquisition of, 142
    characteristics of, *100,* 100–101
    closed, 99
    formation of, 7
    formation with consonants and vowels, 26
    open, 99
    speech rhythm and, 99–101, *100*
    stressed/unstressed, 43–44, 47, 101
Symbol systems, 1–3

T
Teeth. *See* Dentition
Tempo, of speech, 111
Thyroid cartilage, anatomy of, 16, *16, 17*
Tongue
    anatomy of, *13,* 14–15
    in consonant production, 15
        approximant/oral resonant consonants, 82
        fricative consonants, 69, 70, 71
    in vowel production, 15, *27,* 27–28, 30–31
        back vowels, 37–42, *38*
        central vowels, 43–47
        diphthong vowels, *48,* 48–53
        front vowels, 31–36, *32*
Trachea, anatomy of, 18, *19*
Transcription
    broad, defined, 6
    narrow
        of assimilation, 89, *89*
        defined, 6
        diacritic markings for, 87, *88,* 91
        of speech sound disorders, 136, *137*
        of voiceless stops, 93–94, *94*
    phonemic, defined, 6

Transliteration, 108
Trough, in speech sonority, 99

V
Velopharnygeal port, 15
    anatomy of, *13,* 14
    in articulation, 23
Velum (soft palate), anatomy of, 1*3,* 14
Vietnamese language, 130, *132*
Vocal folds
    abduction/adduction of, 16, 21
    anatomy of, 16, *18*
    in consonant production, 56
    in phonation, 16, 21–22
Vocal prominence, 101
Vocal tract construction, in consonant and vowel production, 27
Voice
    fundamental frequency of, 21
    intensity (loudness) of, 22
Voiced sounds, 16
Voiceless sounds, 16
Voice quality
    distinctive nature of, 15
    resonation and, 22–23
Voice training, 147
Voicing
    effect of assimilation on, 86–87, 90–92
    intervocalic, 91
Vowels. *See also* Diphthong vowels; Monophthong vowels
    in African-American English, 127
    age of acquisition, 142
    alphabet-sound agreement of, *4*
    articulatory processes for, 15, 23, *27,* 27–28, 30–31
    back, 30–31, 37–43
    central, 30–31, 43–47
    classification, *27,* 27–30, *29*
    close (height), 30
    differentiated from consonants, 26–30
    duration of, 94–95
    front, 30–37
    high, 30
    International Phonetic Alphabet (IPA) symbols for, *2, 2*–3
    low, 30
    middle, 30
    nasalization of, 92, *92*
    nature of, 30–31

open (height), 30
orthographic system for, 5
resonances of, 23
rounded, 31
schwa, 45
schwar, 47
in Spanish-influenced English, *128,* 128–129

in syllable formation, 26
tense, 31
traditional analysis of, 30–54
voiced, 16

W
Word stress. *See* Accent